T0310105

Graphic
Anaesthesia

Essential diagrams, equations **2nd**
and tables for anaesthesia **Edition**

Feedback, errors and omissions

We are always pleased to receive feedback (good and bad) about our books – if you would like to comment on any of our books, please email info@scionpublishing.com.

We've worked really hard with the authors to ensure that everything in the book is correct. However, errors and ambiguities can still slip through in books as complex as this. If you spot anything you think might be wrong, please email us and we will look into it straight away. If an error has occurred, we will correct it for future printings and post a note about it on our website so that other readers of the book are alerted to this.

Thank you for your help.

Graphic
Anaesthesia

Essential diagrams, equations and tables for anaesthesia

2nd Edition

Dr Tim Hooper FRCA FFICM
Consultant in Intensive Care Medicine and Anaesthesia
Raigmore Hospital, Inverness, UK

Dr James Nickells FRCA
Consultant in Anaesthesia
Southmead Hospital, Bristol, UK

Dr Sonja Payne FRCA
Consultant in Anaesthesia
University of Western Ontario, London, Canada

Dr Annabel Pearson FRCA
Consultant in Anaesthesia
Bristol Royal Hospital for Children, Bristol, UK

Dr Benjamin Walton MCP FRCA FFICM
Consultant in Intensive Care Medicine and Anaesthesia
Southmead Hospital, Bristol, UK

Scion

© **Scion Publishing Limited, 2023**

Second edition published 2023
First edition published 2015

All rights reserved. No part of this book may be reproduced or transmitted, in any form or by any means, without permission.

A CIP catalogue record for this book is available from the British Library.

ISBN 9781914961304

Scion Publishing Limited

The Old Hayloft, Vantage Business Park, Bloxham Road, Banbury OX16 9UX, UK

www.scionpublishing.com

Important Note from the Publisher
The information contained within this book was obtained by Scion Publishing Ltd from sources believed by us to be reliable. However, while every effort has been made to ensure its accuracy, no responsibility for loss or injury whatsoever occasioned to any person acting or refraining from action as a result of information contained herein can be accepted by the authors or publishers.

Readers are reminded that medicine is a constantly evolving science and while the authors and publishers have ensured that all dosages, applications and practices are based on current indications, there may be specific practices which differ between communities. You should always follow the guidelines laid down by the manufacturers of specific products and the relevant authorities in the country in which you are practising.

Although every effort has been made to ensure that all owners of copyright material have been acknowledged in this publication, we would be pleased to acknowledge in subsequent reprints or editions any omissions brought to our attention. Registered names, trademarks, etc. used in this book, even when not marked as such, are not to be considered unprotected by law

Typeset by Medlar Publishing Solutions Pvt Ltd, India
Printed in the UK
Last digit is the print number: 10 9 8 7 6 5 4 3

Contents

Preface xiii
About the authors xiii
Abbreviations xiv

SECTION 1   PHYSIOLOGY

1.1   Cardiac

1.1.1   Cardiac action potential – contractile cells 1
1.1.2   Cardiac action potential – pacemaker cells 2
1.1.3   Cardiac action potential – variation in pacemaker potential 3
1.1.4   Cardiac cycle 4
1.1.5   Cardiac output equation 5
1.1.6   Central venous pressure waveform 6
1.1.7   Central venous pressure waveform – abnormalities 7
1.1.8   Einthoven triangle 8
1.1.9   Ejection fraction equation 9
1.1.10   Electrocardiogram 10
1.1.11   Electrocardiogram – cardiac axis and QTc 11
1.1.12   Fick method for cardiac output studies 12
1.1.13   Frank–Starling curve 13
1.1.14   Oxygen flux 14
1.1.15   Pacemaker nomenclature – antibradycardia 15
1.1.16   Pacemaker nomenclature – antitachycardia
            (implantable cardioverter-defibrillators) 16
1.1.17   Preload, contractility and afterload 17
1.1.18   Pulmonary artery catheter trace 18
1.1.19   Systemic and pulmonary pressures 19
1.1.20   Valsalva manoeuvre 20
1.1.21   Valsalva manoeuvre – clinical applications and physiological abnormalities . . 21
1.1.22   Vaughan–Williams classification 22
1.1.23   Ventricular pressure–volume loop – left ventricle 23
1.1.24   Ventricular pressure–volume loop – right ventricle 24

1.2   Circulation

1.2.1   Blood flow and oxygen consumption of organs 25
1.2.2   Blood vessel structure 26
1.2.3   Hagen–Poiseuille equation 27
1.2.4   Laminar and turbulent flow 28
1.2.5   Laplace's law 29
1.2.6   Ohm's law 30
1.2.7   Starling forces in capillaries 31
1.2.8   Starling forces in capillaries – pathology 32
1.2.9   Systemic vascular resistance 33

1.3	**Respiratory**	
1.3.1	Alveolar gas equation	34
1.3.2	Alveolar partial pressure of oxygen and blood flow	35
1.3.3	Bohr equation	36
1.3.4	Carbon dioxide dissociation curve and Haldane effect	37
1.3.5	Closing capacity	38
1.3.6	Dead space and Fowler's method	39
1.3.7	Diffusion	40
1.3.8	Dynamic compression of airways	41
1.3.9	Fick principle and blood flow	42
1.3.10	Forced expiration curves	43
1.3.11	Functional residual capacity of the lungs	44
1.3.12	Lung and chest wall compliance	45
1.3.13	Lung pressure–volume loop	46
1.3.14	Lung volumes and capacities	47
1.3.15	Oxygen cascade	48
1.3.16	Oxygen dissociation curve and Bohr effect	49
1.3.17	Pulmonary vascular resistance	50
1.3.18	Pulmonary vascular resistance and lung volumes	51
1.3.19	Respiratory flow–volume loops	52
1.3.20	Shunt	53
1.3.21	Ventilation–perfusion ratio	54
1.3.22	Ventilatory response to carbon dioxide	55
1.3.23	Ventilatory response to oxygen	56
1.3.24	West lung zones	57
1.3.25	Work of breathing	58
1.4	**Neurology**	
1.4.1	Action potential	59
1.4.2	Cerebral blood flow and blood pressure	60
1.4.3	Cerebral blood flow variation with ventilation	61
1.4.4	Cerebrospinal fluid	62
1.4.5	Electroencephalogram waveforms	63
1.4.6	Gate control theory of pain	64
1.4.7	Glasgow Coma Scale	65
1.4.8	Intracranial pressure–volume relationship	66
1.4.9	Intracranial pressure waveform	67
1.4.10	Neuron	68
1.4.11	Neurotransmitters – action	69
1.4.12	Neurotransmitters – classification	70
1.4.13	Reflex arc	71
1.4.14	Synaptic transmission	72
1.4.15	Types of nerve	73
1.4.16	Visual pathway	74
1.5	**Renal**	
1.5.1	Autoregulation of renal blood flow	75
1.5.2	Clearance	76

1.5.3	Glomerular filtration rate	77
1.5.4	Loop of Henle	78
1.5.5	Nephron	79
1.5.6	Renin–angiotensin–aldosterone system	80

1.6 Gut

| 1.6.1 | Bile | 81 |
| 1.6.2 | Mediators of gut motility | 82 |

1.7 Acid–base

1.7.1	Acid–base disturbances	83
1.7.2	Anion gap	84
1.7.3	Buffer solution	85
1.7.4	Dissociation constant and pKa	86
1.7.5	Henderson–Hasselbalch equation	87
1.7.6	Lactic acidosis	88
1.7.7	pH	89
1.7.8	Strong ion difference	90

1.8 Metabolic

1.8.1	Krebs cycle	91
1.8.2	Liver lobule	92
1.8.3	Nutrition and energy	93
1.8.4	Vitamins – sources and function	94
1.8.5	Vitamins – toxicity and deficiency	95

1.9 Endocrine

1.9.1	Adrenal gland	96
1.9.2	Adrenergic receptor actions	97
1.9.3	Catecholamine synthesis	98
1.9.4	Hypothalamic–pituitary–adrenal axis – anatomy	99
1.9.5	Hypothalamic–pituitary–adrenal axis – hormones	100
1.9.6	Vitamin D synthesis	101

1.10 Body fluids

1.10.1	Body fluid composition	102
1.10.2	Fluid compartments	103
1.10.3	Intravenous fluid composition	104

1.11 Haematology

1.11.1	Blood groups	105
1.11.2	Coagulation – cascade (classic) model	106
1.11.3	Coagulation – cell-based model	107
1.11.4	Complement cascade	108
1.11.5	Haemoglobin	109
1.11.6	Prostanoid synthesis	110

1.12   Cellular
1.12.1   Cell 111
1.12.2   Cell membrane 112
1.12.3   G-proteins 113
1.12.4   Ion channels 114
1.12.5   Sodium/potassium–ATPase pump 115

1.13   Immunity
1.13.1   Antibody 116
1.13.2   Hypersensitivity 117
1.13.3   Innate and adaptive immunity 118

1.14   Muscle
1.14.1   Actin–myosin cycle 119
1.14.2   Golgi tendon organ 120
1.14.3   Muscle spindle 121
1.14.4   Muscle types 122
1.14.5   Neuromuscular junction 123
1.14.6   Sarcomere 124
1.14.7   Skeletal muscle structure 125

1.15   Pregnancy and paediatrics
1.15.1   Fetal circulation 126
1.15.2   Paediatric differences I 127
1.15.3   Paediatric differences II 128
1.15.4   Physiological changes in pregnancy I 129
1.15.5   Physiological changes in pregnancy II 130

SECTION 2   ANATOMY

2.1   Functional anatomy
2.1.1   Abdominal wall 131
2.1.2   Antecubital fossa 132
2.1.3   Autonomic nervous system 133
2.1.4   Base of skull 134
2.1.5   Brachial plexus 135
2.1.6   Bronchial tree 136
2.1.7   Cardiac vessels – cardiac veins 137
2.1.8   Cardiac vessels – coronary arteries 138
2.1.9   Circle of Willis 139
2.1.10   Cranial nerves 140
2.1.11   Cross-section of neck at C6 141
2.1.12   Cross-section of spinal cord 142
2.1.13   Dermatomes 143
2.1.14   Diaphragm 144
2.1.15   Epidural space 145
2.1.16   Femoral triangle 146

2.1.17	Intercostal space	147
2.1.18	Internal jugular vein	148
2.1.19	Laryngeal innervation	149
2.1.20	Larynx	150
2.1.21	Limb muscle innervation (myotomes)	151
2.1.22	Lumbar plexus	152
2.1.23	Nose	153
2.1.24	Orbit	154
2.1.25	Rib	155
2.1.26	Sacral plexus	156
2.1.27	Sacrum	157
2.1.28	Spinal nerve	158
2.1.29	Thoracic inlet and first rib	159
2.1.30	Vertebra	160

2.2   Anatomy for regional anaesthesia

2.2.1	Axillary	161
2.2.2	Femoral	162
2.2.3	Interscalene	163
2.2.4	Popliteal	164
2.2.5	Sciatic	165
2.2.6	Supraclavicular	166

SECTION 3   PHARMACODYNAMICS AND KINETICS

3.1	Clearance	167
3.2	Compartment model – one and two compartments	168
3.3	Compartment model – three compartments	169
3.4	Dose–response curves	170
3.5	Elimination	171
3.6	Elimination kinetics	172
3.7	Half-lives and time constants	173
3.8	Meyer–Overton hypothesis	174
3.9	Target-controlled infusions	175
3.10	Volume of distribution	176
3.11	Wash-in curves for volatile agents	177

SECTION 4   DRUGS

4.1	Alpha-2 adrenoceptor agonists	179
4.2	Anaesthetic agents – etomidate	180
4.3	Anaesthetic agents – ketamine	181
4.4	Anaesthetic agents – propofol	182
4.5	Anaesthetic agents – thiopentone	183
4.6	Anticoagulants	184
4.7	Antiemetics	185

4.8	Antiplatelets	186
4.9	Benzodiazepines	187
4.10	Blood products	188
4.11	Direct-acting oral anticoagulants	189
4.12	Intralipid	190
4.13	Local anaesthetics – mode of action	191
4.14	Local anaesthetics – properties	192
4.15	Neuromuscular blockers – mode of action	193
4.16	Neuromuscular blocking agents – depolarizing	194
4.17	Neuromuscular blocking agents – non-depolarizing	195
4.18	Opioids – mode of action	196
4.19	Opioids – properties	197
4.20	Paracetamol and NSAIDs	198
4.21	Reversal agents	199
4.22	Tranexamic acid	200
4.23	Volatile anaesthetic agents – mode of action	201
4.24	Volatile anaesthetic agents – physiological effects	202
4.25	Volatile anaesthetic agents – properties	203

SECTION 5   PHYSICS

5.1	Avogadro's law	205
5.2	Beer–Lambert law	206
5.3	Critical temperatures and pressure	207
5.4	Diathermy	208
5.5	Doppler effect	209
5.6	Electrical safety	210
5.7	Electricity	211
5.8	Exponential function	212
5.9	Fick's law of diffusion	213
5.10	Gas laws – Boyle's law	214
5.11	Gas laws – Charles' law	215
5.12	Gas laws – Gay-Lussac's (Third Perfect) law	216
5.13	Gas laws – ideal gas law and Dalton's law	217
5.14	Graham's law	218
5.15	Heat	219
5.16	Henry's law	220
5.17	Humidity	221
5.18	Laser	222
5.19	Metric prefixes	223
5.20	Power	224
5.21	Pressure	225
5.22	Raman effect	226
5.23	Reflection and refraction	227
5.24	SI units	228

5.25   Triple point of water and phase diagram 229
5.26   Types of flow 230
5.27   Wave characteristics 231
5.28   Wheatstone bridge 232
5.29   Work 233

SECTION 6   CLINICAL MEASUREMENT

6.1   Bourdon gauge 235
6.2   Clark electrode 236
6.3   Damping 237
6.4   Depth of anaesthesia monitoring 238
6.5   Fuel cell 239
6.6   Monitoring of neuromuscular blockade 240
6.7   Oximetry – paramagnetic analyser 241
6.8   pH measuring system 242
6.9   Pulse oximeter 243
6.10   Severinghaus carbon dioxide electrode 244
6.11   Temperature measurement 245
6.12   Thermocouple and Seebeck effect 246

SECTION 7   EQUIPMENT

7.1   Bag valve mask resuscitator 247
7.2   Breathing circuits – circle system 248
7.3   Breathing circuits – Mapleson's classification 249
7.4   Bronchoscope 250
7.5   Cleaning and decontamination 251
7.6   Continuous renal replacement therapy – extracorporeal circuit 252
7.7   Continuous renal replacement therapy – modes 253
7.8   Gas cylinders 254
7.9   Glucometer 255
7.10   Humidifier 256
7.11   Intra-aortic balloon pump 257
7.12   Laryngoscopes 258
7.13   Oxygen delivery systems – Bernoulli principle and Venturi effect 259
7.14   Piped gases 260
7.15   Scavenging 261
7.16   Ultrasound 262
7.17   Vacuum-insulated evaporator 263
7.18   Vaporizer 264
7.19   Ventilation – pressure-controlled 265
7.20   Ventilation – volume-controlled 266
7.21   Viscoelastic tests of clotting 267

SECTION 8   STATISTICS

8.1   Mean, median and mode 269
8.2   Normal distribution 270
8.3   Number needed to treat 271
8.4   Odds ratio 272
8.5   Predictive values 273
8.6   Sensitivity and specificity 274
8.7   Significance tests 275
8.8   Statistical variability 276
8.9   Type I and type II errors 277

SECTION 9   CLINICAL PREDICTION

9.1   ASA classification 279
9.2   Clinical frailty scale 280
9.3   Cormack and Lehane classification 281
9.4   Mallampati classification 282
9.5   Scoring systems 283

Preface

This book is a compendium of the diagrams, graphs, equations and tables needed for anaesthetic practice. It has been written with the FRCA examinations in mind, although it is equally well suited for revision at any stage of an anaesthetic practitioner's career. Senior anaesthetists will find this book useful as an aide-memoire when teaching and examining trainee colleagues. Additionally it is hoped it will prove useful to anyone who is looking for short and clear explanations of the fundamental principles surrounding anaesthesia.

Each page contains a separate topic with the relevant diagram, graph, equation or table succinctly described for rapid review and assimilation. The diagrams and graphs have been specifically drawn to allow them, in the main, to be easily reproduced and the ability to draw diagrams and graphs remains a useful tool for learning and retaining important information. As with the first edition, a simple standardized colour palette has been used throughout the book to allow anyone with a 4-colour pen to draw the diagrams clearly and accurately.

The explanations are purposely short (250–300 words) but have been carefully written to provide enough up to date detail to effectively explain the illustration, equation, graph or table. Although the text is centred on an explanation of the basic sciences related to the topic, where appropriate the clinical applications of the principles are also discussed.

Many anaesthetic textbooks have good diagrams and detailed explanations but few, if any, have all the diagrams needed for anaesthetic practice and the FRCA examinations. The first edition of this book was born out of that need. Eight years on from its original publication, this second edition remains true to its origins and has been thoroughly revised with 35 new topics added to ensure it remains comprehensive and up-to-date. We hope you will find it useful and stimulating.

Tim Hooper, James Nickells, Sonja Payne,
Annabel Pearson and Ben Walton

About the authors

Lead author Tim Hooper, anaesthetist and intensivist, had the original idea for the book and has again coordinated this second edition. Artist and anaesthetist James Nickells has provided original artwork for both editions of the book. Sonja Payne and Annabel Pearson, both anaesthetists, provided the majority of the content for the first edition and have been instrumental in providing new content for this edition. Anaesthetist and intensivist Ben Walton has also provided new content. All authors continue to provide anaesthesia and, while this collaboration originated in Bristol, some have now moved further afield to develop their practice.

Abbreviations

AAG	α-1-acid glycoprotein		ECF	extracellular fluid
ACA	anterior cerebral artery		ECG	electrocardiogram
ACE	angiotensin-converting enzyme		EDPVR	end-diastolic pressure–volume relationship
Ach	acetylcholine			
ACOM	anterior communicating artery		EDV	end-diastolic volume
ADH	antidiuretic hormone		EEG	electroencephalogram
ALP	alkaline phosphatase		EMI	electromagnetic interference
ANP	atrial natriuretic peptide		ERAD	extreme right axis deviation
ANS	autonomic nervous system		ERV	expiratory reserve volume
APL	adjustable pressure limiting		ESPVR	end-systolic pressure–volume relationship
ARDS	acute respiratory distress syndrome			
ARR	absolute risk reduction		ESV	end-systolic volume
ATP	adenosine triphosphate		FEF	forced expiratory flow
AV	atrioventricular		FEV_1	forced expiratory volume in 1 second
BDZs	benzodiazepines		FFP	fresh frozen plasma
BVM	bag valve mask		FGF	fresh gas flow
CBF	cerebral blood flow		FICB	fascia iliaca compartment block
CC	closing capacity		FNB	femoral nerve blockade
CFS	Clinical Frailty Scale		FRC	functional residual capacity
CGM	continuous glucose monitoring		FVC	forced vital capacity
CI	confidence interval		GABA	gamma-aminobutyric acid
CMR	central metabolic rate		GFR	glomerular filtration rate
CMV	controlled mechanical ventilation		GI	gastrointestinal
CNS	central nervous system		GPCR	G-protein coupled receptor
CO	cardiac output		GTO	Golgi tendon organ
COPD	chronic obstructive pulmonary disease		Hb	haemoglobin
CPP	cerebral perfusion pressure		hCG	human chorionic gonadotrophin
CRRT	continuous renal replacement therapy		IA	intrinsic activity
CSF	cerebrospinal fluid		IC	inspiratory capacity
CTZ	chemoreceptor trigger zone		ICA	internal carotid artery
CV	closing volume		ICD	implantable cardioverter-defibrillator
CVP	central venous pressure		ICF	intracellular fluid
CVS	cardiovascular system		ICP	intracranial pressure
CVVH	continuous veno-venous haemofiltration		IQR	interquartile range
CVVHD	continuous veno-venous haemodialysis		IRV	inspiratory reserve volume
CVVHDF	continuous veno-venous haemodiafiltration		ISF	interstitial fluid
			IVC	inferior vena cava
DBS	double-burst stimulation		$IV_{ol}C$	isovolumetric contraction
DCT	distal convoluted tubule		$IV_{ol}R$	isovolumetric relaxation
DL	direct laryngoscope		LAP	left atrial pressure
DOACs	direct-acting oral anticoagulants		LBBB	left bundle branch block

LCNT	lateral cutaneous nerve of the thigh	RLN	recurrent laryngeal nerve
MAC	membrane attack complex	RMP	resting membrane potential
MAC	minimum alveolar concentration	RR	relative risk
MAP	mean arterial pressure	RTD	resistance temperature detector
MBL	mannose-binding lectin	RV	residual volume
MCA	middle cerebral artery	SA	sinoatrial
MHC	major histocompatibility complex	SBE	standardized base excess
MPAP	mean pulmonary artery pressure	SCM	sternocleidomastoid
M_v	minute ventilation	SCUF	slow continuous ultrafiltration
NADH	nicotinamide adenine dinucleotide	SD	standard deviation
NMB	neuromuscular blockade	SID	strong ion difference
NMBD	neuromuscular blocking drug	SLN	superficial laryngeal nerve
NMJ	neuromuscular junction	SNS	sympathetic nervous system
NMS	neuroleptic malignant syndrome	STP	standard temperature and pressure
NNH	number needed to harm	SV	spontaneous ventilation
NNT	number needed to treat	SV	stroke volume
NPV	negative predictive value	SVP	saturation vapour pressure
NSAIDs	non-steroidal anti-inflammatory drugs	SVR	systemic vascular resistance
OR	odds ratio	SVT	supraventricular tachycardia
PAH	pulmonary arterial hypertension	TBW	total body water
PAMPs	pathogen-associated molecular patterns	TCI	target-controlled infusion
PCA	posterior cerebral artery	TEB	thoracic electrical bioimpedance
PCOM	posterior communicating artery	TENS	transcutaneous electrical nerve stimulation
PCV	pressure-controlled ventilation		
PCV–VG	pressure-controlled ventilation with volume guarantee	TIVA	total intravenous anaesthesia
		TLC	total lung capacity
PCWP	pulmonary capillary wedge pressure	TMP	transmembrane pressure
PEEP	positive end-expiratory pressure	TOF	train of four
PEFR	peak expiratory flow rate	TPN	total parenteral nutrition
PNS	peripheral nervous system	TSH	thyroid-stimulating hormone
PONV	post-operative nausea and vomiting	TV	tidal volume
PPV	positive predictive value	TXA	tranexamic acid
PRRs	pathogen recognition receptors	VC	vital capacity
PRT	platinum resistance thermometer	VCV	volume-controlled ventilation
PVR	pulmonary vascular resistance	VET	viscoelastic test
RA	right atrium	VGCC	voltage-gated calcium channels
RAD	right axis deviation	VIE	vacuum-insulated evaporator
RBBB	right bundle branch block	VL	video laryngoscope
RBCs	red blood cells	VTE	venous thromboembolism
RBF	renal blood flow	vWF	von Willebrand factor

1.1.1

Cardiac action potential – contractile cells

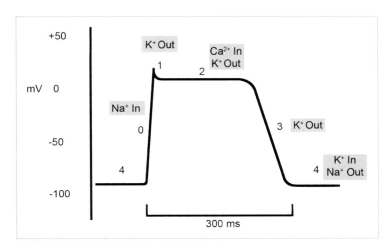

The cardiac action potential differs significantly depending on the function of the cardiac myocyte (i.e. excitatory/pacemaker or contractile). The action potential of contractile cardiac myocytes has 5 phases characterized by a stable resting membrane potential and a prolonged plateau phase.

- Phase 0 – rapid depolarization as membrane permeability to potassium decreases and fast sodium channels open.
- Phase 1 – early rapid repolarization as sodium permeability decreases.
- Phase 2 – plateau phase. A continued influx of calcium through L-type (long opening, voltage-gated) calcium channels maintains depolarization for approximately 300 ms.
- Phase 3 – rapid repolarization due to inactivation of calcium channels and ongoing efflux of potassium.
- Phase 4 – restoration of ionic concentrations, thereby restoring the resting membrane potential of approximately −90 mV.

For the majority of the action potential, contractile myocytes demonstrate an absolute refractory period (beginning of phase 0 until close to end of phase 2). During this time no stimulus, regardless of the magnitude, can incite further depolarization. A relative refractory period exists during phase 3. A supramaximal stimulus during this period will result in an action potential with a slower rate of depolarization and smaller amplitude, producing a weaker contraction.

Anti-arrhythmic drugs and the myocardial action potential

Anti-arrhythmic drugs (see *Section 1.1.22 – Vaughan–Williams classification*) that alter ion movement are used to alter action potentials to prevent or terminate arrhythmias.

- In contractile cells, sodium channel blockers (Vaughan–Williams Class 1) reduce the slope of phase 0 and the magnitude of depolarization. They also prolong the refractory periods by delaying the reactivation of sodium channels.
- Potassium channel blockers (Vaughan–Williams Class 3) delay phase 3 repolarization. This lengthens the duration of the action potential and the refractory periods.

1.1.2

Cardiac action potential – pacemaker cells

The pacemaker potential is seen in cells of the cardiac excitatory system, namely the sinoatrial (SA) and atrioventricular (AV) nodes. Action potentials of cardiac pacemaker myocytes have 3 phases (named out of numerical order to coincide with contractile myocyte action potentials) and are characterized by automaticity, due to an unstable phase 4, and a lack of plateau phase.

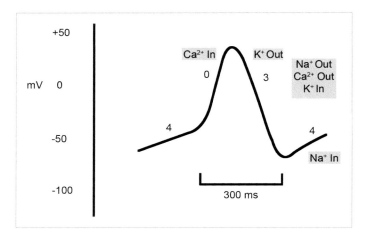

- Phase 4 – spontaneous depolarization. Sodium moves into myocytes via 'funny' voltage-gated channels that open when the cell membrane potential becomes more negative, immediately after the end of the previous action potential. Calcium also enters the cell via T-type channels (T for transient).
- Phase 0 – rapid depolarization occurs once the threshold potential (approximately −40 mV) is reached. L-type calcium channels open and calcium enters the cell.
- Phase 3 – repolarization occurs as potassium permeability increases, resulting in potassium efflux.

Compared to contractile myocytes, pacemaker myocyte action potentials:
- are slow response
- have a less negative phase 4 membrane potential
- have a less negative threshold potential
- have a less steep slope of rapid depolarization (phase 0).

Regulation by the autonomic nervous system

The cardiac excitatory system demonstrates inherent pacemaker activity. The rate of depolarization and duration of action potential are influenced by the autonomic nervous system. In the denervated heart, the SA node depolarizes at a rate of 100 bpm. At rest, parasympathetic activity dominates and reduces SA nodal depolarization. Parasympathetic activation leads to an increase in potassium efflux while reducing sodium and calcium influx. These alterations in ionic conductance result in a more negative phase 4 membrane potential, a decrease in the slope of phase 4 and, overall, an increase in the time to reach the threshold potential. Conversely, sympathetic activation increases the rate of pacemaker depolarization by reducing potassium efflux and increasing sodium and calcium influx.

1.1.3

Cardiac action potential – variation in pacemaker potential

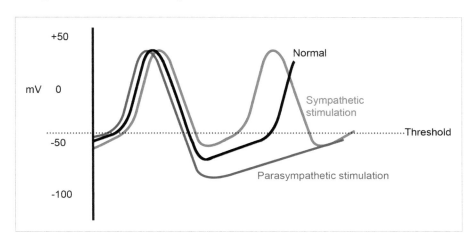

The pacemaker potential is seen in cells in the SA and AV nodes. It is a slow positive increase from the resting potential that occurs at the end of one action potential and before the start of the next. The pacemaker action potential differs from those seen in other cardiac cells because it lacks phases 1 and 2 and has an unstable resting potential. This unstable resting potential allows for spontaneous depolarization and gives the heart its autorhythmicity. It is the rate of change, or gradient, of the resting potential that determines the onset of the next action potential and therefore the discharge rate. The characteristics of the pacemaker potential are predominantly under the control of the autonomic nervous system.

An increase in the gradient of the slope of phase 4 will reduce the amount of time taken for the cell to reach threshold potential, causing depolarization to occur more rapidly. This occurs with sympathetic stimulation (red trace) via β1 adrenoreceptors which results in an increase in cyclic-AMP levels, allowing the opening of calcium channels and thereby increasing the discharge rate of the cell.

Conversely, a decrease in the slope of phase 4 will increase the time taken to reach threshold potential and depolarization, causing a reduced discharge rate. This occurs with parasympathetic stimulation (blue trace). The vagus nerve acts to slow the discharge rate by hyperpolarizing the cell membrane through increased permeability to potassium. The membrane potential is therefore more negative so will take longer to reach threshold potential and to discharge.

1.1.4

Cardiac cycle

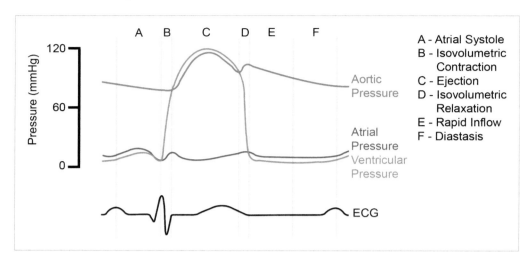

A - Atrial Systole
B - Isovolumetric Contraction
C - Ejection
D - Isovolumetric Relaxation
E - Rapid Inflow
F - Diastasis

The diagram depicts events that occur during one cardiac cycle. It is a graph of pressure against time and includes pressure waveforms for the left ventricle, aorta and central venous pressure (CVP), with the electrocardiogram (ECG) and heart sound timings superimposed.

There are five phases.

- Phase 1 (A). Atrial contraction – 'P' wave of the ECG and 'a' wave of the CVP trace. Atrial contraction (or 'atrial kick') contributes to about 30% of ventricular filling.
- Phase 2 (B). Ventricular isovolumetric contraction ($IV_{ol}C$) – marks the onset of systole and coincides with closure of the mitral and tricuspid valves (first heart sound). The pressure in the ventricle rises rapidly from its baseline, while blood volume remains constant, since both inlet and outlet valves are closed. The 'c' wave of the CVP trace represents tricuspid valve bulging as the right ventricle undergoes $IV_{ol}C$.
- Phase 3 (C). Systole – as the ventricular pressure exceeds that in the aorta and pulmonary arteries, the aortic and pulmonary valves open and blood is ejected. The aortic pressure curve follows that of the left ventricle, but at a slightly lower pressure, depicting the pressure gradient needed to allow forward flow of blood. At the end of this phase, ventricular repolarization is represented by the 't' wave on the ECG.
- Phase 4 (D). Ventricular isovolumetric relaxation ($IV_{ol}R$) – once the aortic and pulmonary valves close (second heart sound), the ventricular pressure rapidly falls to baseline with no change in volume. Aortic valve closure is seen on the aortic pressure trace as the dicrotic notch, after which the pressure in the aorta exceeds that in the ventricle.
- Phase 5 (E and F). Ventricular filling – passive filling of the ventricle during diastole. As ventricular pressure falls below atrial pressure (and CVP), the tricuspid and mitral valves open allowing forward flow of blood. This filling is initially rapid (E), followed by a slower filling phase known as diastasis (F), before atrial contraction occurs and the cycle starts again. The 'y' descent on the CVP trace occurs as the atrium empties.

1.1.5

Cardiac output equation

$$Q = HR \times SV$$

Q = cardiac output (ml.min^{-1})

HR = heart rate (beats.min^{-1})

SV = stroke volume (ml.beat^{-1})

Cardiac output (CO) is defined as volume of blood pumped by the heart per minute; it is equal to the product of heart rate and stroke volume. In considering this equation there are four determinants of CO: heart rate, preload, afterload and contractility. Changes in each variable do not occur in isolation but will impact the remaining variables. Therefore, depending on the magnitude of change, each variable may positively or negatively impact CO.

CO monitoring is frequently used as a means of optimizing tissue oxygenation and guiding treatment. Historically, the gold standard for CO measurement was invasive pulmonary artery catheterization. However, due to the specialist skill required for insertion and the potential for complications, its use has been superseded by less invasive methods.

- Pulse contour analysis (e.g. PiCCO, LiDCO) – algorithms relate the contour of the arterial pressure waveform to stroke volume and systemic vascular resistance. Research demonstrates good agreement with the gold standard. Limitations include the necessity for an optimal arterial pressure trace and potential for error (arrhythmias, aortic regurgitation).
- Oesophageal Doppler – estimates CO through measurement of blood velocity in the descending aorta (see *Section 5.5 – Doppler effect*).
- Transpulmonary thermodilution – based on the classical dilution method (dilution of known concentration of indicator injectate is measured within the arterial system over time) and is coupled with pulse contour analysis in the PiCCO system. Thermodilution is utilized to calibrate the PiCCO system and to provide measurements of volumetric parameters (e.g. global end-diastolic index) and extravascular lung water.
- Thoracic electrical bioimpedance (TEB) – a small electrical current is passed through electrodes applied to the neck and chest. The pulsatile flow of blood leads to fluctuations in current allowing calculation of CO from the impedance waveform. Studies have shown poor correlation between CO values derived via TEB and those derived via thermodilution methods.

1.1.6

Central venous pressure waveform

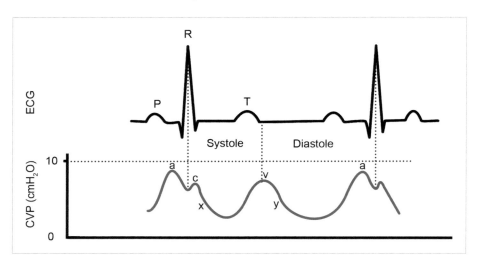

The central venous pressure (CVP) waveform reflects the pressure at the junction of the vena cavae and the right atrium. It consists of three peaks and two descents:
- 'a wave' – the most prominent wave, represents right atrial contraction
- 'c wave' – interrupts 'a wave' decline, due to bulging of the tricuspid valve into the right atrium during right ventricular isovolumetric contraction ($IV_{ol}C$)
- 'x descent' – decline of right atrial pressure during ongoing right ventricular contraction
- 'v wave' – increase in right atrial pressure due to venous filling of the right atrium during late systole
- 'y descent' – decline of right atrial pressure as the tricuspid valve opens.

Alignment with the ECG trace may aid identification of the CVP waveform components.
- Onset of systole marked by ECG R wave; onset of diastole marked by end of ECG T wave.
- Three systolic components – 'c wave', 'x descent' and 'v wave'.
- Two diastolic components – 'y descent' and 'a wave'.

Potential errors in CVP measurement

Sampling errors: positioning of both the central venous catheter and the pressure transducer are important for accurate and precise measurement. Due to the narrow clinical range of CVP, small variations in the transducer reference point may have a disproportionally large effect on CVP measurement.

Interpretation errors: the effects of ventilation on CVP measurement must be considered. All vascular pressures should be measured at end-expiration, because pleural pressure is closest to atmospheric pressure. In positive pressure ventilation, low PEEP results in minimal error by only increasing the observed value by 1–2 mmHg. With high PEEP, error may be more difficult to predict.

1.1.7

Central venous pressure waveform – abnormalities

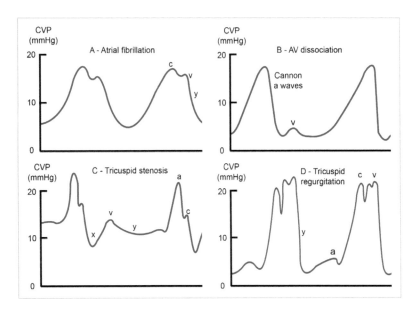

Examination of the CVP waveform may aid diagnosis of various pathophysiological conditions.

Cardiac arrhythmias

A – Atrial fibrillation is characterized by an absent 'a wave'. The 'c wave' is more prominent due to a greater than normal right atrial volume at the end of diastole.

B – In isorhythmic AV dissociation, the atria and ventricles beat independently of each other but at the same rate. As such, the atria contract against a closed tricuspid valve producing an enlarged 'a wave' termed a 'cannon a wave'.

Other arrhythmias also affect the CVP waveform. Sinus tachycardia is characterized by a shortening of diastole and therefore alters the diastolic waveform components (shortening of 'y descent' with merger of the 'v' and 'a' waves). In contrast, sinus bradycardia leads to increased distinction between the three waves.

Valvular disease

C – Tricuspid stenosis is a diastolic abnormality impeding right atrial emptying. As the right atrium contracts against a narrowed tricuspid valve, a prominent 'a wave' is produced. Right atrial pressure remains elevated for longer than normal, attenuating the 'y descent'.

D – In tricuspid regurgitation, systolic flow of blood back into the right atrium through an incompetent valve leads to a persistent elevation of right atrial pressure. As such, the 'c' and 'v' waves gradually merge over time with subsequent loss of the 'x descent'.

Elevation of CVP may be observed with raised intrathoracic pressure (positive-pressure ventilation), cardiac dysfunction (cardiac tamponade, cardiac failure) and circulatory overload.

Reduction in CVP may occur in association with reduced venous return (hypovolaemia, vasodilatation) and a reduction in intrathoracic pressure (spontaneous inspiration).

1.1.8
Einthoven triangle

Bipolar leads (I, II, III) electrically form an equilateral triangle named after Willem Einthoven, the scientist who developed the ECG. These leads, combined with unipolar augmented leads (aVL, aVR, aVF) examine the heart in the frontal plane. Rearranging these six limb leads, allowing an intersection representing the heart, forms the hexaxial reference system. The arrows represent the normal path of electrical current for each lead. This graphical representation of cardiac electrical activity aids interpretation of ventricular axis in the frontal plane.

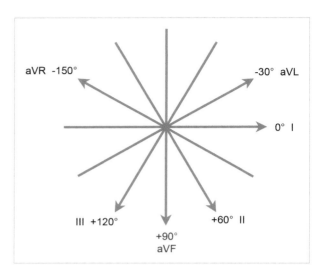

Frontal ventricular axis determination

Normal cardiac electrical activity progresses systematically from the SA node, via internodal fibres to the AV node. Conduction continues via the bundle of His, through right and left bundle branches to Purkinje fibres, resulting in ventricular contraction. Depolarization towards a positive electrode produces a positive deflection on the ECG. When viewing the heart in the frontal plane, mean ventricular depolarization (as denoted by the QRS complex) lies between −30° and +90°. Ventricular axis may be determined using the limb leads. The simplest approach is the quadrant method, examining leads I and aVF. These perpendicular limb leads outline the majority of the normal axis.

- Normal axis – positive QRS complex in both leads.
- Extreme right axis deviation – negative QRS complex in both leads.
- Right axis deviation – negative complex in lead I, positive complex in aVF.
- Left axis deviation – positive complex in lead I, negative complex in aVF. However, as the normal axis ranges from −30° to +90°, this average vector may represent a normal axis. Examination of lead II is also required; if QRS complex is positive the axis is normal (ranging from 0° to −30°).

An alternative equiphasic approach exists, founded on the principle that depolarization travelling perpendicular to a lead produces an equiphasic QRS complex.

1.1.9
Ejection fraction equation

$$EF = \frac{SV}{EDV} \times 100$$

$$SV = EDV - ESV$$

EF = ejection fraction

EDV = end-diastolic volume

ESV = end-systolic volume

SV = stroke volume

The ejection fraction simply describes the amount of blood that is ejected from the ventricle during systolic contraction (stroke volume) as a proportion of the amount of blood that is present in the ventricle at the end of diastole (end-diastolic volume). A 70 kg individual would normally have a stroke volume of about 70 ml and an end-diastolic volume of about 120 ml.

The ejection fraction equation is used to calculate the stroke volume as a percentage of the end-diastolic volume. It gives an indication of the percentage of the ventricular volume that is ejected during each systolic contraction. It can be applied to the left or the right ventricles, with normal values being 50–65%. Right and left ventricular volumes are roughly equal and therefore ejection fractions are broadly similar.

In clinical practice, it can be calculated using echocardiography, pulmonary artery catheterization, nuclear cardiology or by contrast angiography.

In aortic stenosis, the ventricle will compensate for the increased obstruction to outflow by hypertrophy. This will initially maintain the ejection fraction and the pressure gradient across the valve. As the disease progresses and the valve area narrows, the hypertrophied ventricle becomes stiff and less compliant and will no longer be able to compensate. A reduction in the stroke volume (and ejection fraction) is seen, resulting in a fixed reduced cardiac output. The myocardium will eventually fail as compliance continues to worsen.

1.1.10

Electrocardiogram

An electrocardiogram (ECG) is a non-invasive, transthoracic interpretation of cardiac electrical activity over time. Thorough assessment requires a systematic approach including rate, rhythm, axis (normal axis is −30° to +90°), and wave morphology/interval.

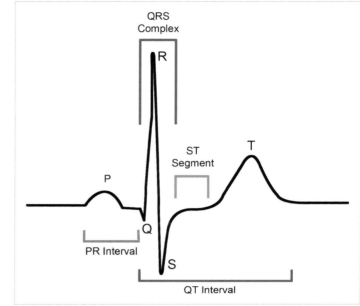

Morphology and intervals

- P wave – represents atrial depolarization. A positive deflection should be present in all leads except aVR.
- PR interval – from the start of the P wave to the end of the PR segment. Normal value 0.12–0.2 s (3–5 small squares). This interval is rate-dependent; as heart rate increases, the PR interval decreases.
- QRS wave – represents ventricular depolarization. The normal duration is ≤0.12 s. A Q wave in leads V1–V3 is abnormal.
- ST segment – from the junction of the QRS complex and the ST segment to the beginning of the T wave. A normal ST segment is isoelectric.
- T wave – represents repolarization of the ventricles.
- QT interval – from the start of the QRS complex to the end of the T wave. This interval represents the time for ventricular activation and recovery. Heart rate variability occurs and therefore a corrected QT interval (QTc) can be calculated (normal value is <0.44 s).

ECG changes associated with acute coronary syndromes and myocardial infarction

- Acute coronary syndromes – include non-ST-elevation myocardial infarction and unstable angina. The primary ECG changes observed are ST segment depression and T wave flattening or inversion.
- Myocardial infarction – early evidence of transmural ischaemia and myocardial infarction includes hyperacute T waves followed by ST elevation. Q wave formation may begin within 1 hour of infarction. Inverted T waves are a later sign within 72 hours of cell death. Stabilization of the ST segment usually occurs within 12 hours, although ST elevation may persist for more than 2 weeks.

1.1.11

Electrocardiogram – cardiac axis and QTc

Division of the hexaxial reference system into four quadrants allows further interpretation of the cardiac ventricular axis (for calculation see *Section 1.1.8 – Einthoven triangle*).

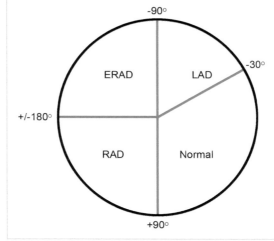

- The normal QRS axis ranges from −30° of left axis deviation (LAD) to +90°.
- LAD is defined as an axis between −30° and −90°. This may be an isolated finding or can be associated with pathology. Causes include: left ventricular hypertrophy, left bundle branch block (LBBB), left anterior fascicular block, myocardial infarction, and mechanical shifts of the heart (e.g. pneumothorax).
- Right axis deviation (RAD) is defined as an axis between +90° and +180°. Causes include: physiological variant in infants and children, right ventricular hypertrophy, myocardial infarction, left posterior fascicular block, chronic lung disease, dextrocardia, and ventricular arrhythmias.
- Extreme right axis deviation (ERAD) is defined as an axis of −90° to +180°. This is a rare finding associated with dextrocardia, ventricular arrhythmias or a paced rhythm.

Precordial axis

Assessment of the precordial leads, V1–V6, enables determination of the precordial axis as described by R wave progression. Normal R wave progression is characterized by a primarily negative QRS complex in V1 and a primarily positive QRS complex in V6. Transition between negative and positive complexes occurs between the V2 and V4 leads.

- Early R wave progression is characterized by much more positive QRS complexes in leads V1 and V2. This observation is always pathological and may be due to posterior myocardial infarction (with the positive QRS complexes representing reciprocal Q waves), right ventricular hypertrophy, RBBB, or Wolff–Parkinson–White syndrome.
- Poor R wave progression is characterized by a predominance of negative QRS complexes through the transitional precordial leads. This late transition can be a normal variant but may also be associated with anterior myocardial infarction, left ventricular hypertrophy, LBBB, or lung disease.

1.1.12

Fick method for cardiac output studies

$$Q = \frac{VO_2}{C_a - C_v}$$

Q = cardiac output (ml.min⁻¹)

VO_2 = volume of oxygen consumed (ml.min⁻¹)

C_a = oxygen content of arterial blood (ml O_2.ml blood⁻¹)

C_v = oxygen content of venous blood (ml O_2.ml blood⁻¹)

The Fick principle states that blood flow to an organ may be calculated using a marker substance if the amount of the marker taken up by the organ per unit time and the arteriovenous difference in marker concentration are known. This principle has been applied to the measurement of cardiac output (CO) where the organ is the entire body and the marker substance is oxygen.

- Direct Fick method – a minimum of 5 minutes of spirometry is required to determine resting oxygen consumption. During this time a peripheral arterial blood sample is obtained to calculate arterial oxygen content. Cardiac catheterization is required to calculate mixed venous oxygen content using a blood sample from the right ventricle/pulmonary trunk. A peripheral venous sample is insufficient because peripheral oxygen content varies markedly between tissues. This method is therefore time consuming and invasive. Validity is limited to the steady-state, prohibiting the use of this method during periods of changing CO such as exercise or other physiological stress.

- Indirect Fick method – application of the Fick principle through carbon dioxide rebreathing avoids invasive measurement of mixed venous oxygen content. Rebreathing techniques estimate arterial and venous carbon dioxide content through measurements of end-tidal partial pressure of carbon dioxide during normal breathing and intermittent rebreathing. Automated systems have eliminated much of the technical difficulty in performing this method.

- Thermodilution – based on the Fick principle, thermodilution is a minimally invasive method for CO measurement. The marker substance is a cold bolus of fluid and the arteriovenous difference is determined by a change in temperature. Thermodilution methods have been studied extensively and shown to correlate well with the direct Fick method. In addition to the minimally invasive nature of this method, other advantages over the direct method include validity during exercise and improved time resolution.

1.1.13

Frank–Starling curve

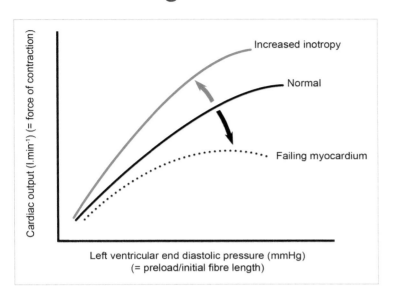

The Frank–Starling curve is used to represent the Frank–Starling law. It states that the ability of the cardiac muscle fibre to contract is dependent upon, and proportional to, its initial fibre length.

As the load experienced by the cardiac muscle fibres increases (within the heart this is the end-diastolic pressure, or preload) so the initial fibre length increases. This results in a proportional increase in the force of contraction due to the overlap between the muscle filaments being optimized. This intrinsic regulatory mechanism occurs up to a certain point. Past this, regulation is lost and contractility does not improve despite increasing fibre length, with eventual muscle fibre failure occurring.

A change in end-diastolic pressure (preload) will cause a patient to shift along the same curve. Increasing preload will cause the patient to shift up along the curve, resulting in increased cardiac output with each contraction. A reduction in preload will cause the opposite.

The whole curve can also be shifted as a result of inotropy or failure of the myocardium. An increased inotropy will cause a greater cardiac output for any given preload and therefore will shift the curve up and to the left. Failure of the myocardium will result in the curve shifting downwards and to the right, demonstrating that for any given preload the cardiac output will be reduced. There is a more exaggerated fall in cardiac output at higher preloads as the fibres become overstretched, with the curve falling off towards the baseline at the far right.

1.1.14

Oxygen flux

$$O_2 \text{ flux (ml.min}^{-1}) = CO \times [(1.34 \times [Hb] \times SpO_2) + (P_aO_2 \times 0.0225)]$$

CO = cardiac output
[Hb] = haemoglobin concentration (g.dl^{-1})
1.34 = maximal O_2 carrying capacity of 1 g of Hb measured *in vivo* (Hüfner's constant) (ml.g^{-1})
SpO_2 = arterial haemoglobin oxygen saturation (%)
P_aO_2 = arterial oxygen tension (kPa)
0.0225 = ml of O_2 dissolved per 100 ml plasma per kPa

Oxygen flux is defined as the amount of oxygen delivered to the tissues per unit time. Oxygen delivery to the tissues is governed by two fundamental elements: cardiac output and arterial oxygen content. Arterial oxygen content comprises the sum of oxygen bound to haemoglobin and oxygen dissolved in plasma. The normal clinical range for oxygen flux is 850–1200 ml.min^{-1}, with measurement requiring pulmonary artery (PA) catheter insertion.

Oxygen flux may be optimized, without invasive PA pressure measurement, if the modifiable variables are considered.
- Cardiac output (CO) – determined by heart rate, preload, contractility and afterload. These factors may be negatively affected by pathological states and drugs (e.g. anaesthetic agents, vasopressors). Optimization may include heart rate control, correction of volume status and administration of vasoactive medications. Direct treatment of disease states should also be implemented.
- Haemoglobin concentration – correction of anaemia will result in an increase in arterial oxygen content. Paradoxically, this may have a deleterious effect on oxygen flux due to the changing rheology of blood in the vascular compartment.
- Haemoglobin oxygen saturation (SpO_2) – may be adversely affected by hypoxia due to hypoventilation, diffusion impairment and ventilation/perfusion inequality. Carbon monoxide poisoning and methaemoglobinaemia should be considered where appropriate. Optimization should focus on the use of supplemental oxygen to maximize alveolar oxygen tension (although the effect will be minimal in shunt) and specific treatment of the cause.
- Arterial oxygen tension – influences SpO_2 and volume of oxygen dissolved in plasma. Increasing P_aO_2 has a finite effect on SpO_2 once maximal saturation is reached. Dissolved arterial oxygen increases proportionally with an increase in P_aO_2. This increase becomes clinically significant at hyperbaric pressures.

1.1.15

Pacemaker nomenclature – antibradycardia

I	II	III	IV	V
Chamber(s) paced	Chamber(s) sensed	Response to sensing	Rate modulation	Multi-site pacing
O = none	O = none	O = none	O/no letter = none	O/no letter = none
A = atrium	A = atrium	I = inhibited	R = rate modulation	A = atrium
V = ventricle	V = ventricle	T = triggered		V = ventricle
D = dual (A + V)	D = dual (A + V)	D = dual (I + T)		D = dual (A + V)

The pacemaker code has five positions.
- Position I – chamber paced.
- Position II – chamber sensed (detection of spontaneous cardiac depolarization).
- Position III – response to sensing on subsequent pacing stimuli.
- Position IV – presence or absence of an adaptive-rate mechanism in response to patient activity. The previous pacemaker code included a programmability hierarchy (i.e. simple vs. multi), which is now deemed unnecessary.
- Position V – presence and location of multisite pacing. This is defined as stimulation sites in both atria, both ventricles, more than one stimulation site in a single chamber or any combination of these.

Pacemakers and diathermy

If possible, diathermy should be avoided in patients with pacemakers. However, if diathermy is required, bipolar is safer (as the current travels between the two instrument electrodes). This should be used in short bursts at the lowest energy settings.

When diathermy is used intra-operatively, a variety of untoward events may occur. These include inappropriate pacemaker inhibition (failure to pace), system reprogramming, and permanent pacemaker damage. With the design of newer units, these events are becoming increasingly rare. The most frequent interaction is pacemaker inhibition caused by misinterpretation of diathermy electrical activity as intrinsic cardiac activity. If the pacemaker has a 'D' or 'I' in position III, the pacemaker becomes inhibited and does not pace. The clinical effect depends on the duration of electrical stimulus, the underlying cardiac rhythm and the degree of dependency on the pacemaker. Ideally, to avoid adverse diathermy interaction, pacemakers should be evaluated by a clinical electrophysiologist prior to surgery to develop a perioperative device management plan. This plan should consider re-programming to a fixed-rate mode, whether (and how) a magnet could be used and recommendation for follow-up post-operatively.

1.1.16

Pacemaker nomenclature – antitachycardia (implantable cardioverter-defibrillators)

I	II	III	IV
Chamber(s) shocked	Antitachycardia pacing chamber(s)	Tachycardia detection	Antibradycardia pacing chamber(s)
O = none	O = none	E = electrogram	O = none
A = atrium	A = atrium	H = haemodynamic	A = atrium
V = ventricle	V = ventricle		V = ventricle
D = dual (A + V)	D = dual (A + V)		D = dual (A + V)

The implantable cardioverter-defibrillator (ICD) code has four positions.
- Position I indicates the chamber shocked.
- Position II indicates the antitachycardia pacing chamber.
- Position III indicates the method of antitachycardia detection. Haemodynamic detection includes sensing of blood pressure or transthoracic impedance.
- Position IV indicates the antibradycardia pacing chamber, in case defibrillation results in bradycardia.

Perioperative considerations in patients with ICDs
- Preoperative – a multidisciplinary approach is essential. Perioperative management of an ICD should ideally be developed in collaboration with the cardiology and surgical teams, however, this may not always be feasible. In the out-of-hours setting, review of the patient's information card and/or medical records should provide helpful information such as indication for treatment and functionality of the device. A CXR will help in determining the type of implantable cardiac device and if all leads are intact.
- Intraoperative – identification of potential sources of electromagnetic interference (EMI) is important to minimize device malfunction. Commonly encountered factors associated with EMI include electrocautery (diathermy), evoked potential monitors, nerve stimulators, and fasciculations. Generation of EMI may cause inappropriate defibrillation. To minimize this risk, antitachycardia functions should be suspended. Variability observed with magnet application to ICDs is less than that observed with pacemakers. For the majority of ICD devices, magnet application temporarily inhibits arrhythmia detection and discharge, with rapid resumption of antitachycardia functions with magnet removal. However, the use of a magnet, by non-experts, with certain devices may result in unanticipated results such as permanent programming changes, changes to antibradycardia functions or no change in function at all. Best practice advises perioperative input from an electrophysiologist or cardiologist. Continuous intraoperative haemodynamic monitoring and immediate availability of an external defibrillator are essential.
- Post-operative – continuous monitoring and external defibrillator availability must be continued until ICD function is resumed. A review by an electrophysiologist is recommended prior to termination of cardiac monitoring.

1.1.17
Preload, contractility and afterload

	Definition	Measurement
Preload	The tension in the wall of the ventricle at the end of ventricular relaxation (diastole)	Can be inferred from ventricular end-diastolic pressure
	Related to initial stretch of muscle fibres with filling of the ventricle in diastole	Central venous pressure (right ventricle)
	Quantitatively calculated using Laplace's law	Pulmonary capillary wedge pressure (left ventricle)
Contractility	Intrinsic ability of the myocardium to contract with a given preload and afterload	Often represented by cardiac output, stroke volume, stroke index or stroke work
	Increases as a result of increased actin and myosin binding, which is proportional to calcium ion concentration	
Afterload	Tension required in ventricle wall in order to eject the stroke volume during systole	Often equated to the systemic vascular resistance
	Altered by changes in the ventricle itself or in the circulation	

The definitions of preload, contractility and afterload were developed from experiments looking at isolated muscle fibres *in vitro*, allowing individual definitions to be produced. *In vivo,* these factors are interlinked, being dependent upon and affected by each other, making measuring them individually more difficult.

The stroke volume is determined by all three variables: preload, contractility and afterload. These, together with the heart rate, determine myocardial performance. Preload can also give an indication of how well a myocardium is performing. A heart requiring a higher preload to generate a cardiac output is not performing as well as one that is generating the same cardiac output with a lower preload.

In vivo, direct measurement of initial myocardial fibre length is not possible and therefore preload cannot be determined. As such, various surrogate markers have to be used. The volume in the ventricle at the end of diastole gives an indication of fibre stretch just before the onset of contraction. This can be measured by echocardiography and is called the end-diastolic volume.

The pressure generated in the heart chambers for a given volume is dependent on the chamber's compliance, with the end-diastolic pressure often being referred to as the 'filling pressure'. The right atrial pressure can be inferred from the CVP giving an indication of the filling pressure of the right side of the heart. The left-sided pressures are more difficult to measure and require a pulmonary artery catheter to obtain their values.

Contractility is difficult to define in isolation, being affected by all the factors that affect myocardial performance. Most factors that increase contractility do so by increasing the intracellular calcium concentration. Inotropy is often used synonymously with contractility.

Afterload can be represented by the mean arterial pressure during systole, or by measurement of the end-systolic pressure.

1.1.18

Pulmonary artery catheter trace

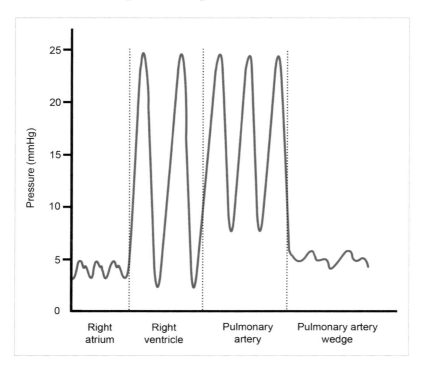

A pulmonary artery catheter is a balloon-tipped, flow-directed multi-lumen catheter, initially inserted through a central venous introducer sheath. During its placement a trace is produced demonstrating the pressures as the catheter moves through the chambers of the right heart and into the pulmonary circulation. The pulmonary capillary wedge pressure (PCWP) is used as a surrogate for the left atrial pressure.

Continuous pressure monitoring is used, via the distal lumen of the catheter, to guide correct insertion and produce the trace seen above. The balloon is inflated once the catheter has reached the right atrium and is allowed to float with the flow of blood to reach the pulmonary circulation. The right atrium pressure waveform is similar to the CVP waveform. On reaching the right ventricle the wave will oscillate between 0–5 mmHg and 20–25 mmHg. The catheter will then pass through the pulmonary valve and enter the pulmonary artery. The systolic pressure will remain the same as the right ventricle, but the diastolic pressure will rise to about 10–15 mmHg owing to the presence of the pulmonary valve. A PCWP is obtained by allowing the catheter's balloon to occlude a pulmonary vessel. The trace will look similar to the CVP waveform, but with a range of 6–12 mmHg. The measurement should ideally be taken in West Zone 3 of the lung (where the pulmonary artery pressure is greater than both the alveolar and pulmonary venous pressures, ensuring a continuous column of blood to the left atrium) and at the end of expiration.

Pulmonary artery catheters can also be used to measure cardiac output (by means of an integral thermistor), mixed venous oxygen saturations, right-sided heart pressures and the right ventricular ejection fraction. It can also be used to derive systemic and pulmonary vascular resistances and the cardiac index.

1.1.19

Systemic and pulmonary pressures

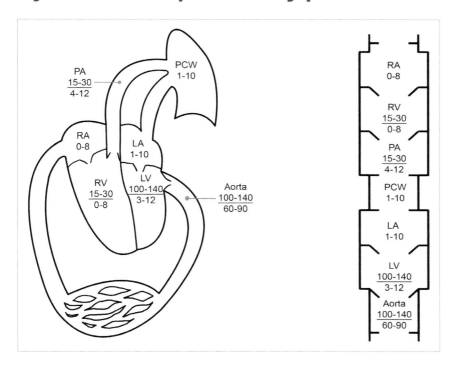

The heart consists of two pumps in parallel: the low pressure right side that pumps into the pulmonary circulation, and the higher pressure left side that pumps into the systemic circulation.

The CVP approximates to the pressure in the right atrium and oscillates between 0 and 5 mmHg. In the right ventricle, the systolic pressure increases to 20–25 mmHg, with the diastolic pressure remaining similar to that in the right atrium. The presence of the pulmonary valve increases the diastolic pressure in the pulmonary artery to 10–15 mmHg, while the systolic pressure remains the same. The pulmonary capillary pressures are 6–12 mmHg, creating a pressure gradient that allows forward flow of blood from the pulmonary artery into the pulmonary circulation. The pulmonary capillary (wedge) pressure is often used as a surrogate for left atrial pressure and, in the presence of a normal mitral valve, left ventricular end-diastolic pressure. A pulmonary artery catheter allows accurate measurement of these pressures (see *Section 1.1.18 – Pulmonary artery catheter trace*).

The pressures in the left side of the heart are higher than the right due to the higher vascular resistance in the systemic circulation. To generate these higher pressures it therefore has a larger muscle bulk than the right. Left atrial pressure measures between 1 and 10 mmHg. During systole, the left ventricular pressure will rise to about 120 mmHg to generate forward flow. As blood passes through the aortic valve, the diastolic pressure will rise to about 60–80 mmHg with the systolic pressure remaining the same. Arterial cannulation can be performed to measure systemic pressures continuously. Peripheral cannulation will produce higher peak systolic and lower diastolic pressures than more central cannulation due to the differences in impedance and harmonic resonance. However, mean arterial pressure will remain broadly similar.

1.1.20

Valsalva manoeuvre

A Valsalva manoeuvre is performed by attempted expiration against a closed glottis. This results in an abrupt but transient increase in intrathoracic pressure and vagal tone. The normal physiological response to this manoeuvre consists of four phases.

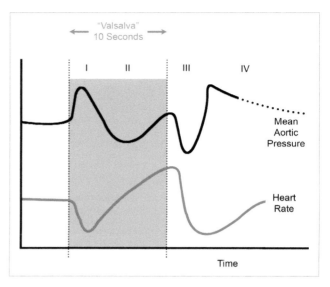

- **Phase I** – sudden rise in intrathoracic pressure compresses capacitance thoracic vessels, increasing return of blood from the lungs to left atrium. A sudden, but transient, increase in systemic blood pressure is observed in accordance with the Frank–Starling law of the heart, coupled with direct compression of the thoracic aortic arch. Aortic arch baroreceptors are activated, initiating a compensatory reduction in heart rate.

- **Phase II** – venous return of systemic blood is impeded by sustained increase in intrathoracic pressure. This reduction in preload leads to a fall in cardiac output, once again, in accordance with the Frank–Starling law. A progressive reduction in blood pressure is observed. Baroreceptor activity is reduced, resulting in a sympathetically mediated gradual increase in heart rate, systemic vasoconstriction and a restoration of blood pressure.

- **Phase III** – sudden release of the intrathoracic pressure leads to an abrupt reduction of systemic blood pressure as compression of the aortic arch and thoracic capacitance vessels ceases. Baroreceptor activity is reduced, thereby maintaining heart rate elevation.

- **Phase IV** – an increase in blood pressure occurs with rapid restoration of the cardiac output as venous return suddenly increases. Systolic blood pressure exceeds the resting value ('overshoot') as blood is ejected into a constricted peripheral vascular system, as mediated by sympathetic activation in phase II. This rise in blood pressure results in baroreceptor activation and a compensatory bradycardia. Phase IV is not considered complete until the blood pressure has stabilized at its resting value. This may take up to 90 seconds and an 'undershoot' of blood pressure is often observed.

1.1.21

Valsalva manoeuvre – clinical applications and physiological abnormalities

- Test of autonomic integrity – the Valsalva manoeuvre is a simple, non-invasive tool to aid assessment of the autonomic nervous system. A sustained increase in intrathoracic pressure should incite autonomically mediated cardiovascular responses. Phases II and IV are of particular importance for the evaluation of autonomic baroreceptor activity.

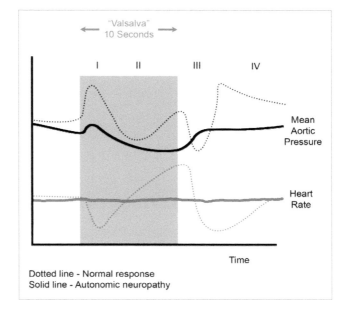

Dotted line - Normal response
Solid line - Autonomic neuropathy

- Acquired autonomic neuropathies are most commonly observed as secondary features of systemic disease. Causes may be classified as metabolic (diabetes mellitus, uraemic neuropathy), toxic/drug-induced (alcohol-mediated, secondary to chemotherapeutic agents), infectious (HIV, Lyme disease) or autoimmune (Guillain–Barré syndrome, rheumatoid arthritis, systemic lupus erythematosus). Clinical presentation of autonomic neuropathy is as variable as its aetiology. For anaesthetists, cardiovascular autonomic neuropathy is likely to be the most important clinically due to its association with a variety of adverse outcomes (intraoperative cardiovascular lability, increased cardiac-related mortality).
- The abnormal Valsalva response observed in autonomic neuropathy is secondary to failure of baroreceptor activation. The diagram demonstrates the excessive reduction of blood pressure in phase II, which remains low until the intrathoracic pressure is released. The compensatory changes in heart rate are blunted and the overshoot in phase IV is absent.
- Termination of supraventricular tachycardia (SVT) – the Valsalva manoeuvre may be used as an initial, non-invasive means for termination of SVT. Activation of the baroreceptor reflex in phase I leads to an increase in parasympathetic tone, and subsequent increase in refractoriness of the AV node.
- Intraoperative use – a Valsalva manoeuvre may be generated intraoperatively by the anaesthetist for a variety of reasons, largely for associated mechanical benefits. These include assessment of haemostasis (e.g. thyroid or spinal surgery) and re-expansion of the lung (following one-lung anaesthesia or lung collapse). A pressure of 40 mmHg is commonly used and should be performed with care, appreciating the possible resultant cardiovascular effects.

1.1.22

Vaughan–Williams classification

Class	Mechanism of action	Effect on conduction	Drugs
Ia	Sodium channel blockade	Prolongs refractory period	Quinidine, procainamide, disopyramide
Ib		Shortens refractory period	Lidocaine, phenytoin, mexiletine
Ic		No effect	Flecainide, propafenone
II	Beta-adrenoceptor blockade	Slows AV conduction	Propanolol, atenolol, esmolol
III	Potassium channel blockade	Slows AV conduction	Amiodarone, sotalol
IV	Calcium channel blockade	Prolongs refractory period	Verapamil, diltiazem
V	Other or unknown	Varied	Adenosine, digoxin, magnesium

The Vaughan–Williams classification was traditionally used to classify anti-arrhythmic drugs into groups depending on their primary mechanism of action. There were originally 4 groups, with a 5th group added later to include drugs with multiple or alternative mechanisms of action.

- Class I agents are grouped by their action on the sodium channel. They act by binding to the alpha subunit and thereby reduce the maximal rate of contraction during phase 0 of the cardiac action potential. They are divided into three further groups depending on their effect on cardiac conduction and are often described as having membrane stabilizing effects.
- Class II agents are beta-adrenoceptor blockers and act by reducing the effect of catecholamines at the beta-1 receptors in the heart. They increase the refractory period of the AV node and therefore can be useful in treating SVTs.
- Class III agents block potassium channels and therefore prolong repolarization and slow AV conduction. This also has the effect of extending the Q–T interval and hence can cause torsade de pointes in susceptible individuals.
- Class IV agents block calcium channels and decrease conduction through the AV node. They also reduce cardiac contractility and therefore can have adverse effects in heart failure.
- Class V includes drugs that do not fit neatly into the above classes due to multiple or alternative mechanisms of action. Amiodarone has class I, II, III and IV actions and sotalol has class I, II and III actions. Drugs acting by alternative mechanisms include adenosine (alpha-1 receptors), digoxin (Na^+/K^+-ATPase pump) and magnesium (calcium antagonist).

1.1.23

Ventricular pressure–volume loop – left ventricle

A. Isovolumetric contraction – onset of left ventricular (LV) contraction results in closure of the mitral valve as LV pressure exceeds left atrial (LA) pressure. As the LV contracts against the closed mitral and aortic valves, the LV pressure increases without an increase in volume.

B. Ejection – once LV pressure exceeds aortic diastolic pressure, the aortic valve opens and ejection begins. LV pressure continues to increase to peak systolic pressure and then decrease as LV relaxation begins. During this phase, LV volume decreases.

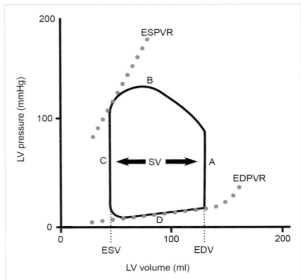

C. Isovolumetric relaxation – begins with closure of the aortic valve as LV pressure falls below aortic pressure. Both valves are closed, leading to a decrease in pressure, while volume remains constant.

D. LV filling – once LV pressure falls below LA pressure, the mitral valve opens and LV filling begins. A further decrease in LV pressure occurs despite filling as the LV relaxes completely. Both LV pressure and volume rise to end-diastolic values before the cycle commences again.

The width of the pressure–volume loop is the difference between the end-diastolic (EDV) and end-systolic volumes (ESV). In the normal heart of a healthy 70 kg male, this stroke volume (SV) is approximately 70 ml. The area within the loop is the work done by the LV to eject the SV into the aorta; known as stroke work.

End-diastolic pressure–volume relationship (EDPVR) describes the passive filling curve for the LV. The slope of the EDPVR at any point along the curve is the reciprocal of ventricular compliance. End-systolic pressure–volume relationship (ESPVR) describes the maximal pressure that can be achieved by the LV at any given volume. The slope of the ESPVR provides a marker of myocardial contractility. It is an improved index of systolic myocardial function compared to SV, because ESPVR is relatively insensitive to changes in other cardiac output parameters (e.g. preload and afterload).

1.1.24

Ventricular pressure–volume loop – right ventricle

The pressure–volume loop of the right ventricle is characterized by an early peak and rapid decline, giving rise to a more triangular shape compared to the rounded left ventricular loop. This is largely secondary to poorly defined isovolumetric periods. Right ventricular contraction occurs in a peristaltic pattern compared to synchronized contraction of the left ventricle. As such, right ventricular isovolumetric contraction is rapidly superseded by ejection. As the pulmonary vascular bed offers a resistance one-tenth the systemic

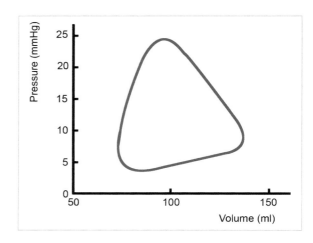

circulation, right ventricular end-systolic pressure (15–30 mmHg) is dramatically lower compared to the left ventricle (90–140 mmHg). A period of isovolumetric relaxation is equally ill-defined due to a 'hangout period': the ongoing ejection of blood despite falling right ventricular pressure. It is probably due to the high capacitance of the pulmonary vascular bed. Despite dramatic differences in pressures generated by the ventricles, stroke volumes are approximately equal. Low impedance offered by the pulmonary circulation demands that the right ventricle use only one-fifth the energy of the left, demonstrated by a smaller loop area denoting stroke work done.

Factors affecting right heart function

- Preload of the right heart is determined by venous return and ventricular compliance. Preload is significantly influenced by the mechanics of breathing. During spontaneous inspiration a reduction in intrapleural pressure causes an increase in venous return, with the converse observed during expiration. This leads to fluctuations in stroke volume during the respiratory cycle.
- Afterload of the right heart is determined by impedance of the pulmonary vascular bed. Resistance remains low while vascular recruitment is possible. Once pulmonary capacitance is exhausted a modest increase in pulmonary resistance leads to reduction in right ventricular cardiac output.
- Ventricular interdependence describes the effect of contralateral ventricular contraction. Studies have shown approximately 30% of right ventricular systolic pressure results from left ventricular contraction.

1.2.1

Blood flow and oxygen consumption of organs

Organ	Cardiac output	Blood flow		Oxygen consumption	
	(%)	(ml.min^{-1})	(ml.100 g^{-1}.min^{-1})	(ml.min^{-1})	(ml.100 g^{-1}.min^{-1})
Heart	5	250	80	30	10
Brain	15	700	50	50	3
Kidneys	20	1200	400	20	6

Cardiac output is distributed between the major organs of the body as shown above. The blood flow to an organ is proportional to the perfusion pressure and inversely proportional to the vascular resistance of the supplying vessels.

The heart has the highest oxygen consumption per 100g of tissue of all of the organs in the body. The total coronary blood flow at rest is about 250 ml.min^{-1}, representing about 5% of the cardiac output. At rest, the myocardium normally extracts about 70% of the oxygen content of the arterial blood, therefore any increase in oxygen demand must be met by an increase in coronary blood flow; during exercise this may increase five-fold. Blood flow occurs mostly during diastole, therefore any increase in heart rate reduces time for diastole and so reduces perfusion time. In patients with hypertension, the left ventricle will hypertrophy in order to overcome the increase in afterload. This will increase myocardial work and oxygen demand whilst also decreasing flow.

The brain receives about 15% of the resting cardiac output; the overall blood flow is about 700 ml.min^{-1} (50 ml.100 g^{-1}.min^{-1}). This shows regional variation; the more metabolically active grey matter receives 70 ml.100 g^{-1}.min^{-1}, compared to the white matter that receives 30 ml.100 g^{-1}.min^{-1}. The cerebral metabolic rate for oxygen is high (3 ml.100 g^{-1}.min^{-1}), leaving the jugular venous blood about 65% saturated. Neurons produce energy almost entirely by oxidative metabolism with very little capacity for anaerobic metabolism, and they can therefore withstand only very short periods of ischaemia.

The kidneys receive about 20% of the cardiac output, but only represent about 0.5% of body weight; the blood flow per 100 g of tissue is therefore high. This abundant blood flow not only supports the metabolic demands of the organ, but also functions to maintain the glomerular filtration rate.

1.2.2

Blood vessel structure

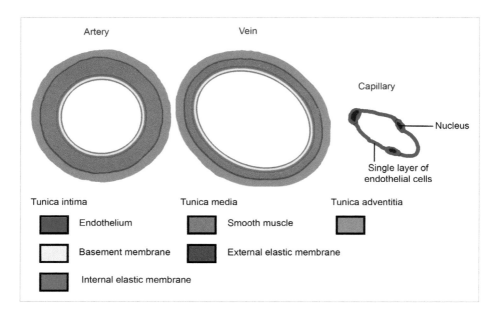

A blood vessel comprises a layered wall surrounding a central lumen. The wall has three concentric layers.

- Tunica intima (innermost) – single layer of endothelial cells and underlying basement membrane. The intima reduces friction between the vessel wall and blood.
- Tunica media (middle) – circularly arranged smooth muscle cells and sheets of elastin. Smooth muscle facilitates regulation of blood flow through vasoconstriction and vasodilatation. Elastin allows distensibility and recoil to accommodate pulsatile flow of blood.
- Tunica externa/adventitia (outermost) – collagen fibres protect the vessel and anchor it to surrounding structures. This layer also contains sympathetic vasomotor nerves that release noradrenaline which diffuses into the media to act on smooth muscle.

Arterial system – arterial walls possess a thicker tunica media than veins to accommodate higher pressures. Arteries may be classified according to size and function.

- Large elastic arteries (e.g. aorta) – elastin is abundant within the media to absorb high pressures produced by the left ventricle. During diastole, vessels recoil, propelling blood forward.
- Medium muscular arteries (e.g. coronary arteries) – rich in smooth muscle, adjustments in vessel diameter allow control of regional blood flow.
- Small arterioles (e.g. in visceral organs) – the tunica media is abundant in smooth muscle.

Capillaries – an exception to the layered structure, these vessels consist of a single layer of endothelial cells on a basement membrane. This arrangement facilitates exchange of oxygen, nutrients and other substances between blood and tissues.

Venous system – capillaries unite to form venules, which join to form veins. The tunica media is much thinner due to less smooth muscle and elastin; therefore, veins are more distensible than arteries, contributing capacitance to the circulation. Reduced elastic recoil necessitates contraction of surrounding muscles or respiratory pressure gradients to propel blood forward. Valves prevent reversal of flow.

1.2.3

Hagen–Poiseuille equation

$$\text{Flow} = \frac{\Delta P r^4 \pi}{8l\eta}$$

ΔP = pressure difference

r = radius

l = length

η = viscosity

The Hagen–Poiseuille equation is used to describe the factors that affect laminar flow of Newtonian fluids through a tube. It includes those factors contributed by the tube itself (length, radius and pressure gradient across it) and by the fluid (viscosity).

A Newtonian fluid is one in which the viscosity of the fluid does not change despite changes in flow rate, an example being water. Blood is a non-Newtonian fluid because its viscosity decreases with increasing flow rate. However, the Hagen–Poiseuille equation is often used to describe blood flow through the circulation.

Flow is directly proportional to the pressure gradient across a tube and to the fourth power of the radius. As the pressure difference increases flow will increase and, likewise, as the radius of a tube increases the flow will greatly increase: doubling the radius will result in a 16-fold increase in flow rate. This explains the use of a pressure bag for rapid infusion of fluid through a large bore cannula to a patient requiring resuscitation.

Flow is inversely proportional to the length of the tube and to the viscosity of the fluid, meaning that flow rates will decrease as the length of the tube and the viscosity of the fluid increases. This explains the increased flow seen through a short peripheral cannula compared to a 15 cm central line lumen of the same gauge. A more viscous fluid (e.g. blood) will have a slower flow rate when compared to a less viscous fluid (e.g. crystalloid) infused through the same giving set. Importantly, viscosity only applies to laminar flow, with density becoming more important when the flow becomes turbulent.

1.2.4

Laminar and turbulent flow

Flow is defined as the volume of a fluid passing a point per unit time (ml.min⁻¹). Flow may be described as laminar, turbulent or mixed. Generally, blood flow within blood vessels is laminar, characterized by organized movement of concentric layers of blood. Ideal conditions favouring laminar flow include straight blood vessels of small diameter. According to the equation for Reynolds number (see *Section 5.26 – Types of flow*), flow becomes turbulent with increasing vessel diameter, increasing blood velocity and decreasing blood viscosity.

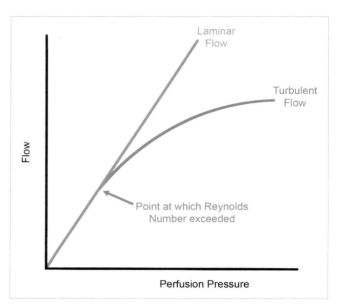

This disorganized flow may also be observed at vessel branch points and with lumenal irregularity. For a given perfusion pressure, laminar flow achieves a greater flow rate compared to turbulent flow, as demonstrated in the pressure–flow graph above.

Blood flow in coronary atherosclerotic disease

Narrowing of blood vessels secondary to the formation of atheromatous plaques is associated with turbulent blood flow. In accordance with the laws of fluid dynamics (see *Section 7.13 – Oxygen delivery systems — Bernoulli principle and Venturi effect*), the velocity of a fluid must increase as it passes through a constriction. This increase in velocity along with irregularity of the vessel lumen predispose to turbulent flow. Turbulent blood flow reduces perfusion pressure distal to the stenosis because kinetic energy is lost as friction. Therefore, to maintain a constant rate of coronary blood flow perfusion pressure must increase. This increase in perfusion pressure is achieved through local autoregulation by metabolic, myogenic and endothelial mechanisms, leading to microvascular vasodilatation. Autoregulation can compensate for up to approximately 70% diameter reduction, thereby maintaining normal resting coronary blood flow. However, with an increase in oxygen requirements, usually associated with exertion, the myocardium is at risk of ischaemia unless coronary blood flow can be maintained. First-line treatment of angina includes the use of nitrates, which improve coronary blood flow through coronary vasodilatation.

1.2.5
Laplace's law

For a cylinder:

$$P = \frac{T}{r}$$

For a sphere:

$$P = \frac{2T}{r}$$

P = transmural pressure

T = tension in the wall

r = radius

Pierre-Simon Laplace was a French scientist of the 18th and early 19th century. His law states that for a hollow distensible structure, the transmural pressure gradient is given by the wall tension in each direction, divided by the radius. In a cylinder there is only one radius (the other being infinity) and therefore transmural pressure is proportional to the wall tension and inversely proportional to the radius. On the other hand, in a sphere, there are two radii that are equal, so the relationship becomes two times the wall tension divided by the radius.

Vessels, such as the arterioles, are effectively cylinders and obey Laplace's law. It is proposed as one theory of autoregulation – as the intraluminal pressure changes, the muscular wall tension varies in order to maintain a constant radius and therefore blood flow.

Similarly, the ventricle of the heart is rather like a sphere. When the heart is dilated, i.e. has an increased radius, it must generate a greater wall tension in order to maintain the same pressure. This explains the benefit of reducing the preload to a failing heart, thereby reducing its starting radius and the force it needs to generate to maintain the same pressure; this reduces the work of the myocardium.

1.2.6

Ohm's law

$$V = IR$$

$$Q = \frac{\Delta P}{R}$$

$$CO = \frac{MAP}{SVR}$$

V = voltage

I = current

R = resistance (to blood flow)

Q = flow

ΔP = pressure difference between a proximal and distal point in circulatory system

CO = cardiac output

MAP = mean arterial pressure

SVR = systemic vascular resistance

Ohm's law was originally developed to describe the flow of electrons within an electrical circuit. The law states that for a given resistance, the potential difference (voltage) across an ideal conductor is directly proportional to the current through it. A modification of this principle describes the haemodynamic relationship between blood flow, resistance and pressure. When applied to the circulation as a whole, Ohm's law defines a simplified relationship between cardiac output (CO), mean arterial pressure (MAP) and systemic vascular resistance (SVR).

Haemodynamic determinants of systemic hypertension

Based on the modified Ohm's law equation, systemic hypertension requires an increase in CO and/or SVR. Typically, in established systemic hypertension, SVR is increased in the presence of a normal or reduced CO. Associated haemodynamic changes include a central shift of blood volume and a reduction in arterial compliance. Persistent systemic hypertension leads to structural remodelling of both the heart and blood vessels in accordance with Laplace's law (see *Section 1.2.5 – Laplace's law*). As pressure within the left ventricle (due to a rise in afterload) and blood vessels is chronically increased, wall thickness also increases to minimize wall tension.

Recommendations for first-line treatment of essential hypertension include angiotensin-converting enzyme inhibitors (ACEi) and calcium channel blockers, depending on age and ethnicity. Both of these pharmaceutical agents aim to reduce systemic blood pressure, at least in part, through peripheral vasodilatation and a reduction in SVR.

1.2.7

Starling forces in capillaries

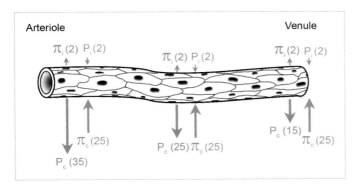

Net fluid movement = outward forces − inward forces

$$Q = K[(P_c - P_i) - \sigma(\pi_c - \pi_i)]$$

Q = net flow of fluid
K = permeability coefficient (flow rate per unit pressure gradient)
P_c = capillary hydrostatic pressure (mmHg)
P_i = interstitial hydrostatic pressure (mmHg)
σ = reflection coefficient (permeability of the capillary membrane to proteins)
π_c = capillary oncotic pressure (mmHg)
π_i = interstitial osmotic pressure (mmHg)

Ernest Starling is famous not only for his experiments on the heart (see *Section 1.1.13 – Frank–Starling curve*) but also for his proposed explanation for fluid movement across capillaries. He described how the movement of fluid into the interstitial space is encouraged by the hydrostatic pressure gradient and counteracted by the colloid osmotic pressure gradient.

The capillary hydrostatic pressure (P_c) is generated by the column of blood within the capillary. Counteracting this is the interstitial hydrostatic pressure (P_i) exerted by the fluid surrounding the capillary within the interstitial space.

The capillary oncotic pressure (π_c), a form of osmotic pressure generated by plasma proteins, is the pressure needed to prevent movement of water across the capillary membrane. Similarly, the interstitial osmotic pressure (π_i) is the pressure needed to prevent the movement of water across the capillary due to the effect of proteins in the interstitial space; in health this value is low.

1.2.8

Starling forces in capillaries – pathology

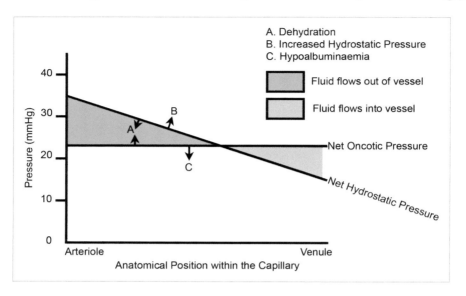

A. Dehydration
B. Increased Hydrostatic Pressure
C. Hypoalbuminaemia

Fluid flows out of vessel

Fluid flows into vessel

In a healthy person, capillary hydrostatic pressure is about 35 mmHg at the arteriolar end, exceeding the capillary oncotic pressure and favouring net fluid flow out of the capillary. At the venous end, where the capillary hydrostatic pressure falls to about 15 mmHg, the opposite happens. In the centre of the capillary the hydrostatic and oncotic pressures are roughly equal and therefore no net fluid movement occurs. In health there is a slight net fluid movement leaving the capillary and this is removed by the lymphatic system.

Altering the balance of these forces will result in changes to fluid movement across the capillary. Dehydration (A) increases the capillary oncotic pressure and favours movement of fluid into the capillary in an attempt to restore circulating volume. Conversely, any reduction in capillary oncotic pressure, e.g. hypoalbuminaemia (C), or increases in capillary hydrostatic pressure (B), from venous congestion perhaps, will cause net filtration of fluid out of the capillaries causing tissue oedema.

1.2.9
Systemic vascular resistance

$$CO = \frac{MAP}{SVR}$$

$$SVR = 80 \times \frac{MAP - CVP}{CO}$$

CO = cardiac output (l.min⁻¹)

MAP = mean arterial pressure (mmHg)

SVR = systemic vascular resistance (dyn.s.cm⁻⁵)

CVP = central venous pressure (mmHg)

Systemic vascular resistance (SVR) is the resistance to blood flow provided by all the systemic vasculature with the exception of the pulmonary circulation. The SVR may be calculated using a modification of Ohm's law (see *Section 1.2.6 – Ohm's Law*), where blood flow is equal to driving pressure divided by resistance. The numerical constant (80) is used to convert mmHg.min.l⁻¹ to the units used for measuring vascular resistance: dyn.s.cm⁻⁵. Although SVR may be calculated numerically using the equation above, *in vivo* SVR in itself is not determined by mean arterial pressure (MAP) or cardiac output (CO) *per se*. Instead it is influenced by intrinsic and extrinsic factors (see below) and a more appropriate interpretation of this equation is that for a given CO, a high MAP can be attributed, in part, to a high SVR.

Determinants of SVR

The main determinants of SVR include vessel length, vessel radius and blood viscosity. These variables may be related to SVR using the Hagen–Poiseuille equation (see *Section 1.2.3 – Hagen–Poiseuille equation*). The most significant parameter is vessel radius, as denoted by the inverse relationship of resistance to the fourth power of the radius. The majority of SVR is provided by muscular arterioles which act to regulate blood flow to various organs within the body. Despite having a larger radius than capillaries, the arterioles are a higher resistance system. This is explained by the vast number of capillaries organized in parallel, thereby functioning as a system with a large cumulative radius.

SVR is modulated by a balance of vasodilatation and vasoconstriction, achieved through extrinsic and intrinsic means. Extrinsic factors, such as activation of the sympathetic nervous system or renin–angiotensin system, act to increase SVR through vasoconstriction. Other extrinsic mediators, such as prostaglandins and atrial natriuretic peptide, lead to vasodilatation and a reduction in SVR. Intrinsic factors originate from within the blood vessel itself or surrounding tissue, modulating the radius of the blood vessels and hence vascular tone. They include myogenic mechanisms, endothelial mediators (e.g. nitric oxide) and release of local hormones (e.g. prostaglandins, bradykinin).

1.3.1

Alveolar gas equation

$$P_AO_2 = [F_iO_2 \times (P_B - P_AH_2O)] - \frac{P_ACO_2}{R}$$

P_AO_2 = alveolar partial pressure of oxygen
F_iO_2 = fractional inspired concentration of oxygen
P_B = atmospheric or barometric pressure
P_AH_2O = alveolar partial pressure of water (saturated vapour pressure at 37°C)
P_ACO_2 = alveolar partial pressure of carbon dioxide
R = respiratory quotient

The alveolar gas equation is used to calculate the partial pressure of oxygen in an alveolus. This can then be used to determine the alveolar–arterial oxygen difference (using an arterial blood gas sample to measure the arterial oxygen concentration) or in the measurement of shunt.

The fractional partial pressure of inspired gas only applies to the dry portion of the mixture. Therefore, to calculate the inspired partial pressure of oxygen (P_iO_2), the saturated vapour pressure of water is first subtracted from the atmospheric pressure, before multiplying it by the fractional inspired concentration of oxygen.

It is assumed that there is a negligible carbon dioxide gradient between the arterial and alveolar spaces because the alveolar membrane is very thin and carbon dioxide is highly diffusible. The alveolar and arterial partial pressures of carbon dioxide (P_ACO_2 and P_aCO_2 respectively) are therefore assumed to be equal.

The respiratory quotient (R) is a dimensionless number being derived from the expired carbon dioxide divided by the inspired oxygen measurement. It is often used in calculations of basal metabolic rate and is dependent on the energy substrate utilized. A value of 0.8 is often used to represent a normal diet, however, a pure carbohydrate diet would give a value of 1.0 (i.e. for every oxygen molecule used in metabolizing carbohydrate, one molecule of carbon dioxide is produced).

$$P_AO_2 = [0.21 \times (101.3 - 6.3)] - \frac{5.3}{0.8} = 19.95 - 6.6 = 13.35 \text{ kPa}$$

In the above calculation, where normal values have been used, there is very little difference between the alveolar and arterial partial pressure of oxygen. Ventilation-perfusion mismatching and shunt will often lead to a small difference; up to 2 kPa is acceptable.

Interestingly, the alveolar gas equation cannot be used in all circumstances. If a sufficiently low value for F_iO_2 is inserted, then a negative value for the P_AO_2 is achieved – something that is not possible in life.

1.3.2

Alveolar partial pressure of oxygen and blood flow

Under normal conditions passive factors such as lung volume, alveolar and intrapleural pressures, gravity and cardiac output will determine pulmonary vascular resistance and therefore blood flow. However, the lungs also demonstrate an active response to hypoxia known as hypoxic pulmonary vasoconstriction.

This is a local response in hypoxic regions of the lung. Smooth muscle contraction in the arteriolar walls diverts blood away to preferentially perfuse those areas that

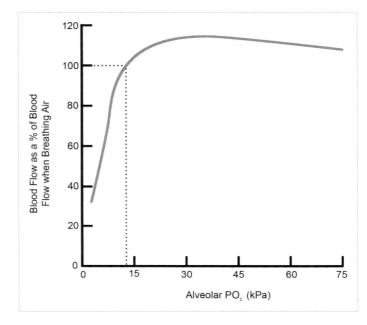

are better oxygenated. However, the mechanism by which this occurs is unclear. The response is independent of central control (as excised lung demonstrates the same response) with local factors likely playing a part. One theory is that inhibitors of nitric oxide (also known as endothelium-derived relaxing factors) are up-regulated in hypoxic conditions.

Interestingly, it is the alveolar, rather than the arterial, concentration of oxygen that causes the response. If the lung is perfused with well-oxygenated blood, but the alveolar oxygen concentration is kept low, the response still occurs. The response is also non-linear; there is little change in blood flow at higher alveolar oxygen concentrations, but when reduced below a certain point marked vasoconstriction occurs. At very low levels blood flow is almost abolished.

The following examples illustrate the response.
- Fetal pulmonary vascular resistance is very high, partly due to hypoxic pulmonary vasoconstriction, resulting in only a small portion of the cardiac output being directed to the pulmonary vascular bed. With the first breath at birth, the vascular resistance falls dramatically due to oxygenation of the alveoli, and pulmonary blood flow increases greatly.
- In pulmonary oedema, diversion of blood to the upper lobes is often seen on the patient's chest X-ray. This demonstrates preferential blood flow diversion to vessels supplying the better oxygenated upper portion of the lungs and away from the oedematous, hypoxic lower regions of the lung.

1.3.3

Bohr equation

$$\frac{V_d}{V_t} = \frac{P_A CO_2 - P_E CO_2}{P_A CO_2}$$

V_d = physiological dead space volume

V_t = tidal volume

$P_A CO_2$ = alveolar partial pressure of carbon dioxide

$P_E CO_2$ = expired partial pressure of carbon dioxide

The Bohr equation is used to derive physiological dead space (V_d); the sum of anatomical and alveolar dead space (see *Section 1.3.6 – Dead space and Fowler's method*). The basis of this equation is that total expired carbon dioxide comes exclusively from alveolar gas with no contribution from dead space. The amount of carbon dioxide diffusing into the alveoli from the pulmonary capillaries is diluted by carbon dioxide depleted air from alveoli that are not perfused (alveolar dead space) and by air in the conducting systems (anatomical dead space). For ease of measurement, $P_A CO_2$ is substituted with arterial partial pressure of carbon dioxide. In health and at rest, the normal ratio of V_d to V_t is in the range of 0.2–0.35. In this setting, physiological and anatomical dead space are approximately equal.

Physiological dead space in disease

In health, anatomical dead space accounts for the majority of V_d. In disease, there is little change in the volume of the conducting airways and therefore changes in V_d are primarily influenced by changes in alveolar dead space.

Acute changes: a rapid increase in alveolar dead space often results from changes in pulmonary blood flow and a subsequent reduction in alveolar perfusion. The most common cause of an acute increase in V_d is a reduction in cardiac output. Other causes include obstruction to pulmonary blood flow. This may be secondary to a thrombotic/embolic event or an abrupt increase in pulmonary vascular resistance.

Chronic changes: chronic pulmonary disease may predispose to irreversible changes in the alveolar/pulmonary capillary relationship. In advanced COPD (chronic obstructive pulmonary disease), V_d is increased due to an underlying ventilation/perfusion mismatch. This problem may be exacerbated with oxygen administration by relieving hypoxic pulmonary vasoconstriction.

Therapeutic manipulations: administration of positive-pressure ventilation may increase alveolar dead space through a reduction in venous return and cardiac output.

1.3.4

Carbon dioxide dissociation curve and Haldane effect

The carbon dioxide dissociation curve illustrates the relationship between partial pressure of carbon dioxide (PCO_2) and total concentration of carbon dioxide in the blood. Carbon dioxide is transported within blood from the tissues to the lungs in three forms: dissolved in plasma, as

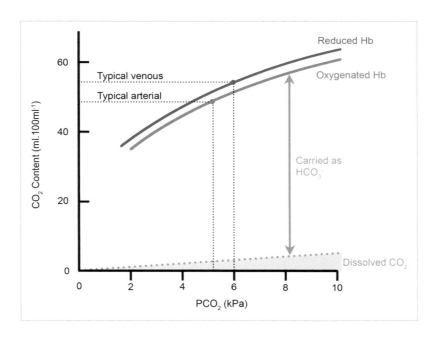

bicarbonate and bound to proteins. Carbon dioxide is 20 times more soluble in solution than oxygen. As such, dissolved carbon dioxide provides a significant means of transport.

The Haldane effect describes the effect of oxygen concentration on carbon dioxide transport. At any given PCO_2, carbon dioxide content of oxygenated blood is less than that of deoxygenated blood. This phenomenon is explained by two mechanisms.

- Reduced (deoxygenated) Hb is less acidic than oxygenated Hb, providing significant buffering capacity for hydrogen ions. An intracellular reaction of carbon dioxide and water forms carbonic acid, with subsequent dissociation into bicarbonate and hydrogen ions. Whilst bicarbonate ions diffuse freely out of the red blood cell, the red blood cell membrane is relatively impermeable to hydrogen ions. A rise in intracellular hydrogen ions would slow further conversion of carbon dioxide and water, limiting carbon dioxide transport. However, reduced Hb avidly binds hydrogen ions, therefore allowing further carbon dioxide uptake.
- Reduced Hb is 3.5 times more effective than oxygenated Hb at combining with carbon dioxide to form carbaminohaemoglobin.

The Haldane effect facilitates carbon dioxide uptake in tissues where PO_2 is low, and carbon dioxide offload in the lungs where PO_2 is high.

Oxygen administration in severe COPD may lead to oxygen-induced hypercapnia. This is partially explained by the Haldane effect. A rise in oxygenated Hb, with supplemental oxygen administration, reduces carbon dioxide transport and elimination. In patients with severe disease, who are unable to increase minute ventilation, hypercapnia occurs. A further contributing factor to oxygen-induced hypercapnia is an increase in V/Q mismatch: oxygen administration increases physiological dead space through a reduction in hypoxic vasoconstriction.

1.3.5

Closing capacity

$$CC = CV + RV$$

CC = closing capacity

CV = closing volume

RV = residual volume

The closing capacity (CC) describes the lung volume at which airway closure occurs. This occurs in the smallest airways and alveoli, and is due to the fact that they lack cartilage and depend on external factors to keep them open. It is seen most in the dependent parts of the lung.

A capacity is used to describe the sum of two or more volumes: the CC is the sum of the closing volume (CV) and the residual volume (RV). The RV describes the amount of gas that remains in the lung after a maximal forced expiration. The CC is therefore greater than the RV but usually less than the functional residual capacity (FRC, the sum of the RV and expiratory reserve volume). This means that there is normally enough gas in the lung to keep the small airways open during inhalation and exhalation. Airway closure that occurs within the FRC results in shunt.

Factors that increase closing capacity and therefore the potential for airway collapse during normal respiration, include:
- age; CC is broadly equivalent to FRC in neonates and infants, in the supine position in over 40 year olds, and in the upright position in over 70 year olds
- smoking
- disease states that increase intrathoracic pressure such as asthma.

Factors such as obesity, the supine position and anaesthesia may cause the CC to encroach upon a reduced FRC, again leading to the potential for airway closure.

The CV can be measured using a nitrogen washout test, or Fowler's method – the same method used to define anatomical dead space (see *Section 1.3.6 – Dead space and Fowler's method*).

1.3.6

Dead space and Fowler's method

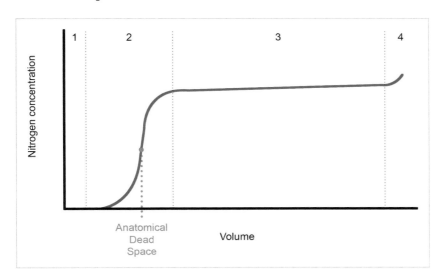

Physiological dead space describes the volume of inspired air not involved in gas exchange (approximately $2\,ml.kg^{-1}$ or 30% of tidal volume). It is calculated using the Bohr equation (see *Section 1.3.3 – Bohr equation*) and divided into anatomical and alveolar dead space.

Anatomical dead space describes the volume of gas found in the conducting airways, i.e. mouth, nose, pharynx and larger airways. It is measured using Fowler's method. Alveolar dead space is the volume of alveoli that are ventilated but not perfused, representing one extreme of ventilation–perfusion mismatch.

Many factors can increase dead space:
- patient factors include increased lung volumes, neck extension, pulmonary or air embolism, decreased lung perfusion and pulmonary disease
- anaesthetic equipment factors include excess circuit tubing length, facemasks and circuit connections; ET tubes and tracheostomies actually reduce dead space.

Fowler's method is a single breath nitrogen washout test. A vital capacity breath of 100% oxygen is taken, and then exhaled to residual volume. The exhaled nitrogen concentration is measured using a rapid-response nitrogen analyser. Four phases are seen.
- Phase 1: dead space gas from conducting airways – pure oxygen.
- Phase 2: dead space and alveolar gas mixture. Anatomical dead space is measured at the mid-point of phase 2.
- Phase 3: alveolar gas – a 'plateau' (with a slight upward gradient, accentuated in lung disease) of pure alveolar gas containing nitrogen that was present in the alveoli before the pure oxygen breath started.
- Phase 4: a final upstroke that occurs at closing capacity. During the vital capacity breath of 100% oxygen, most of the breath will be delivered to the lower, smaller volume, alveoli, since the alveoli at the top of the lung will already be relatively well filled with gas containing nitrogen. When the lower alveoli start to collapse, the nitrogen-rich gas from the upper alveoli is exhaled, giving the upstroke.

1.3.7

Diffusion

$$Q = k_p \times \frac{A}{T} \times (C_1 - C_2)$$

$$k_p \propto \frac{solubility}{\sqrt{molecular\ weight}}$$

Q = rate of diffusion
k_p = permeability (or diffusion) constant
A = area of membrane
T = thickness of membrane
$C_1 - C_2$ = concentration gradient

Diffusing capacity

$$D_{LCO} = k_p \times \frac{A}{T} = \frac{V_{CO}}{P_A CO}$$

D_{LCO} = diffusing capacity of carbon monoxide
V_{CO} = uptake of carbon monoxide
    by the lung per unit time (i.e. Q)
$P_A CO$ = partial pressure of carbon monoxide
    in the alveoli (i.e. C_1)

Diffusion is defined as passive movement of a substance from an area of high concentration to one of low concentration, resulting from random movement of the substance's constituent molecules. The rate of diffusion is determined, in part, by the laws of diffusion (see *Sections 5.9 – Fick's law of diffusion* and *5.14 – Graham's law*).

Diffusing capacity (or transfer factor)

The diffusing capacity (D_L) provides information on gas transfer from alveoli to haemoglobin (Hb) within the pulmonary capillaries. Carbon monoxide is currently the most commonly used gas for measuring pulmonary diffusion properties. Due to the high affinity of carbon monoxide with Hb, the partial pressure of carbon monoxide within the pulmonary capillaries is negligible when a low concentration of carbon monoxide is inhaled (C_2 in the diffusion equation). Thus, movement of carbon monoxide from the alveoli to Hb is mainly dependent on diffusion across the alveolar membrane, although ventilation and perfusion may affect this process.

The variable D_L represents area and thickness of the alveolar capillary membrane for the lungs as a whole, combined with the diffusion constant. Rearranging the equation for rate of diffusion gives rise to the diffusing capacity. As partial pressure of carbon monoxide in the pulmonary capillary is negligible, the lower concentration variable is not included in this equation. Interpretation should be conducted in conjunction with spirometry measurements.

Diseases that reduce D_{LCO} include:
- absolute or functional loss of lung parenchyma (e.g. emphysema or interstitial lung disease); the D_{LCO} is largely unchanged in chronic bronchitis
- pulmonary inflammation or congestion (e.g. acute pneumonitis or severe cardiac failure)
- vascular abnormalities (e.g. pulmonary embolus)
- anaemia may cause a reduction because the capacity for carbon monoxide binding with Hb is reduced.

Diseases that increase D_{LCO} due to an increased volume of blood exposed to inspired gases include:
- alveolar haemorrhage (e.g. Goodpasture's syndrome)
- intracardiac left–right shunt
- polycythaemia.

Dynamic compression of airways

On an expiratory flow–volume curve, there is an initial rapid rise in flow as the lungs start to empty. A peak is reached and then flow decreases in a steady linear fashion over the majority of expiration (A). Despite varying the way in which expiration is achieved, either forced, with a reduced overall effort (B) or a slower initial phase (C), the descending portion of the flow–volume curve takes a similar path. This suggests that something is limiting expiratory flow and that the flow rate is independent of effort. This limitation of flow is caused by dynamic compression of the airways.

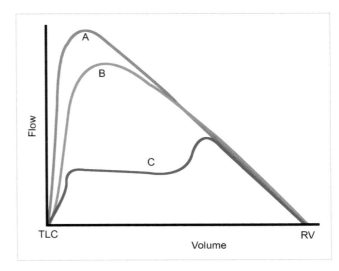

Airways are held open by the pressure difference between the airways (intraluminal pressure) and surrounding tissue (effectively intrapleural pressure). At pre- and end-inspiration, when there is no net flow of air, and during inspiration, the intraluminal pressure is greater than the intrapleural pressure and the airways are held open. During forced expiration both pressures increase, but the intrapleural pressure generated becomes greater than the intraluminal pressure, causing the airways to become compressed, limiting flow. With increased expiratory effort, more compression will occur; when intrapleural pressures are considerably greater than airway pressures, small airway closure will occur. The point at which collapse occurs is called the equal pressure point. As expiration progresses, and lung volume reduces, this point moves more distally due to increasing airway resistance and reduced intraluminal pressure.

Certain conditions will exaggerate this situation. In obstructive lung diseases, loss of elastic recoil and increased airway resistance leads to decreased intraluminal pressures, generating the classic flow–volume curve of reduced flow rates and a 'scooped out' pattern of the descending limb. In a variable intrathoracic obstruction (e.g. tumours or tracheomalacia), the flow rates will be further reduced during forced expiration as the positive intrathoracic pressure generated exacerbates the obstruction, increasing airway compression.

1.3.9

Fick principle and blood flow

$$\text{Pulmonary blood flow} = \frac{O_2 \text{ consumption per minute}}{(C_aO_2 - C_vO_2)}$$

C_aO_2 = arterial oxygen concentration
C_vO_2 = mixed venous oxygen concentration

The Fick principle is a way of calculating blood flow to an organ and, when applied to the lungs, can be used to calculate cardiac output.

The Fick principle states that organ blood flow per unit time is equal to the amount of a marker substance taken up by that organ divided by the concentration difference of the marker substance entering and leaving the organ. In Fick's original experiments, the organ in question was the whole body and oxygen was used as the marker substance.

The amount of blood passing through the lungs per minute (i.e. cardiac output) can be calculated using the Fick principle. Applied to the lung, this states that the volume of blood passing through the lungs per minute is equal to the oxygen consumption per minute divided by the difference between the arterial and mixed venous oxygen concentrations. The oxygen consumption is calculated by using a spirometer to measure the oxygen concentration in an expired gas sample. Mixed venous blood is taken from a catheter in the pulmonary artery and the arterial sample is taken from a brachial or radial arterial blood sample.

Blood flow within the lung is not homogenous; it decreases almost linearly from the bottom to the top of the lung with the patient in the upright position. This will subsequently change with posture, so that if the patient lies down, the blood flow will be greatest in the posterior dependent parts of the lung with the distribution of flow being more even from cephalad to caudad. These regional differences are due to the effect of gravity on the hydrostatic pressure within the blood vessels. During exercise, these regional differences become less marked with the flow increasing throughout the lung.

Forced expiration curves

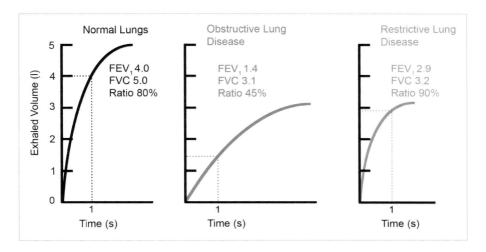

Forced expiration is a simple reproducible test of pulmonary function. A single forced expiration yields the following variables:

- forced vital capacity (FVC) – total volume forcibly exhaled following maximal inspiration
- forced expiratory volume in 1 second (FEV_1) – volume of gas forcibly exhaled in 1 second following maximal inspiration.

Normal values vary with age and sex. The FEV_1 and FVC may be expressed as a percentage of predicted normal for a person of the same sex, age and height. The FEV_1 is commonly reported as a ratio with FVC, expressed as a percentage, with a normal value of FEV_1/FVC being 80%. These variables are useful in differentiating normal ventilation from pathological changes in pulmonary function. A combination of obstructive and restrictive patterns are frequently seen in disease states.

In obstructive lung disease, such as asthma and COPD, FEV_1 is reduced due to an increase in resistance to expiratory flow. The FVC may be reduced due to premature airway closure (gas-trapping), but to a lesser extent than FEV_1, leading to an overall reduction of the FEV_1/FVC ratio.

In restrictive lung disease, such as pulmonary fibrosis, FEV_1 and FVC are both reduced in similar proportions. In some cases, FEV_1 may be reduced to a lesser extent as early expiration is affected less by disease. Overall, a normal or slightly increased FEV_1/FVC is observed.

Forced expiration and COPD

COPD is characterized by airflow obstruction that is not fully reversible. The severity of airflow obstruction correlates to the degree of FEV_1 reduction. According to the National Institute for Health and Care Excellence (NICE), measurements of forced expiration should be used to define COPD as follows:

- FEV_1/FVC <70% indicates airflow obstruction
- if FEV_1 is >80% predicted, COPD should be diagnosed only in the presence of respiratory symptoms.

1.3.11

Functional residual capacity of the lungs

$$V_2 = \frac{V_1(C_1 - C_2)}{C_2}$$

C_1 = initial concentration of helium present

C_2 = concentration of helium present after equilibrium is reached

V_1 = volume of the spirometer

V_2 = lung volume (FRC)

The function residual capacity (FRC) describes the volume of gas left in the lung after normal exhalation during normal tidal volume breathing. It is the sum of the residual volume (RV) and the expiratory reserve volume (ERV). Neither the RV nor the FRC can be measured with simple spirometry and therefore need an alternative method to determine their volumes.

Helium dilution is one of the ways to measure FRC. After a normal tidal volume breath is exhaled, the subject breathes from a spirometer of known volume (V_1) containing a known concentration of helium (C_1). After some breaths, equilibrium is reached and the helium concentration becomes equal in both the spirometer and the lung (C_2). Carbon dioxide is absorbed using soda lime and oxygen is replaced in the gas mixture as the subject uses it. Helium is virtually insoluble in the blood and therefore the amount present at initiation is equal to the amount present after equilibrium is reached. The volume of the FRC (V_2) can therefore be calculated as seen in the equation.

A similar principle can be applied to calculate the FRC using a nitrogen washout test (see *Section 1.3.6 – Dead space and Fowler's method*). It can also be calculated with a body plethysmograph using Boyle's law (see *Section 5.10 – Gas laws – Boyle's law*). The helium dilution and nitrogen washout tests do not include those areas of the lung that are collapsed or have poor air entry, whereas the body plethysmograph measures the total volume in the lung, trapped or not. By using a combination of helium dilution or nitrogen washout and body plethysmography, an indication of the degree of airway collapse or hypoventilation can be obtained.

1.3.12

Lung and chest wall compliance

$$\frac{1}{C_{total}} = \frac{1}{C_{lung}} + \frac{1}{C_{chest\ wall}}$$

C_{total} = total lung compliance

C_{lung} = lung compliance

$C_{chest\ wall}$ = chest wall compliance

Compliance is defined as the change in volume for a unit change in pressure and gives an indication of how easily distensible a structure is. In the respiratory system compliance has two components: the lung and the chest wall. Total thoracic compliance is calculated using the equation shown. Normal lung compliance and chest wall compliance are both about 1.5–2.0 l.kPa^{-1} (150–200 ml.cm H$_2$O^{-1}) and total compliance is therefore 1.0 l.kPa^{-1} (100 ml.cm H$_2$O^{-1}).

A pressure–volume curve (see *Section 1.3.13 – Lung pressure–volume loop*) can be used to represent lung compliance and

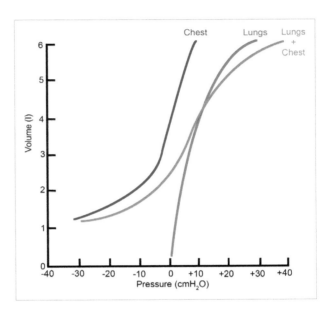

give an idea of compliance at different lung volumes. Compliance can be measured as static or dynamic depending on whether gas flow continues during the measurement. Static compliance is obtained by applying distending pressures to the lung and measuring the change in volume; the patient expires in increments and intrapleural pressure is measured when there is no gas flow. To measure dynamic compliance, a pressure–volume loop is produced throughout the respiratory cycle. Measurements for static compliance tend to be higher than for dynamic compliance because the lung has time to equilibrate.

Factors affecting compliance include the following.
- FRC – compliance is reduced if FRC is either higher or lower than normal. In order to account for this, specific compliance can be measured where the compliance is divided by the FRC.
- ARDS and pulmonary oedema reduce total compliance by reducing lung compliance.
- Circumferential burns or restrictive chest wall disease reduce total compliance by reducing chest wall compliance.
- Posture – the lungs exhibit greater compliance in the upright position.
- Obesity reduces compliance due to both raised intra-abdominal pressure reducing FRC and lung compliance. Increased soft tissue mass also causes reduced chest wall compliance.

1.3.13

Lung pressure–volume loop

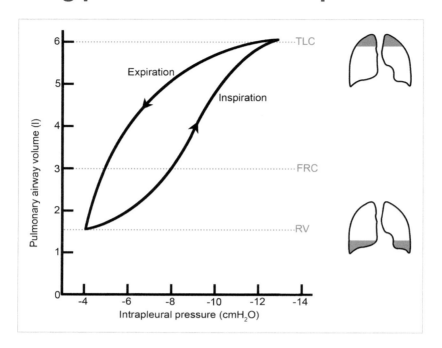

The pressure–volume loop is used to depict compliance of the lung. In spontaneous ventilation the pressure values on the x-axis should be negative, whereas for positive pressure ventilation, positive pressure values are used.

The curve depicts a vital capacity breath. The inspiratory portion of the graph shows how, at normal tidal volumes, the line is steep and approximately linear, demonstrating a highly compliant lung. The lower portion of the curve is flatter demonstrating the increased pressure needed to overcome collapsed alveoli and increase the volume of the lung. The higher portion of the curve is again seen to flatten as the maximum elastic limit of the alveoli is reached and compliance reduces. The expiratory curve is initially flat due to the low compliance seen at high volumes and then becomes steeper as it returns to baseline.

Inspiration and expiration do not follow the same path – a demonstration of hysteresis, where the value changes depending on whether it is increasing or decreasing. This implies absorption of energy; the area inside the loop represents the amount of energy lost as elastic tissues stretch and then recoil and as airway resistance is overcome.

The lung schematics represent regional differences in the compliance of the alveoli. Those at the top of the lung sit at the high end of the inspiratory curve because they are already fully expanded at the beginning of a vital capacity breath and therefore need higher pressures to increase their volume (i.e. poorly compliant). On the other hand, alveoli at the bottom of the lung have a relatively small volume initially and expand easily. In mechanically ventilated patients, both these values shift down the curve so that the alveoli at the top of the lung become relatively more compliant and those at the bottom, less so.

1.3.14

Lung volumes and capacities

Lung volumes and capacities are functional, not anatomical, volumes. Figures provided are approximate values for an average 70 kg adult.

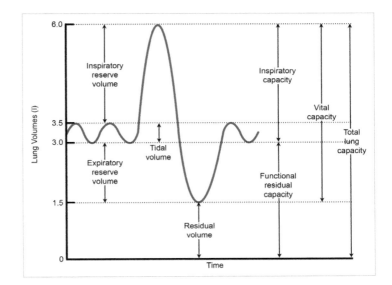

Volumes

- Tidal volume (TV) – volume of air inspired during normal breathing; 500 ml.
- Inspiratory reserve volume (IRV) – volume of additional air forcibly inspired following inspiration of a normal TV; 2500 ml.
- Expiratory reserve volume (ERV) – volume of additional air forcibly exhaled following exhalation of a normal TV; 1500 ml.
- Residual volume (RV) – volume of air remaining in the lungs following exhalation of ERV; 1500 ml.

The TV, IRV and ERV may be measured directly via spirometry. Measurement of RV requires a helium dilution technique.

Capacities are the sum of 2 or more lung volumes

- Total lung capacity (TLC) – volume of air in the lungs following maximal inflation; sum of all lung volumes; 6000 ml.
- Vital capacity (VC) – volume of air that can be exhaled following maximal inflation; sum of TV, IRV and ERV; 4500 ml.
- Inspiratory capacity (IC) – maximum volume of air that may be inspired following exhalation of a normal TV; sum of TV and IRV; 3000 ml.
- Functional residual capacity (FRC) – volume of air remaining in the lungs following exhalation of normal TV; sum of ERV and RV; 3000 ml.

The TLC and FRC may be calculated using body plethysmography.

Lung volume/capacity changes in pregnancy

- The TV increases by up to 45% at term.
- The FRC is reduced by 20–30% at term due to a reduction in ERV and RV. As such, the closing capacity encroaches upon FRC, leading to an increase in ventilation–perfusion mismatch. This is particularly evident in the supine position.
- The VC remains largely unchanged despite a reduction in FRC as IC increases by 15% at term.

1.3.15

Oxygen cascade

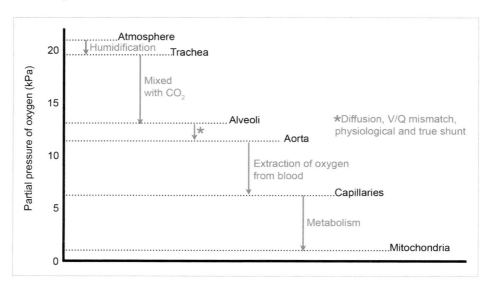

The oxygen cascade or oxygen flux diagram depicts the delivery of oxygen from the air to the tissues. At each step, there are factors which act to reduce the oxygen concentration that is finally delivered to the mitochondria.

The fractional oxygen concentration of dry air is approximately 21% and therefore the partial pressure of oxygen is 21 kPa at atmospheric pressure ($PO_2 = F_iO_2 \times P_{ATM}$). When air is inspired, it mixes with water vapour in the upper airways and trachea reducing the partial pressure of oxygen ($PO_2 = F_iO_2 (P_{ATM} - P_{H_2O})$). The partial pressure will again reduce when it reaches the alveoli as oxygen is absorbed and carbon dioxide expired, represented by the alveolar gas equation ($P_AO_2 = [F_iO_2 (P_{ATM} - P_{H_2O})] - (P_ACO_2/R)$; see *Section 1.3.1 – Alveolar gas equation*).

In the pulmonary capillaries, a further very small drop in partial pressure will have occurred due to diffusion across the alveolar–capillary membrane (almost negligible for oxygen). It reduces again in the pulmonary veins due to mixing of physiological shunt blood from less well ventilated areas of lung (V/Q mismatch) and in the left side of the heart from anatomical shunt blood being added. Anatomical, or true, shunt comprises blood from some of the bronchial veins that drain either into the pulmonary veins or left atrium, and from a few Thebesian veins that drain blood from the myocardium into the left atrium. These sources produce an alveolar–arterial gradient (A–a gradient) of usually less than 2 kPa.

Extraction of oxygen from this blood then causes the end-capillary partial pressure of oxygen to be about 6–7 kPa. In the mitochondria themselves, the partial pressure varies from 1 to 5 kPa. The Pasteur point describes the threshold below which oxidative phosphorylation cannot occur (and therefore anaerobic respiration starts); it is about 0.15–0.3 kPa.

1.3.16

Oxygen dissociation curve and Bohr effect

The sigmoid shape of the oxyhaemoglobin dissociation curve results from cooperative binding of oxygen to haemoglobin (Hb) and has several physiological advantages. A small reduction in P_aO_2 at normal levels results in minimal change in Hb saturation (plateau phase).

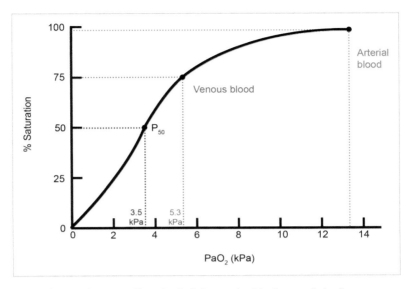

In health, a relatively large reduction in P_aO_2 of inspired air is required before a clinically significant decline in Hb saturation is observed. A small reduction in P_aO_2 at lower levels results in a significant change in Hb saturation (steep phase), facilitating sufficient oxygen unloading at the tissues.

Factors affecting dissociation curve

Shifting of the curve relates to rightwards or leftwards movement of P50; the P_aO_2 at which Hb is 50% saturated.
- A rightwards shift depicts a reduction in oxygen avidity of Hb, favouring unloading of oxygen. This occurs with an increase in P_aCO_2, hydrogen ion concentration, 2,3-DPG concentration and temperature.
- A leftwards shift depicts an increase in avidity of oxygen for Hb. This occurs in settings opposite to those leading to a rightwards shift. In addition, fetal Hb, carboxyhaemoglobinaemia and methaemoglobinaemia result in a leftwards shift.

Bohr effect

The Bohr effect describes how carbon dioxide and hydrogen concentrations affect affinity of Hb for oxygen. Carbon dioxide combines with water, forming carbonic acid, subsequently dissociating into bicarbonate and hydrogen ions. As blood pH decreases, hydrogen ions directly interact with Hb amino acids to reduce the affinity for oxygen. This facilitates oxygen unloading in metabolically active tissues.

Double Bohr effect

The double Bohr effect describes the reciprocal exchange of oxygen and carbon dioxide in the placenta. At the maternal–fetal interface, fetal blood releases carbon dioxide into the maternal circulation resulting in a reduced oxygen affinity of maternal Hb, promoting oxygen release (the Bohr effect). Fetal blood becomes more alkaline with the release of carbon dioxide, leading to a reciprocal increase in fetal Hb oxygen affinity.

1.3.17

Pulmonary vascular resistance

$$PVR = 80 \times \frac{(MPAP - PCWP)}{CO}$$

PVR = pulmonary vascular resistance (dyn.s.cm^{-5})

MPAP = mean pulmonary artery pressure (mmHg)

PCWP = pulmonary capillary wedge pressure (mmHg)

CO = cardiac output (l.min^{-1})

Pulmonary vascular resistance (PVR) is resistance provided by the pulmonary circulation against which the right ventricle must eject. As with systemic vascular resistance, PVR may be calculated using a modification of Ohm's law (see *Section 1.2.6 – Ohm's law*), where blood flow is equal to driving pressure divided by resistance. In this instance, driving pressure is the difference between mean pulmonary artery pressure (MPAP) and left atrial filling pressure. Pulmonary capillary wedge pressure is used as an indirect measure of left atrial pressure (LAP). The numerical constant (80) is used to convert mmHg.min.l^{-1} into the units used to measure vascular resistance: dyn.s.cm^{-5}.

Pulmonary hypertension

Pulmonary hypertension is defined as a MPAP >25 mmHg at rest, with a PCWP >12 mmHg. The World Health Organization has classified pulmonary hypertension as follows.

- Pulmonary arterial hypertension (PAH) – causes include connective tissue diseases (e.g. scleroderma), congenital cardiac abnormalities (e.g. left–right shunt) and idiopathic pulmonary hypertension. Clinically, PAH is characterized by a rise in MPAP without an increase in LAP. Regardless of the cause of PAH, pathogenesis involves an imbalance of endogenous vascular mediators (e.g. nitric oxide) which ultimately lead to vessel vasoconstriction, thrombosis and inflammation.
- Pulmonary hypertension associated with left heart disease – represents the most common cause of pulmonary hypertension, including chronic left ventricular failure and chronic mitral valve disease. A rise in LAP results in a passive increase in resistance to pulmonary venous drainage.
- Pulmonary hypertension associated with lung disease or hypoxaemia – causes include COPD, obstructive sleep apnoea and chronic high altitude exposure. Chronic hypoxic pulmonary vasoconstriction results in an increase in PVR. This leads to a rise in MPAP and similar pathophysiological changes observed with PAH.
- Pulmonary hypertension due to chronic thrombotic and/or embolic disease – obstruction of a pulmonary artery gives rise to an increase in MPAP.
- Miscellaneous – includes sarcoidosis and pulmonary veno-occlusive disease.

1.3.18
Pulmonary vascular resistance and lung volumes

Passive extravascular factors have a significant effect on pulmonary vascular resistance (PVR) due to the high distensibility of the vessels, the small amount of smooth muscle in the vessel walls and the low intravascular pressures. These passive factors include lung volume, alveolar and intrapleural pressures, gravity and cardiac output.

Lung volume has a significant affect on the PVR as the vasculature is found largely within the lung parenchyma. PVR is lowest at functional residual capacity (FRC) and increases both with higher and lower lung volumes.

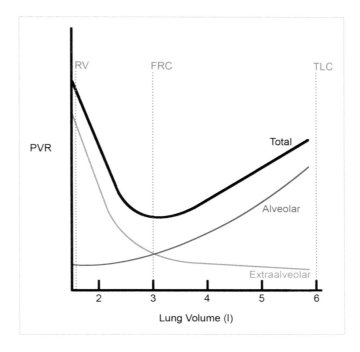

At volumes above FRC, pulmonary vessels outside the alveoli are distended and their resistance falls. However, the septal capillaries in the alveolar walls are stretched longitudinally causing a reduction in their diameter and therefore an increase in their resistance. The overall effect is an increased pulmonary resistance as the septal capillaries have the dominant effect.

At volumes below FRC, pulmonary vessels outside the alveoli are no longer held open by traction of the surrounding lung tissue, leading to collapse and an increase in resistance. There is also direct vessel compression by the lung causing a reduction in their diameter. As the alveoli get smaller there is a reduction in the longitudinal stretch of the septal capillaries and resistance falls. However, this effect is small and overall there is an increase in PVR due to the dominant effect from the increased resistance in the extra-alveolar vessels.

Drugs that cause contraction of smooth muscle will lead to an increase in PVR. These include serotonin, histamine and noradrenaline, with their effect being more marked at lower lung volumes when expanding traction forces on the vessels are weak. Drugs that relax smooth muscle and lead to a reduced PVR include acetylcholine and isoprenaline.

1.3.19

Respiratory flow–volume loops

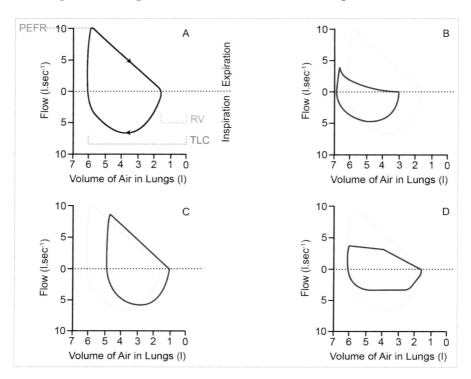

Flow–volume loops are obtained via forced spirometry to measure airflow and lung volumes simultaneously. They offer the advantage of assessing if airflow is appropriate for a particular lung volume (i.e. airflow is normally slower at low lung volumes) and may be used to differentiate between types of pulmonary disease, characterize severity and assess therapeutic response. Note that lung volumes (x-axis) are presented in a descending order and inspiration is represented by a downward deflection on the y-axis.

A. **Normal**: the plot begins following maximal inspiration, total lung capacity (TLC), when airflow is zero. Forced expiration produces a rapid, linear increase in airflow to a peak expiratory flow rate (PEFR). Airflow decreases in a linear fashion until the residual volume (RV) is reached. The portion of the expiratory limb between 25% and 75% expiration, forced expiratory flow 25–75 (FEF 25–75), is effort independent and represents small airway function. Maximal inspiration produces an inspiratory limb that is symmetrical and convex.

B. **Obstructive disease** (e.g. asthma, emphysema): PEFR is reduced due to general airflow limitation. The expiratory limb is concave with a low FEF 25–75. Premature airway closure leads to an increase in RV. The inspiratory limb has a smaller amplitude demonstrating a reduction in airflow. The TLC exceeds the normal volume in health due to dynamic hyperinflation and a loss of elastic recoil of lung parenchyma.

C. **Restrictive disease** (e.g. interstitial lung disease): the loop is narrowed due to a reduction in both TLC and RV. Airflow is greater than normal at comparable lung volumes due to an increase in elastic recoil.

D. **Fixed upper airway obstruction** (e.g. tracheal mass, goitre): both the expiratory and inspiratory limbs are flattened, demonstrating constant reduction in airflow throughout the respiratory cycle. Depending on the degree of obstruction, TLC may be decreased with an increase in RV.

1.3.20

Shunt

$$\frac{Qs}{Qt} = \frac{\left(C_cO_2 - C_aO_2\right)}{\left(C_cO_2 - C_vO_2\right)}$$

Qs = shunted blood

Qt = total cardiac output

C_cO_2 = oxygen content in capillary blood

C_aO_2 = oxygen content in arterial blood

C_vO_2 = oxygen content in venous blood

Shunt is the fraction of mixed venous blood bypassing oxygenation in the lungs. Physiological shunt comprises the following.
- Intrapulmonary shunt – areas with a low ventilation/perfusion (V/Q) ratio demonstrate an imbalance whereby pulmonary perfusion exceeds ventilation. In health, dependent lung regions exhibit some shunt owing to a low V/Q ratio. This is exaggerated in pathophysiological states such as atelectasis and airway obstruction.
- Anatomical shunt – a structural channel facilitating blood to bypass alveoli, often called a right-to-left shunt. In health, cardiac (i.e. Thebesian veins) and bronchial circulations demonstrate anatomical shunt as venous blood empties directly into the left heart and pulmonary vein, respectively. Pathophysiological causes of anatomical shunt include atrial and ventricular septal defects.

The shunt equation is used to calculate shunt magnitude. This equation is an application of the Fick principle (see *Section 1.1.12 – Fick method for cardiac output studies*) using a two compartment model.
- Ideal compartment – perfect V/Q matching and ideal gas exchange.
- Shunt compartment – pulmonary capillaries have no exposure to alveoli.

The shunt fraction is the proportion of cardiac output that travels through the shunt compartment (normally 2–5%). However, the shunt compartment is an artificial concept and therefore the shunt equation provides only a gross estimate of pulmonary oxygen exchange dysfunction. Shunt is, classically, refractory to supplemental oxygen because increasing the alveolar partial pressure of oxygen will not improve V/Q matching. However, administration of 100% oxygen may increase dissolved oxygen content.

Shunt in acute respiratory distress syndrome

Severe hypoxaemia is a hallmark of ARDS and develops due to formation of protein-rich alveolar oedema causing an increase in intrapulmonary shunt. Invasive ventilation is frequently required and high levels of positive end-expiratory pressure (PEEP) have become a cornerstone of ARDS management. PEEP improves oxygenation, in part, via splinting open collapsed alveoli and reducing intrapulmonary shunt.

1.3.21

Ventilation–perfusion ratio

The alveolar partial pressures of oxygen (P_AO_2) and carbon dioxide (P_ACO_2) are determined by the ratio of alveolar ventilation (V) to pulmonary capillary blood flow (Q). P_AO_2 is determined by the rate at which oxygen is added to the alveoli and its removal rate by capillary blood flow. P_ACO_2 is determined by the rate at which carbon dioxide diffuses into the alveoli from capillary blood and its removal rate via ventilation. The global V/Q ratio of the normal lung is approximately 0.8.

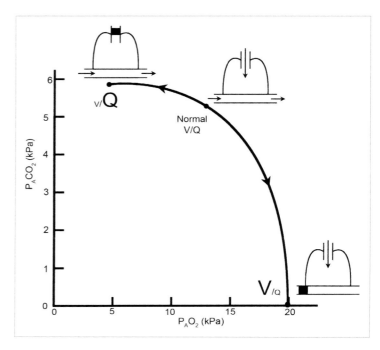

- As V/Q ratio increases, oxygen is added to the alveoli at a rate greater than its removal, resulting in a rise in P_AO_2. Conversely, carbon dioxide is removed from the alveoli at a rate greater than that delivered by the blood, causing P_ACO_2 to fall. This is most commonly observed in the upper region of the normal lung where ventilation exceeds perfusion (V/Q ratio approximately 3 at lung apex). At its extreme, a V/Q ratio of infinity represents ventilation without perfusion; dead space.
- A decrease in the V/Q ratio is most commonly observed in the lower region of the normal lung (V/Q ratio approximately 0.3 at lung base) and results in a reduction in P_AO_2 and an increase in P_ACO_2. At its extreme, a V/Q ratio of zero represents perfusion without ventilation; shunt.

Measurement of V/Q mismatch

V/Q mismatch impairs oxygen uptake and carbon dioxide elimination. Chemoreceptor-mediated increases in ventilatory drive normalize arterial partial pressure of carbon dioxide (P_aCO_2) with only a modest increase in arterial partial pressure of oxygen (P_aO_2). Global V/Q mismatch may be estimated via the alveolar–arterial (A–a) oxygen difference. The P_AO_2 is calculated using the alveolar gas equation and P_aO_2 is measured directly. In health, the A–a gradient is less than 2 kPa when breathing air. Assessment of regional V/Q mismatch involves radioisotope scanning of ventilation and pulmonary perfusion.

1.3.22

Ventilatory response to carbon dioxide

A change in the partial pressure of carbon dioxide in the alveoli (P_ACO_2), and therefore in arterial partial pressure of carbon dioxide (P_aCO_2), is detected primarily by the central chemoreceptors. These are found on the anterolateral surface of the medulla and are sensitive to a rise in hydrogen ion concentration. An increase in P_aCO_2 will lead to an increased amount of carbon dioxide diffusing across the blood–brain

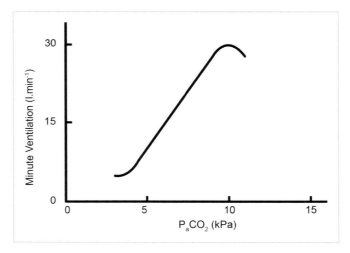

barrier, increasing the hydrogen ion concentration and reducing the CSF pH. This will stimulate the chemoreceptors, sending a message to the external intercostal muscles and diaphragm via the intercostal nerves and phrenic nerve, respectively; this leads to a rise in the minute ventilation (increased respiratory rate and depth) in order to restore the CSF pH to normal.

A respiratory acidosis affects the ventilatory response more than a metabolic acidosis of the same value due to the increased permeability of the blood–brain barrier to carbon dioxide compared to hydrogen ions. The response is linear over normal clinical conditions; if the P_aCO_2 doubles, the minute ventilation increases four-fold. Outside of this range, above 10–11 kPa, a depression of ventilation is demonstrated by the graph falling away due to CO_2 narcosis. At the lower end of the graph, the curve flattens out but will not reach zero. The slope will vary between individuals and is affected by certain disease states, drugs (such as opiates), hormones and P_AO_2.

In chronic lung disease, the central chemoreceptors become less sensitive to raised carbon dioxide levels and therefore hypoxaemia becomes the main driver for ventilation. During anaesthesia, the response to hypoxaemia and hypercapnia are markedly depressed. Opiates act as powerful central respiratory depressants. Respiratory stimulants, such as doxapram, act at peripheral chemoreceptors to increase minute ventilation.

1.3.23

Ventilatory response to oxygen

The control of ventilation is coordinated by three main factors:

- by centres within the central nervous system
- by receptors in the respiratory muscles and lung
- by other specialized chemoreceptors such as the carotid and aortic bodies.

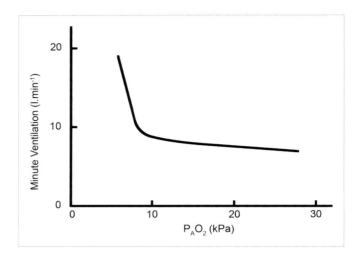

Hypoxaemia is primarily detected by peripheral chemoreceptors found in the carotid and aortic bodies. The chemoreceptors responsible for detecting changes in blood gases are called glomus cells. The aortic body chemoreceptors detect changes in blood oxygen and carbon dioxide concentrations but not changes in pH, whereas the carotid bodies detect all three. The aortic bodies give feedback to the medulla oblongata via afferent branches of the vagus nerve; the medulla in turn regulates breathing and blood pressure.

The carotid bodies are small structures (2–3 mg) found above the carotid bifurcation bilaterally and have the highest blood flow per 100 g tissue in the body (0.04 ml.blood^{-1}.min^{-1}; equivalent to 2 l.100 g tissue^{-1}.min^{-1}). They have an afferent nerve supply to the brainstem regulatory centres via the glossopharyngeal nerve. Their rate of discharge is increased by reduced oxygen delivery (either reduced P_aO_2 or reduced cardiac output) or by impaired utilization of oxygen (e.g. cyanide poisoning). This response, however, is non-linear because, although they are sensitive to a P_aO_2 <65 kPa, they show little response until the P_aO_2 is <13 kPa. Under normal conditions, the minute volume will remain constant until the P_AO_2 falls below around 8 kPa. At this point there will be a sharp rise in the peripheral chemoreceptor discharge rate, due to a fall in P_aO_2, and therefore minute ventilation will increase.

The discharge rate of the chemoreceptors is also increased by a rise in P_aCO_2 or a fall in arterial pH, although the central chemoreceptors play a more significant role in relation to P_aCO_2 (see *Section 1.3.22 – Ventilatory response to carbon dioxide*).

1.3.24

West lung zones

Perfusion of the lung is not uniform. In the upright position, blood flow increases in a largely linear fashion from top to bottom. This inequality may be explained by pulmonary vessel hydrostatic forces combined with alveolar pressures. Conceptually, the lung may be divided into three zones representing a gravitational model of pulmonary perfusion.

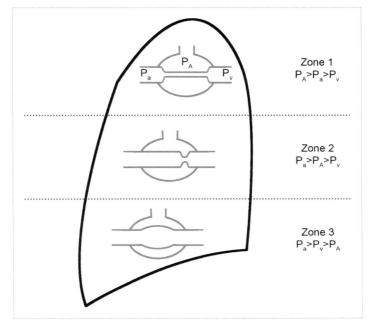

Zone 1
$P_A>P_a>P_v$

Zone 2
$P_a>P_A>P_v$

Zone 3
$P_a>P_v>P_A$

- Zone 1 – may occur at the top, in which pulmonary arterial pressure (P_a) falls below alveolar pressure (P_A). Pulmonary capillaries are compressed, and no flow occurs. This is not observed in health but may exist with reduced P_a (e.g. major haemorrhage) or raised P_A (e.g. intermittent positive pressure ventilation). This region represents alveolar dead space; ventilated but not perfused.
- Zone 2 – the region where P_a exceeds P_A, with pulmonary venous pressure (P_v) remaining low. Pulmonary perfusion is dependent on the pressure gradient between P_a and P_A. Unlike usual blood flow dynamics, P_v has no influence on flow. Because pulmonary arterial hydrostatic pressure increases from top to bottom of zone 2, due to the effects of gravity, blood flow increases accordingly.
- Zone 3 – this region occurs at the base of the lung and demonstrates the greatest blood flow. Both P_a and P_v exceed P_A. Blood flow is dependent on the arterial–venous pressure gradient while P_A has no influence.

This gravitational model, published in 1964, fails to adequately explain the heterogeneity in perfusion. Studies have demonstrated perfusion inequalities within horizontal planes, in addition to the well known vertical gradient. Extensive evidence supports the role of pulmonary vascular architecture in the determination of blood flow variation. Branching of the pulmonary vessels is asymmetric: at each bifurcation, the diameter and length of subsequent branches are unlikely to be identical in size. Blood flow dynamics may therefore be greatly affected considering there are approximately 28 generations of pulmonary vessels.

1.3.25

Work of breathing

The work of breathing is the work required by the respiratory muscles to overcome the impedance to respiration caused by the lung, chest wall and abdominal contents. It can be calculated from the product of the pressure change across the lung and the volume of gas that is moved with respiration. In order for respiration to occur, both elastic forces and flow resistance must be overcome.

On the graph above, the shaded area represents the work needed for inspiration. The area B + C represents the work done in inspiration to overcome elastic forces of the tissue and area A

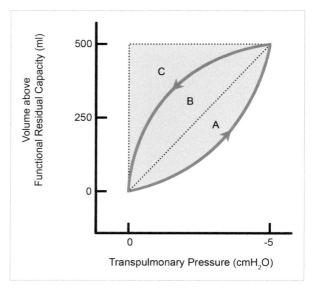

represents the extra work done overcoming viscous resistance and friction (in both airway and tissue). Area B is the work done against resistance during expiration. This area is enclosed within the shaded area for inspiration demonstrating that the energy needed for expiration can be provided from stored energy in the elastic tissues during inspiration. Area C represents the energy lost as heat.

During normal respiration, the work done in inspiration is mainly to overcome the elastic forces of the thorax and lung and the resistance of the airways and non-elastic tissues. The work done in expiration uses the potential energy stored within the elastic tissues generated during inspiration; expiration is therefore normally passive.

An increase in tidal volume will require a greater work of breathing to overcome the increased elastic recoil (larger area of B + C). Similarly, if the respiratory rate increases so will the flow rate and the work of breathing will increase to overcome the increased resistance experienced (larger area A). The work required for expiration may change in certain pathological conditions, such as during airway obstruction, where the work of breathing required increases and expiration becomes active.

1.4.1

Action potential

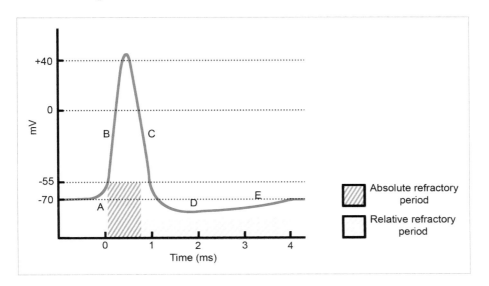

An action potential describes transient, sequential changes in transmembrane potential, resulting in transmission of an electrical impulse.

Resting membrane potential

RMP describes differential distribution of charged particles across the cell membrane, resulting in the interior of the cell being negatively charged relative to the exterior. Distribution of each ion is dependent upon its own permeability across the membrane, active transport (e.g. Na^+/K^+-ATPase pump), and distribution of other particles (development of an uneven charge occurs in the presence of charged substances that are unable to cross the membrane – the Gibbs–Donnan effect). In excitable cells, RMP is −70 mV for nerves and −90 mV for muscle fibres.

Neuron action potential sequence

A. Depolarization to threshold potential – a stimulus, received by dendrites, opens transmembrane sodium (Na^+) channels. As Na^+ moves into the cell, the membrane potential becomes more positive. If the membrane potential rises to −55 mV, the threshold potential, the process continues.

B. Rapid depolarization – Na^+ conductance increases suddenly due to further opening of Na^+ channels. Influx of Na^+ down its electrochemical gradient drives the interior of the cell to +40 mV. Potassium (K^+) channels also open but the process is slower, allowing time for depolarization to occur.

C. Repolarization – Na^+ channels close whilst K^+ channels remain open. Rapid efflux of K^+ lowers the membrane potential towards RMP. The absolute refractory period, during which the neuron is totally unresponsive to any stimulus, occurs between the threshold potential being reached and when repolarization is one-third complete.

D. Hyperpolarization – repolarization typically leads to an overshoot of RMP to approximately −90 mV. A period of hyperpolarization results in a relative refractory period whereby the neuron would require a supranormal stimulus to initiate a subsequent action potential.

E. Restoration of RMP – normal ion distribution is restored via the Na^+/K^+-ATPase pump.

1.4.2

Cerebral blood flow and blood pressure

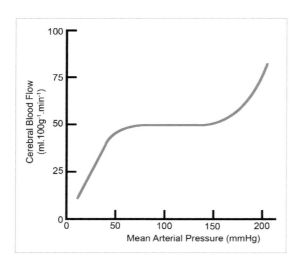

$$CPP = MAP - (ICP + CVP)$$

CPP = cerebral perfusion pressure
MAP = mean arterial pressure
ICP = intracranial pressure
CVP = central venous pressure

Cerebral blood flow (CBF) is affected by many factors but is autoregulated so that flow is maintained despite changes in its perfusing pressure. It normally equates to about 15% of the cardiac output, approximating 700 ml.min^{-1} or 50 ml.100 g^{-1}.min^{-1}. Factors affecting it include MAP, partial pressures of oxygen and carbon dioxide (see *Section 1.4.3 – Cerebral blood flow variation with ventilation*), drugs and temperature.

The cerebral perfusion pressure (CPP) can be calculated from the equation shown. The CVP is often omitted from the equation, because its contribution is not significant under normal conditions. Note that in patients with raised intracranial pressure (ICP), the MAP must increase in order to maintain CPP.

Between a MAP of about 50–150 mmHg, the CBF is maintained at about 50 ml.100g^{-1}.min^{-1}; this is known as the autoregulatory range. Outside of these pressures autoregulation is lost and CBF becomes proportional to MAP. In patients with hypertension, this autoregulatory range may be 'reset' and the curve will shift to the right. In certain disease states, such as subarachnoid haemorrhage, stroke or head injury, autoregulation may be lost altogether and blood flow will become pressure dependent. Autoregulation mechanisms are thought to include myogenic (arteriolar smooth muscle responds to transmural blood pressure changes), metabolic (cerebral metabolism releases vasoactive substances to maintain adequate oxygen delivery) and neurogenic (autonomic nervous system affects arteriolar resistance).

Temperature affects CBF by altering the cerebral metabolic rate for oxygen (CMRO$_2$). The relationship is non-linear; at 37°C a 1°C drop in temperature reduces the CMRO$_2$ by 6–7%, whereas at 15°C the same 1°C drop in temperature only decreases it by 1%.

All inhalational anaesthetic agents cause a dose-dependent vasodilatation and loss of autoregulation of CBF. Propofol, thiopental, etomidate and the benzodiazepines all reduce CBF, whereas ketamine causes an increase in flow.

1.4.3

Cerebral blood flow variation with ventilation

The partial pressure of carbon dioxide (P_aCO_2) has an important linear effect on cerebral blood flow. It can be seen in the graph that cerebral blood flow will approximately double for a doubling of P_aCO_2 due to vasodilatation of cerebral blood vessels. No further increase in flow is possible at high levels of P_aCO_2 because the arterioles are maximally dilated. Similarly, flow will reduce with hypocapnia due to vasoconstriction of blood vessels. Below about 3.5 kPa, maximal arteriolar vasoconstriction occurs and can lead to tissue hypoxia. These effects are mediated via a complex pathway of interrelated mediators. The initial stimulus is a decrease in brain pH, further mediated by nitric oxide, potassium channels, prostanoids, cyclic nucleotides and a decrease in intracellular calcium as the final common pathway.

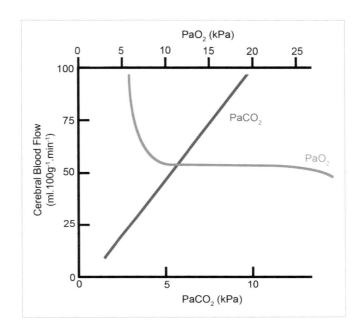

This vascular response to P_aCO_2 can be utilized in ventilated patients with raised intracranial pressure. Increasing ventilation will reduce the P_aCO_2 and cause vasoconstriction of the cerebral vessels. This will therefore reduce cerebral blood volume and intracranial pressure. This effect may be lost in areas of injured brain. If reduced too much, the vasoconstriction can reduce flow causing worsening cerebral ischaemia. A low–normal P_aCO_2 is therefore the aim. This beneficial response will be lost after prolonged periods of hyperventilation.

Arterial partial pressure of oxygen (P_aO_2) has little effect on cerebral blood flow above 8 kPa, with flow remaining constant. Below 8 kPa, there is a sharp increase in blood flow due to vasodilatation. This vasodilatory effect of hypoxia will override any other reflexes to maintain tissue oxygenation. Hypoxia acts directly on the brain tissue to promote the release of adenosine and some prostanoids to cause vasodilatation. It can also act directly on the vascular smooth muscle, causing hyperpolarization, reduced calcium uptake and therefore vasodilatation.

1.4.4

Cerebrospinal fluid

Constituent	CSF	Plasma
Sodium	Comparable	136 –148 mmol.l^{-1}
Chloride	123–128 mmol.l^{-1}	95–105 mmol.l^{-1}
Potassium	2.0–3.0 mmol.l^{-1}	3.8–5.0 mmol.l^{-1}
Calcium	1.1–1.3 mmol.l^{-1}	2.2–2.6 mmol.l^{-1}
Glucose (fasting)	60% of plasma	3.0–5.0 mmol.l^{-1}
Protein	0.2–0.4 g.l^{-1}	60–80 g.l^{-1}
pH	Comparable	7.35–7.45
Osmolality	Comparable	275–295 mOsm.kg^{-1}

Cerebrospinal fluid (CSF) is a specialized extracellular fluid that exists within the ventricles of the brain and the subarachnoid space. The functions of CSF are many and include:
- physical protection by buoyancy
- provision of a chemically stable environment for neuronal activity
- distribution of nutrients to neural tissue and facilitation of removal of waste products
- involvement in acid–base regulation for control of respiration.

Characteristic CSF findings in major CNS infections

	Bacterial meningitis	Partially-treated bacterial meningitis	Viral meningitis
Cell count	↑ Predominantly polymorphs	↑ Predominantly lymphocytes	↑ Predominantly lymphocytes (although polymorphs common in first 24–36 h)
Protein	↑↑ (1–5 g.l^{-1})	↑	↑ (0.5–1 g.l^{-1})
Glucose	↓ (CSF/plasma ratio <0.4)	↓ to normal	Usually normal
Microbiology stain	High yield	Reduced yield by 20%	Nil (PCR testing may be useful for herpes simplex infection)

- Gross examination of CSF may reveal turbidity which can be attributed to an elevated cell count (either red and/or white blood cells), high bacterial or fungal load, or epidural fat aspirated at the time of lumbar puncture.
- A raised white blood cell count is most commonly caused by infection (meningitic or encephalitic processes). Other causes may include subarachnoid haemorrhage, intrathecal drugs, cerebral infarction or Guillain–Barré syndrome.
- A normal glucose CSF/plasma ratio is approximately 0.6 (with a ratio of 0.4 in patients with diabetes due to a lag in glucose transport). A ratio lower than this may be caused by bacterial infection, subarachnoid haemorrhage or meningeal infiltration by neoplasms.
- Raised protein levels are observed with meningitis. However, other causes include cerebrovascular disease (thrombosis and haemorrhage), demyelinating disease and status epilepticus.

1.4.5

Electroencephalogram waveforms

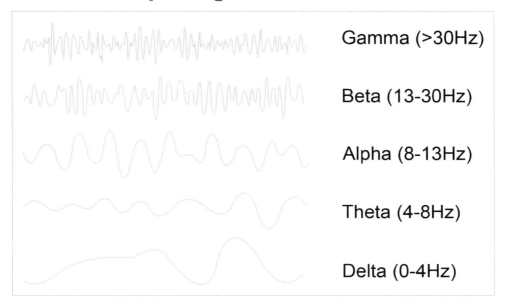

Gamma (>30Hz)

Beta (13-30Hz)

Alpha (8-13Hz)

Theta (4-8Hz)

Delta (0-4Hz)

Electroencephalography (EEG) is a method of recording spontaneous electrical activity of the brain, usually measured via surface electrodes.

EEG waveforms are commonly classified into bands which correspond to different behaviours and cognitive states. For example, the highest frequency waveforms (gamma) are associated with high-level information, processing and integrated thoughts. In health, the lowest frequency waveforms (delta) occur during deep sleep.

The EEG signal is the combination of many waveforms from different neural networks occurring at different frequencies. EEG data are complex signals due to the presence of a mixture of different frequencies occurring at the same time. Fourier transformation allows reformatting of the data into the component frequency bands.

Morphology describes the shape of a single waveform or set of waves. Single waves may be monophasic, biphasic or polyphasic. A series of waves can be monomorphic or polymorphic.

EEG monitoring in anaesthesia and critical care

Multiple commercial devices are available that measure and process EEG signals as a representation of anaesthetic depth (see *Section 6.4 – Depth of anaesthesia monitoring*).

EEG monitoring may be utilized in the intensive care setting to measure cerebral activity, particularly when clinical neurological examination is difficult or unreliable. Indications include seizure detection, presence of cerebral ischaemia and prognostication after coma. Raw EEG data requires specialized knowledge and expertise to ensure accurate interpretation.

Specialized epilepsy centres may offer placement of intracranial strip/grid electrodes and stereotactic cerebral depth electrodes to improve EEG signal quality and better guide seizure management. General anaesthesia is required to facilitate electrode implantation. A thorough understanding of epilepsy classification and perioperative considerations is required.

1.4.6

Gate control theory of pain

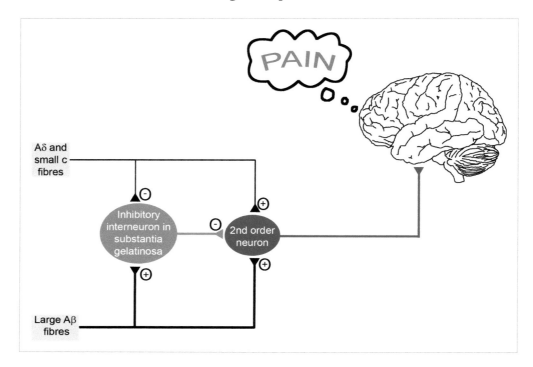

Pain is an unpleasant sensory and emotional experience that is associated with actual or potential tissue damage, or described in terms thereof. Tissue damage is detected peripherally by nociceptors and transmitted via small c fibres (slow pain, e.g. pressure) and small Aδ fibres (fast pain, e.g. sudden heat) to the CNS where they are interpreted and perceived by the brain. It is suggested that within the CNS there are circuits that can modulate incoming pain information; the gate control theory is one such example.

In the mid-1960s, Melzack and Wall proposed a theory that the transmission of a peripheral painful stimulus to the CNS occurs via a 'gate' at the spinal cord level. The concept is that a non-painful input closes the 'gate' to the painful input, thereby preventing further transmission of the painful stimulus and suppressing the perception of pain. The gate is thought to be an inhibitory interneuron in the substantia gelatinosa of the dorsal horn of the spinal cord. It can be stimulated or inhibited presynaptically by different non-noxious afferent inputs, e.g. touch or vibration sensation via Aβ fibres.

Clinical applications of this theory include the use of neuromodulatory techniques for chronic pain, such as transcutaneous electrical nerve stimulation (TENS) and spinal cord stimulators. TENS units produce two different current frequencies below the painful threshold in order to produce analgesia via the gate theory mechanism. Following on from the TENS system, Shealy and colleagues proposed the use of spinal cord stimulators to produce a similar effect and they have been used in neuropathic pain, complex regional pain syndrome, angina pectoris and peripheral vascular disease. Aside from their effects related to the gate control theory, they are also thought to have anti-ischaemic effects; the mechanism of which is poorly understood.

1.4.7

Glasgow Coma Scale

	Response	Score
Best eye opening	Spontaneous	4
	To verbal command	3
	To pain	2
	None	1
Best verbal response	Orientated	5
	Disorientated – confused conversation but able to answer questions	4
	Inappropriate responses, words discernible	3
	Incomprehensible speech	2
	None	1
Best motor response	Obeys commands	6
	Purposeful movement to painful stimulus	5
	Withdraws from pain	4
	Abnormal flexion, decorticate posture	3
	Abnormal extension, decerebrate posture	2
	None	1

The Glasgow Coma Scale (GCS) is a scoring system originally developed to obtain an objective clinical measure of brain injury severity. Its use has been widely extrapolated to assess patients with other causes of depressed neurological function. Three aspects of behaviour are graded independently and added together: a maximum of 15, and a minimum of 3, may be scored. If an endotracheal tube or tracheostomy is present the best verbal response is often annotated as a T.

Use of GCS as a prognostic marker of disease outcome

In addition to its use in grading consciousness, the GCS score has been demonstrated to be a prognostic marker of morbidity and mortality for certain diseases.

- **Traumatic brain injury** – prediction of functional outcome and mortality is difficult due to the heterogeneity of pathology and the potential for secondary brain injury. Research has focused on development of prognostic models to identify reliable prognostic factors better. Initial GCS has been demonstrated as an independent predictor of outcome. The motor component yields most of the predictive power of the score. Other prognostic factors include presence of dysautonomia, hyperglycaemia and subdural haematoma.
- **Subarachnoid haemorrhage** – the World Federation of Neurological Surgeons (WFNS) scale combines GCS with the presence/absence of a focal neurological deficit to create a five grade scale. The Prognosis on Admission of Aneurysmal Subarachnoid Haemorrhage (PAASH) scale is also a five grade scale based solely on the GCS. Both of these scales demonstrate good prognostic value for predicting patient outcome.
- **Critically ill** – Acute Physiology and Chronic Health Evaluation (APACHE) and Simplified Acute Physiology Score (SAPS) are predictive scoring systems that have been developed to measure disease severity and predict the mortality of patients in the intensive care unit. The GCS is a clinical variable in both of these scoring systems.

1.4.8

Intracranial pressure–volume relationship

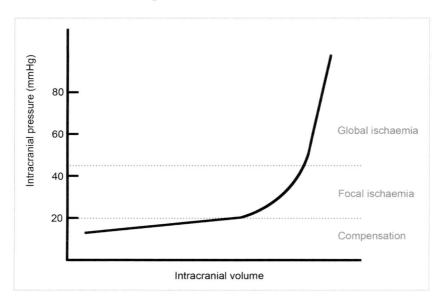

The Monro–Kellie doctrine states that the skull is a rigid container of constant volume and that any change in volume of one of its contents will lead to a reciprocal change in volume of another in order to maintain a constant intracranial pressure (ICP). The intracranial content consists of brain tissue (80–85%), CSF (5–12%) and blood (5–7%).

In an attempt to maintain a constant ICP, compensation will occur in response to an increase in intracranial contents. Initially there is a reduction in venous blood volume, followed by a reduction in CSF volume and then arterial blood volume. An ICP <20 mmHg can be maintained with compensation but, at a threshold level, small changes in volume will cause large increases in intracranial pressure. As ICP rises, CPP and therefore cerebral blood flow will fall; above 20 mmHg focal ischaemia will start to occur and once the intracranial pressure exceeds 45 mmHg global ischaemia will occur.

Treatments for a raised intracranial pressure include the following.

Reduction in blood volume by:
- maintaining a P_aCO_2 of 4–4.5 kPa will prevent vasodilatation, although the effectiveness of this will reduce with time (see *Section 1.4.3 – Cerebral blood flow variation with ventilation*)
- encouraging venous drainage by maintaining a head-up neutral position and avoiding tight endotracheal tube ties
- reducing cerebral metabolic rate using sedative, analgesia and mild hypothermia.

Reduction in brain volume by:
- administering diuretics and corticosteroids (in certain situations) to reduce cerebral oedema
- surgical decompression.

Reduction in CSF volume with:
- drainage via the lateral ventricle using an extra-ventricular drain or lumbar drain.

1.4.9

Intracranial pressure waveform

Intracranial pressure (ICP) describes the pressure exerted by the CSF in the lateral ventricles and has a normal value of 5–15 mmHg. Changes in ICP can be explained using the Monro–Kellie doctrine (see *Section 1.4.8 – Intracranial pressure–volume relationship*). The ICP waveform is similar to an arterial pressure trace and has characteristic waves.

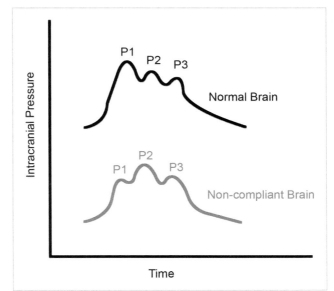

- P1 – the 1st peak, or percussive wave, is the arterial pressure transmitted from the choroid plexus.
- P2 – the 2nd peak, or rebound/ tidal wave, is a measure of brain compliance.
- P3 – the 3rd peak, or dicrotic notch, represents aortic valve closure.

P1 is usually the highest peak, however, in a non-compliant brain P2 may become higher as compliance reduces. The waveform also varies with respiration, reflecting changes in the CVP.

Lundberg proposed three abnormal patterns of ICP waveforms.
- **A waves** – plateau waves, last 2–20 mins and have an amplitude of 50–100 mmHg with a steep rise and then steep fall to baseline. They represent an extreme compromise of brain compliance and may be caused by vasodilatation in response to the CPP falling below the ischaemic threshold, leading to an increased ICP.
- **B waves** – occur every 0.5–2 mins with an amplitude <50 mmHg. These change with ventilation and can reflect reduced compliance, although are unreliable clinically.
- **C waves** – low amplitude (<20 mmHg), occur more frequently at about 4–8 per minute. They are less useful clinically.

In certain clinical situations, such as traumatic brain injury, ICP monitoring may be indicated. The following methods are suitable.
- Subarachnoid bolt – inserted via a burr hole.
- Intracerebral or intraparenchymal transducer – sited within brain tissue (fibreoptic – Camino; strain gauge – Codman).
- External ventricular drain (EVD) – more invasive but can be used to drain CSF.
- Extradural fibreoptic probe – placed via a burr hole.

1.4.10

Neuron

Fibre type	Function	Fibre diameter (μm)	Conduction speed (m.s⁻¹)
Aα	Somatic motor and proprioception	12–20 *Largest	70–120 *Fastest
Aβ	Touch and pressure	5–12	50–70
Aγ	Motor fibres to muscle spindles	3–6	30–50
Aδ	Pain, temperature and touch	2–5	<30
B	Myelinated pre-ganglionic autonomic fibres	1–3	<15
C	Unmyelinated post-ganglionic autonomic fibres, pain and temperature	<1 *Smallest	<2 *Slowest

Neurons are the basic unit of the nervous system. A typical neuron comprises three parts: a cell body and two extensions, a dendrite and an axon. The cell body contains the nucleus and other intracellular organelles. Dendrites transmit incoming information to the cell body, while axons transmit information from it. The axon may be myelinated or unmyelinated. Myelinated axons are surrounded by supporting cells that produce an insulating myelin layer; oligodendrocytes occur in the central nervous system and Schwann cells in the peripheral nervous system. Myelination increases the speed of propagation of a nerve impulse along an axon. The axon divides into terminal branches that end in an enlargement called a terminal button. This contains neurotransmitters which carry the nerve impulse across a synapse to other neurons. Neurons vary in function, diameter and conduction speeds as illustrated in the above table.

Classification of pain

Pain is defined as an unpleasant sensory and emotional experience associated with actual or potential tissue damage.
- **Nociceptive pain** – is a protective process originating in the setting of normal pain pathways. Noxious stimuli activate Aδ or C fibres, with impulses being transmitted via the dorsal horn to higher centres in the brain.
- **Neuropathic pain** – occurs with the abnormal activation of pain pathways caused by a primary lesion or dysfunction of the somatosensory nervous system. Pathological mechanisms are poorly understood. Peripheral changes include sensitization of nociceptors (resulting in a reduced threshold for nerve activation), abnormal neuronal sprouting, and ectopic firing of Aδ and C fibres (due to an increased expression of abnormal sodium and calcium channels). Central changes occur in response to peripheral nerve damage including 'wind-up' of the spinal cord (a progressive, frequency-dependent sensitization process resulting in a more intense response to a constant intensity stimulus) and loss of inhibitory mechanisms.

1.4.11

Neurotransmitters – action

Neurotransmitter	Effect
Noradrenaline (NAdr)	Neurotransmitter in sympathetic nervous system (SNS), ascending reticular activating system and hypothalamus. Stimulates α-adrenoceptors with some β_1 action.
Adrenaline (Adr)	Catecholamine, acting as hormone and neurotransmitter in SNS and brainstem pathways. Stimulates α- and β-adrenoceptors (dose-dependent effect).
Dopamine	Catecholamine and neurotransmitter, found in post-ganglionic sympathetic nerve endings and adrenal medulla, regulates motor behaviour and emotional arousal.
Serotonin (5HT)	Found in gastrointestinal tract and CNS. Regulates appetite, sleep, memory and learning, temperature, mood, muscle contraction and some functions of the CVS and endocrine system.
Glycine	Inhibitory in the spinal cord.
Glutamate	Fast excitatory synapses in CNS.
GABA	Fast inhibitory synapses in CNS.
Substance P	Neuropeptide, involved in pain transmission and also in smooth muscle relaxation.
Acetylcholine (ACh)	Transmitter at neuromuscular junction and in many regions of the brain.

The only direct action of a neurotransmitter is to activate a receptor; the effects depend on the neurons that use the neurotransmitter and the receptor to which it binds.

In general, the amino acids and acetylcholine are involved in fast signalling, whereas the polypeptides, amines and nitric oxide have slower, more diffuse regulatory functions. Many neurotransmitters can be released together and can potentiate each other's actions, e.g. vasoactive intestinal polypeptide and acetylcholine.

Drugs may affect the action of neurotransmitters by:
- Decreasing the rate of neurotransmitter synthesis by affecting enzyme function. This will reduce neurotransmitter availability and therefore activity.
- Blocking or stimulating the release of the neurotransmitter.
- Preventing the storage of neurotransmitter in vesicles.
- Receptor antagonism, e.g. haloperidol, chlorpromazine and clozapine are dopamine receptor antagonists.
- Receptor agonism, e.g. diazepam on the GABA receptor.
- Preventing the deactivation of the neurotransmitter after its release from a receptor, thereby prolonging its action. This is achieved either by blocking reuptake of the neurotransmitter or inhibiting enzymes that are involved in its degradation. Fluoxetine, a selective serotonin reuptake inhibitor, blocks reuptake of serotonin by the presynaptic cell thereby increasing serotonin concentration in the synapse. Neostigmine is an acetylcholinesterase inhibitor that increases the concentration of acetylcholine in the synapse by preventing its breakdown (and hence acts as a reversal agent for non-depolarizing muscle relaxants).

1.4.12

Neurotransmitters – classification

Category	Examples	Metabotropic	Ionotropic
Amines	Noradrenaline (NAdr)	Adrenergic receptor	–
	Adrenaline (Adr)	Adrenergic receptor	–
	Dopamine	Dopamine receptor	–
	Serotonin (5HT)	Serotonin receptor (all but 5HT$_3$)	5HT$_3$ receptor
	Histamine	Histamine receptor	–
Amino acids	Glycine	–	Glycine, NMDA receptors (co-agonist)
	Glutamate	Glutamate receptor	NMDA, AMPA, kianate receptors
	GABA	GABA$_B$ receptor	GABA$_A$ receptor
	Aspartate	–	NMDA receptor
Polypeptides	Substance P	–	–
	Enkephalins	δ opioid receptor	–
	Vasopressin	Vasopressin receptor	–
	Oxytocin	Oxytocin receptor	–
Others	Acetylcholine (ACh)	Muscarinic ACh receptor	Nicotinic ACh receptor
	Nitric oxide	Soluble guanylyl cyclase	–

Neurotransmitters are endogenous chemicals secreted from presynaptic nerve endings that act at the postsynaptic membrane to produce an effect. Neurotransmitters are stored in vesicles clustered beneath the presynaptic membrane in the axon terminal, and which can then be released in response to a threshold action potential or graded electrical potential. On the postsynaptic membrane, they act at specific receptors to either open or close membrane channels; the effect of which may be excitatory or inhibitory. They are only briefly available at the postsynaptic membrane, after which they are rapidly deactivated by either reuptake into the presynaptic terminal or by degradative enzymes in the synaptic cleft.

Neurotransmitters can be classified in a number of ways, although classifying them as excitatory or inhibitory can be confusing because many have both actions, and some may be inhibitory at one synapse and excitatory at another. The most prevalent neurotransmitter is glutamate, which is excitatory in over 90% of synapses in the CNS. The next most prevalent is GABA, which is predominantly inhibitory in action. Acetylcholine is also prevalent and has both excitatory and inhibitory actions.

Another way to classify them is according to their structure, into amines, amino acids, polypeptides and others, as seen in the table. Receptors are divided into metabotropic (those that involve a second messenger system) and ionotropic (those that involve ligand-gated ion channels). It can be seen from the table that some substances that are active as hormones may also have neurotransmitter functions, e.g. vasopressin and oxytocin.

1.4.13

Reflex arc

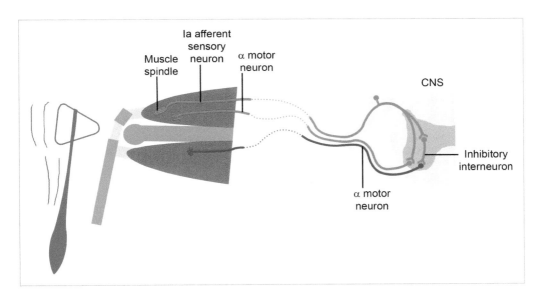

A reflex is an involuntary, automatic response to changes within or outside the body. The anatomical pathway is the reflex arc, where a particular sensory stimulus produces a predictable, and specific response. This neural pathway usually consists of five components:
- receptor – sense organ (e.g. muscle spindle, Golgi tendon organ)
- afferent/sensory neuron – carries impulse towards CNS
- interneuron – carries impulse within CNS
- efferent/motor neuron – carries impulse away from CNS
- effector organ.

Reflex arcs may be characterized as follows.
- Somatic – the effector organ is skeletal muscle.
- Autonomic – the effector organ is smooth muscle or gland cells which regulate visceral function, including involuntary control of breathing, heart rate and blood pressure.

Reflex arcs may also be characterized according to the number of neuronal synapses between the afferent and motor neuron.

Monosynaptic reflex: the simplest reflex arc. The stretch reflex (e.g. knee jerk reflex) is an example of a monosynaptic reflex. A patellar tap stretches the patellar tendon, subsequently stretching the quadriceps muscle. The muscle spindle within the muscle lengthens and activity of associated Ia afferents increases. Within the spinal cord, these afferents synapse with an α motor neuron, leading to quadriceps contraction. Postural muscle tone and balance are maintained via this mechanism.

Polysynaptic reflex: the majority of reflexes demonstrate a more complicated pathway. In conjunction with the monosynaptic stretch reflex, a polysynaptic process occurs. A collateral branch of the afferent neuron synapses with an inhibitory interneuron, which in turn synapses with an antagonist α motor neuron. The effect is relaxation of the antagonist muscle group (e.g. hamstrings) allowing contraction of the stretched muscle (e.g. quadriceps). This is the principle of reciprocal innervation.

1.4.14

Synaptic transmission

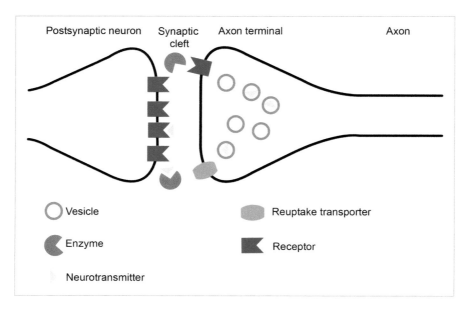

Synaptic, or neuro-, transmission describes the way in which two neurons communicate. This may be electrically via gap junctions where cells are in direct contact, or chemically across a synaptic cleft.

In chemical transmission, a signalling molecule such as a neurotransmitter is released from one neuron (the presynaptic neuron) and binds to a second neuron (the postsynaptic neuron). This allows propagation of an action potential and the firing of subsequent neurons. The synaptic cleft describes the space between the two membranes and is approximately 20 nm wide.

The neurotransmitter is synthesized in the cell body or axon terminal and stored in granules or vesicles in the axon terminal. When an action potential arrives at the axon, calcium enters the axon terminal via voltage-gated calcium channels and binds with calmodulin. This causes release of the neurotransmitter by exocytosis into the synaptic cleft. The neurotransmitter then diffuses across the cleft and binds to receptors on the postsynaptic, or presynaptic, membrane. The receptor channels may produce either a direct (ionotropic) or indirect (metabotropic) response.

The response to binding may be excitatory or inhibitory, causing depolarization or hyperpolarization of the membrane, respectively (see *Section 1.4.12 – Neurotransmitters – classification*). The postsynaptic membrane may receive multiple inputs and may be spatial (multiple presynaptic terminals) or temporal (multiple times from the same terminal). The net effect of these inputs (summation) will influence whether or not the postsynaptic neuron will propagate the action potential and 'fire'.

The neurotransmitter within the synaptic cleft is then deactivated either by enzyme degradation or reuptake into the nerve terminal (for reuse or removal). Autoreceptors on the presynaptic neuron also act as a negative feedback system for neurotransmitter release.

1.4.15

Types of nerve

Functional classification

- Somatic afferent – sensory; carries messages from any organ towards the CNS
- Somatic efferent – motor; carries messages from the CNS to the skeletal muscles
- Autonomic – controls involuntary and semi-voluntary functions of the organs, smooth muscle and glands

Morphological classification

- Pseudo-unipolar – sensory; short axon which quickly divides into two branches (central to spinal cord, peripheral)
- Bipolar – sensory (retina, olfactory epithelium, inner ear); two main extensions (axon and dendrite) of equal length
- Multipolar – most common type; many short dendrites emanating from a cell body with one long axon

The peripheral nervous system (PNS) consists of nerves and ganglia present outside of the brain and spinal cord. The PNS includes the cranial nerves (with the exception of the optic nerve), spinal nerves, peripheral nerves and neuromuscular junctions. The main function of the PNS is to conduct information to and from the CNS.

Perioperative peripheral nerve injury

The aetiology of injuries is varied and may be multifactorial with the following mechanisms possible.
- Direct nerve damage – surgery, needle trauma in regional anaesthesia.
- Stretch and compression – poor padding, tourniquet use or surgical retractors.
- Ischaemia – tourniquet use, prolonged immobility or metabolic abnormalities.
- Toxicity associated with injected solution – injection of a local anaesthetic directly into a nerve fascile, use of neurolytics in certain disease states (e.g. diabetes mellitus).
- Double crush syndrome – pre-existing nerve injury heightens the susceptibility of the nerve to damage elsewhere as impairment of conduction by double compression is cumulative.
- Unknown.

These injuries are largely preventable if risk factors are identified and managed appropriately. Common risk factors include patient co-morbidities (diabetes mellitus, smoking, hypertension), perioperative physiology (hypovolaemia, hypotension, hypothermia and hypoxia), anaesthetic factors (general and regional anaesthesia associated with greater injury compared to sedation), and surgical factors (difficult patient positioning, prolonged surgery, vascular damage).

Perioperative peripheral nerve injuries may be classified as follows.
- Compression injury with the nerve still intact. These injuries usually recover within 6 weeks of nerve insult.
- Crush injury where the continuity of the axon is lost.
- Transection injury with complete disruption of the nerve trunk.

Lower limb injuries are less common than injuries of the upper limb. Ulnar nerve injuries are the most common perioperative peripheral nerve injury due to its superficial nature and close proximity to the bony medial epicondyle.

1.4.16

Visual pathway

Lesion and field loss	Anatomical damage	Cause
A – unilateral field loss	Optic nerve	Trauma, ischaemia, inflammation
B – bitemporal hemianopia	Optic chiasm	Compression from pituitary tumours or aneurysm of anterior communicating artery
C&D – homonymous hemianopia	Optic tract or radiation	Cerebrovascular accident, trauma, tumours
E&F – quadrantanopia	Temporal lobe (upper), parietal lobe (lower)	Cerebrovascular disorders

The visual pathway describes the journey that nerve impulses take from the retina to the visual cortex. It consists of the retina, optic nerve, optic chiasm and tracts, lateral geniculate bodies, optic radiation and the visual cortex.

Light passes through the anterior structures of the eye before reaching the retina. Photoreceptors lie outermost in the retina against the pigment epithelium (away from the lens and vitreous humour) and consist of rods and cones. The rods are evenly spread throughout the retina and are responsible for monochromatic and night vision.

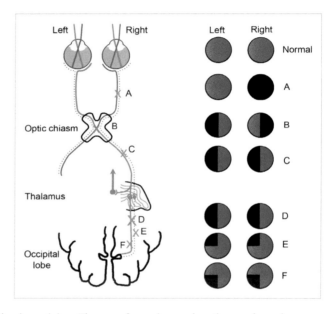

Cones are concerned with bright and colour vision. They are fewer in number than rods and are located primarily around the fovea.

Light reaching the photoreceptors generates an electrical potential. This is transmitted from the photoreceptors to bipolar cells, which then synapse with the ganglion cells. The axons of the ganglion cells converge at the blind spot of the optic disc to form the optic nerve. The optic nerve is covered by pia, arachnoid and dura mater and passes posteriorly to exit the bony orbit through the optic canal in the lesser wing of the sphenoid.

The optic chiasm lies in the floor of the third ventricle, directly above the pituitary gland. The axons from the nasal halves of the retina cross at the optic chiasm, whereas those from the temporal halves remain on the ipsilateral side. The two tracts exit the chiasm backwards to synapse in the lateral geniculate body (a sensory relay nucleus in the thalamus). From here, synaptic connections are made to the primary visual cortex in the occipital lobe, via the optic radiation. Some fibres of the optic tracts also relay to the superior colliculi, and pretectal nucleus, which are involved in eye movements, posture and in the pupillary light reflex.

1.5.1
Autoregulation of renal blood flow

Autoregulation of blood flow is a mechanism whereby an organ or vascular bed intrinsically maintains a relatively constant perfusion pressure independent of changes to systemic blood pressure. This process is clearly demonstrated by those organs that are essential to life: the brain, kidneys and heart.

Renal autoregulation maintains a relatively stable renal blood flow (RBF) through a wide range of mean arterial pressures.

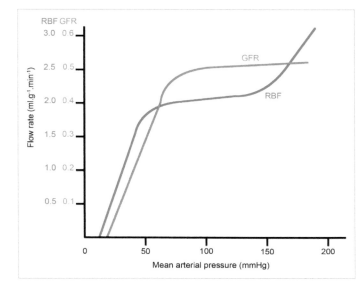

This intrinsic process is not fully understood but appears to be, in part, mediated via myogenic (faster) and tubuloglomerular (slower) feedback mechanisms. Both alter preglomerular vascular resistance via changes in tone of the afferent arteriole. As the effector site for both mechanisms is the preglomerular resistance vessels, a relatively constant glomerular filtration rate (GFR) is also maintained.

- **Myogenic theory** – involves the activation of stretch receptors in response to increases in arteriolar transmural pressure. This induces a direct vasoconstriction and increase in resistance of the afferent arteriole, returning renal blood flow to normal according to Ohm's law (see *Section 1.2.6 – Ohm's law*).
- **Tubuloglomerular feedback** – involves flow-dependent sensing of tubular ion delivery via the macula densa. As tubular flow rate and ion delivery change in response to a change in renal blood flow and GFR, the macula densa alters tone in the adjacent segment of afferent arteriole through the release of extracellular messengers (ATP and/or adenosine).

Abolition of these mechanisms does not completely remove autoregulatory vasoconstriction, implicating the presence of other, yet undefined, physiological mechanisms.

Hypertensive renal injury

Hypertension remains a common aetiology of chronic kidney disease, either in isolation or as part of other disease processes. Hypertensive damage of glomerular capillaries correlates most strongly with oscillating peaks in systolic blood pressure. As the faster myogenic mechanism is capable of compensatory responses at high frequencies (seen with blood pressure oscillations), this mechanism is particularly important in renal protection from barotrauma.

1.5.2

Clearance

$$Cl_x = \frac{[U_x] \times U_{flow}}{[P_x]}$$

$$Cl_{H_2O} = U_{flow} - \left[\frac{U_{osmol} \times U_{flow}}{P_{osmol}} \right]$$

$$= U_{flow} \left[1 - \frac{U_{osmol}}{P_{osmol}} \right]$$

Cl_x = clearance of substance × (ml.min^{-1})

$[U_x]$ = urine concentration (mg.ml^{-1})

U_{flow} = urine flow rate (ml.min^{-1})

$[P_x]$ = plasma concentration (mg.ml^{-1})

Cl_{H_2O} = free water clearance

U_{osmol} = urine osmolality

P_{osmol} = plasma osmolality

Clearance can be defined as the volume of plasma that is cleared of a substance per unit time (measured in ml.min^{-1}). Renal clearance is a measure of the excretion ability of the kidneys or the rate at which substances are cleared from the blood. It can alternatively be defined as the hypothetical plasma volume containing the amount of any substance excreted in the urine per minute. It is a useful way of approximating GFR (see *Section 1.5.3 – Glomerular filtration rate*).

The amount of a substance excreted in the urine can be calculated by multiplying together the urine concentration (U_x) and the urine flow rate (U_{flow}) to give the excretion rate in mg.min^{-1}. This is then divided by the plasma concentration (P_x), which is usually measured from a blood sample, to give the clearance (Cl_x) of a substance in ml.min^{-1}. Clearance is constant in first order kinetics because a constant fraction of the drug is removed per unit time, but is variable in zero-order kinetics because the amount of drug eliminated is dependent on the concentration of the drug in the blood per unit time.

Free water clearance is the volume of plasma that is cleared of water per minute. As plasma is mostly water, this number is low; a value of zero suggests that the plasma is isotonic with the urine. Creatinine clearance gives much larger numbers, about 120 ml.min^{-1}, as creatinine is filtered but is inert to the rest of the tubule. In reality, it is secreted in small amounts so will overestimate the GFR (by 10–20%), but is a useful surrogate. To measure the clearance more accurately, inulin may be used. Inulin is freely filtered, but not secreted, reabsorbed, metabolized or stored, however it is a complex procedure and is only used when a very accurate value is required.

1.5.3

Glomerular filtration rate

$$GFR = K_f \left[\left(P_G + \pi_B \right) - \left(P_B + \pi_G \right) \right]$$

K_f = filtration coefficient
P_G = hydrostatic pressure in the glomerular capillaries
π_B = colloid osmotic pressure in Bowman's capsule
P_B = hydrostatic pressure in Bowman's capsule
π_G = colloid osmotic pressure in the glomerular capillaries

The glomerular filtration rate (GFR) is the volume of plasma filtered by the kidneys per minute, normalized to 1.73 m² body surface area; normally 125 ml.min⁻¹. Filtration is defined as passive movement of water and solutes across a membrane secondary to hydrostatic pressure. Due to its passive nature, physiological determinants of diffusion apply.

- Net filtration pressure – as determined by Starling's forces (see *Section 1.2.7 – Starling forces in capillaries*). P_G is the mechanical pressure exerted on the plasma by the pressure gradient between afferent and efferent arterioles. Unlike the venous end in other capillary beds, the efferent arteriole acts as a second resistance vessel, maintaining a relatively stable hydrostatic pressure along the capillary length. Only small amounts of protein enter Bowman's capsule, effectively eliminating the colloid osmotic pressure.
- Total surface area available for filtration.
- Permeability of filtration membrane – dependent on molecular size, protein binding and charge.

These latter two factors are accounted for by the use of a filtration coefficient (K_f).

Regulation of GFR

In health, surface area and membrane permeability are constant. Therefore, GFR is regulated through changes in net filtration pressure via the following mechanisms.

- Renal autoregulation (see *Section 1.5.1 – Autoregulation of renal blood flow*).
- Hormonal regulation via the renin–angiotensin system (see *Section 1.5.6 – Renin–angiotensin–aldosterone system*), atrial natriuretic peptide (ANP) and aldosterone.
  - Secreted by cardiac muscle cells, ANP increases net filtration pressure through dilatation of the afferent arteriole and constriction of the efferent arteriole. Glomerular mesangial cells relax, leading to a larger surface area for filtration. The overall effect is an increase in GFR.
  - Aldosterone reduces GFR, predominantly via indirect effects resulting in a rise in systemic and intraglomerular blood pressure.
- Neuronal regulation via the autonomic nervous system, predominantly via postganglionic sympathetic fibres. Sympathetic activation causes direct vasoconstriction of the afferent arteriole, decreasing GFR.

1.5.4

Loop of Henle

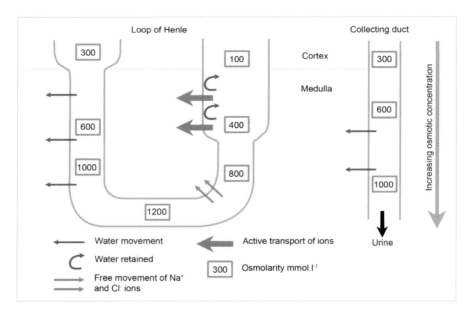

The loop of Henle is the portion of the nephron between the proximal convoluted tubule and the distal convoluted tubule (DCT). Its main function is to create a concentration gradient in the renal medulla to produce concentrated urine.

It has 4 parts.
- **Thin descending loop** – low permeability to ions and urea but highly permeable to water. The fluid entering is isotonic, water moves out along its concentration gradient into the interstitium, so facilitating the concentration of urine in the tubule.
- **Thin ascending loop** – impermeable to water but permeable to ions. The fluid entering is hypertonic, ion transport may still occur so the urine osmolality falls.
- **Thick ascending limb** – also impermeable to water, contains ion pumps to pump electrolytes actively into the interstitium. Sodium (Na^+), potassium (K^+) and chloride (Cl^-) ions are reabsorbed from the urine by the $Na^+/2Cl^-/K^+$ co-transporter. The fluid leaving this limb is hypotonic.
- **Cortical thick ascending limb** – drains urine into the DCT.

This process is assisted by the presence of a blood supply that does not dissipate the concentration gradients produced. The vasa recta are straight capillaries that originate from the cortical efferent arterioles and also have a countercurrent multiplier mechanism. This prevents washout of the solutes from the medulla and maintains the medullary concentration. Water is osmotically drawn from the descending limb and enters the vasa recta. The low blood flow in these capillaries allows time for osmotic equilibration. Flow can be altered by changing the resistance of the efferent arterioles.

The countercurrent system creates a high concentration gradient deep in the medulla between the interstitium and collecting duct. This allows water to move passively through aquaporin channels in the collecting duct, creating more concentrated urine for excretion. The collecting duct is also under the control of antidiuretic hormone (vasopressin).

1.5.5

Nephron

Each adult human kidney contains approximately 1–1.5 million nephrons. There are two sorts: cortical nephrons (85%) that have short loops of Henle and are found in the outer renal cortex, and juxtamedullary nephrons (15%) that have long loops of Henle that descend into the medulla (see *Section 1.5.4 – Loop of Henle*). Only the latter have a significant effect on medullary hypertonicity.

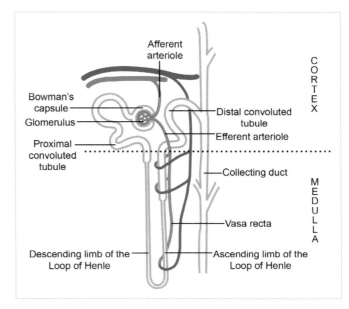

Structure and function

- **Glomerulus**: a dense ball of specialized capillaries fed by blood under high pressure from an afferent arteriole. Movement of substances into the Bowman's capsule depends on their molecular weight and electrical charge. The glomerular capillaries merge and blood exits via an efferent arteriole.
- **Proximal tubule**: divided into two parts, convoluted (PCT) and straight. Extremely metabolically active, being involved in the reabsorption of electrolytes and water, secretion of substances (e.g. drugs) and acid–base balance.
- **Loop of Henle**: allows production of a hypertonic environment within the renal medulla, thus allowing reabsorption of water by osmosis from the collecting ducts that pass in close proximity (see *Section 1.5.4 – Loop of Henle*). The descending limb is permeable to water, the ascending limb impermeable.
- **Distal convoluted tubule (DCT)**: partly responsible for the regulation of K^+, Na^+, Ca^{2+} and pH.
- **Collecting duct**: acted upon by aldosterone and antidiuretic hormone (ADH), the latter exerting its effect via aquaporin channels.
- **Juxtaglomerular apparatus**: an area of the nephron where the afferent arteriole and the initial portion of the DCT are in close contact. It regulates blood pressure and urine production. Within it, specialized smooth muscle cells of the afferent arteriole (granular juxtaglomerular cells) act as mechanoreceptors that monitor blood pressure in the afferent arteriole. These cells secrete renin. In the adjacent part of the DCT, specialized cells within the macula densa act as chemoreceptors that monitor the concentration of Na^+ and Cl^- in the urine.

1.5.6

Renin–angiotensin–aldosterone system

The renin–angiotensin–aldosterone system regulates fluid balance and systemic vascular resistance (SVR). Renin, released from the kidneys, stimulates formation of angiotensin that in turn stimulates the release of aldosterone from the adrenal cortex.

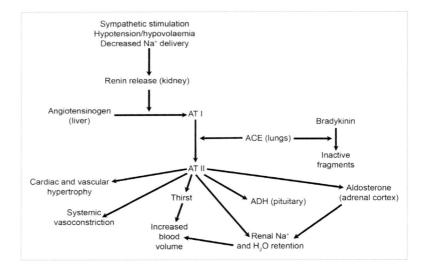

Renin is stored and released from the juxtaglomerular cells of the afferent arterioles. Its release is stimulated by sympathetic stimulation (via β_1-adrenoceptors), renal artery hypotension and reduced sodium delivery to the distal renal tubules (sensed by the macula densa cells). Once released, renin acts on angiotensinogen (released from the liver), which is cleaved to form the decapeptide angiotensin I (AT I). Angiotensin I is then converted by angiotensin-converting enzyme (ACE), found in vascular endothelium particularly in the lung, to form the octapeptide angiotensin II (AT II).

Angiotensin II has many functions.
- Vasoconstriction of arterioles leading to an increase in SVR and arterial pressure.
- Acts directly on the kidneys to increase sodium (Na^+) reabsorption by stimulating Na^+/H^+ exchangers in the proximal tubule and thick ascending limb of the loop of Henle, and Na^+ channels in the collecting ducts.
- Stimulates aldosterone release from the zona glomerulosa of the adrenal cortex, which acts on the DCT and cortical collecting ducts to increase Na^+ and water retention. K^+ is excreted in exchange for Na^+.
- Stimulates ADH release from the posterior pituitary.
- Stimulates thirst centres.
- Enhances sympathetic adrenergic function by facilitating noradrenaline release and inhibiting its reuptake.
- Causes ventricular and vascular hypertrophy.

The pathway is modulated by atrial and brain natriuretic peptides that act in an important counter-regulatory system.

The pathway can be manipulated at several stages to reduce arterial pressure, ventricular afterload, blood volume and preload, and inhibit or reverse cardiac and vascular hypertrophy. ACE inhibitors, AT II receptor antagonists and aldosterone receptor antagonists are used in the treatment of hypertension and cardiac failure.

1.6.1

Bile

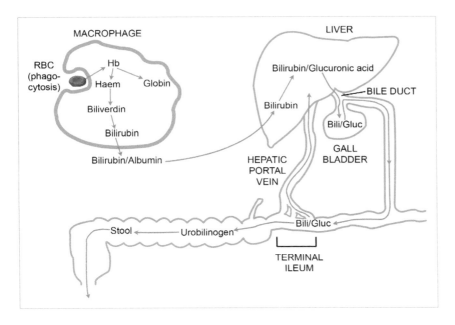

Bile is produced by the liver, stored and concentrated in the gall bladder and released into the small intestine in response to food. Bile is made up of water, bile salts, bilirubin, fats and inorganic salts.

Functions:

- Digestion of lipids – bile salts have hydrophilic and hydrophobic portions. The hydrophobic portion aggregates around droplets of fats to create micelles, with the hydrophilic portions facing outwards. The hydrophilic portions repel each other and prevent the fat reforming into larger droplets, increasing the surface area for the action of pancreatic lipases.
- Absorption of the fat-soluble vitamins (A, D, E and K).
- Excretion of bilirubin.
- Acid neutralization – bile is alkaline and neutralizes excess gastric acid.

Bilirubin is produced when red blood cells are broken down by macrophages in the reticuloendothelial system. Haemoglobin is released and is degraded into haem and globin. Globin is broken down into amino acids and haem into biliverdin and then reduced to form lipid-soluble unconjugated bilirubin (yellow). It crosses the lipid membrane to combine with albumin in the plasma; measured as indirect, or unconjugated, bilirubin in the laboratory.

Bilirubin is conjugated in the liver with glucuronic acid, which is water-soluble. Much of this is then excreted in the bile duct system and into the gall bladder. In normal circumstances a small amount of conjugated bilirubin is released into the plasma and can be measured (direct, or conjugated, bilirubin). Conjugated bilirubin in the gall bladder enters the small intestine and is reabsorbed in the terminal ileum; this is enterohepatic circulation. Any bilirubin not reabsorbed passes to the colon where it is metabolized to water-soluble urobilinogen and then oxidized to form urobilin and stercobilin (brown). A small amount of the urobilinogen may be excreted in the urine (colouring it yellow) and some enters the enterohepatic circulation.

1.6.2

Mediators of gut motility

	Location	Target for secretion	Motility
Gastrin	G cells in antrum of stomach, duodenum and pancreas	Enterochromaffin-like cells, parietal cells	Stimulates gastric contraction
Secretin	S cells of the small intestine (in crypts of Lieberkuhn)	Pancreas and stomach	Inhibits stomach emptying, stimulates gall bladder contraction
Cholecystokinin (CCK)	I cells of small intestine, neurons in brain and gut	Gastric smooth muscle, gall bladder and pancreas	Inhibits stomach emptying, stimulates gall bladder contraction
Motilin	M cells in small intestine	Gastric and duodenal smooth muscle	Stimulates migratory motor complex
Gastric inhibitory polypeptide	K cells of small intestine	Pancreatic beta cells	None
Glucagon-like polypeptide	Small intestine endocrine cells	Pancreatic endocrine cells	Slows gastric emptying

Gastric motility describes the contraction of smooth muscle that serves to move food through the gastrointestinal (GI) tract. The GI tract is divided into four sections by sphincter muscles: the oesophagus, the stomach, the small intestine and the large intestine. Each section has distinct functions requiring different patterns of contraction.

Smooth muscle subunits, found throughout the GI tract, are connected by gap junctions and fire spontaneously in a tonic or phasic way. Tonic contractions are typically seen in the sphincter muscles and describe contractions that are maintained for longer periods. Phasic contractions describe brief periods of both contraction and relaxation and are typically seen in the posterior stomach and small intestine.

There are two distinct patterns of phasic contraction.
• Peristalsis occurs after a meal and consists of contractions in a wave-like propulsive pattern travelling down sections of the GI tract. This pattern is under the influence of hormones, paracrine signals and the autonomic nervous system.
• Segmentation functions to mix the luminal contents. Occurring in an oscillating fashion, small segments of circular smooth muscle contract while the muscle either side relaxes.

Modified smooth muscle cells, called interstitial cells of Cajal, act as pacemaker cells producing slow wave potentials that cause action potentials in the smooth muscle cells. They exist to stimulate spontaneous cycles of contractions. The amplitude and duration of these potentials can be modified by neurotransmitters, hormones and other paracrine signals. Enteroendocrine cells found in the stomach, pancreas and small intestine secrete various GI hormones that control many different functions in the GI tract. They are spread throughout the GI tract and exert both autocrine and paracrine actions.

1.7.1

Acid–base disturbances

Acid–base disturbance occurs when body buffers are unable to maintain pH within the physiological range. Clinical disturbances of acid–base are traditionally defined in terms of the carbon dioxide/bicarbonate (CO_2/HCO_3^-) buffer system. By using the Henderson–Hasselbalch equation (see *Section 1.7.5 – Henderson–Hasselbalch equation*), pH may be calculated if the CO_2 and HCO_3^- concentrations are known. However, it is impractical for bedside assessment and its use is not required with blood gas pH measurement.

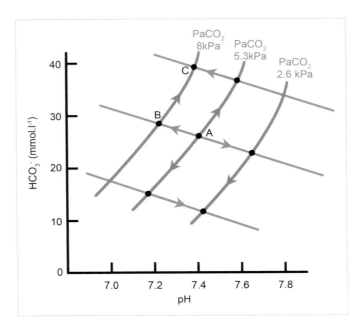

The Davenport diagram is a graphic representation of the Henderson–Hasselbalch equation and demonstrates the relationship between pH, partial pressure of CO_2 (P_aCO_2) and HCO_3^-. Normal values for plasma are illustrated by point A. The green lines on the diagram are buffer lines; their vertical displacement being dependent on the effect of non-CO_2/HCO_3^- buffering systems in the blood. The red lines represent the isopleths for P_aCO_2. Any acute change in P_aCO_2 results in movement along the buffer lines, e.g. line AB illustrates a respiratory acidosis (rise in P_aCO_2). Compensatory changes lead to HCO_3^- retention, returning pH to normal range (line BC).

The middle buffer line depicted (normal buffer line) represents changes in blood pH with normal concentrations of weak acids and bases. The slope of this line is determined by haemoglobin concentration, because haemoglobin acts as a buffer of hydrogen in the blood. Metabolic alterations in pH will shift the normal buffer line up or down the graph, with the slope of the line unchanged. The vertical displacement of the line corresponds to the base excess. For example, a negative base excess (i.e. a base deficit) may occur following the addition of acid to the blood causing consumption of HCO_3^-. This metabolic acidosis, due to a reduction in HCO_3^-, shifts the buffer line down the graph. Respiratory compensation would involve a reduction of P_aCO_2 along this line, returning pH to the physiological range.

1.7.2

Anion gap

$$\text{Anion gap} = ([Na^+] + [K^+]) - ([Cl^-] + [HCO_3^-])$$

The anion gap is the difference between measured serum cations and anions. Routinely measured cations are sodium and potassium, while chloride and bicarbonate are routinely measured anions. Unmeasured cations include calcium and magnesium; unmeasured anions include plasma proteins, phosphate and organic anions (e.g. lactate and ketoacids). The anion gap is founded on the law of electroneutrality, stating that in any aqueous solution in equilibrium, the sum of all cations must equal the sum of all anions. Due to an abundance of unmeasured plasma proteins, predominantly albumin, measured cations exceed measured anions. This produces an anion gap with normal values ranging from 3 to 11 mmol.l^{-1}. An increase in anion gap indicates an increase in the proportion of unmeasured serum anions. A normal anion gap associated with a metabolic acidosis suggests hyperchloraemia.

Approach to acid–base disturbances

- The Siggard–Anderson approach employs assessment of the Henderson–Hasselbalch equation (pH, HCO$_3^-$ and PCO$_2$) and standardized base excess (SBE). Development of SBE acknowledged the importance of buffers other than bicarbonate (e.g. haemoglobin, plasma proteins) in buffering carbon dioxide, the major source of acid in the body. SBE allowed quantification of the metabolic component of acid–base disturbances, independent of PCO$_2$. Limitations of this approach include assumption of normal plasma protein concentration when calculating SBE (rare in critical illness) and inability to differentiate between causes of metabolic acidosis.
- Development of anion gap allowed some differentiation of aetiologies of metabolic acid–base disturbances. Limitations include gross underestimation of anion gap in the presence of hypoalbuminaemia, an unmeasured anion. This may produce misleading results if this reduction is offset by an increase in other unmeasured anions (e.g. lactate).
- The Stewart approach modified the preceding systems in recognition of body fluids, pH and bicarbonate as dependent variables. This model highlights the importance of albumin as a major variable in acid–base physiology (see *Section 1.7.8 – Strong ion difference*).

1.7.3

Buffer solution

$$HA \leftrightarrow H^+ + A^-$$

$$CO_2 + H_2O \leftrightarrow H_2CO_3 \leftrightarrow H^+ + HCO_3^-$$

HA = weak acid

A⁻ = weak base

H_2CO_3 = carbonic acid

H⁺ = hydrogen ion (proton)

HCO_3^- = bicarbonate ion

The Bronsted–Lowry theory defines an acid as a proton (hydrogen ion – H⁺) donor and a base as a H⁺ acceptor. Acid–base reactions are more appropriately thought of as a dynamic equilibrium of proton transfer. A buffer is a conjugate acid–base pair that acts to resist changes in pH. The pKa of a buffer system defines the pH at which it acts most efficiently. A buffer system usually consists of a weak acid (HA) and its conjugate base (A⁻).

Many important buffer systems exist in the body:
- bicarbonate buffer system
- haemoglobin
- plasma proteins
- phosphate buffer system.

Buffer solutions achieve their resistance to pH change because of the equilibrium represented in the equation. When an acid is added to the solution the equilibrium is shifted to the left and, because of this, the H⁺ concentration increases by less than the amount expected. A similar but opposite effect occurs with the addition of an alkali.

Bicarbonate is the main extracellular buffer system. Carbonic anhydrase catalyses a reaction between carbon dioxide (CO_2) and water to form carbonic acid. This dissociates into H⁺ and bicarbonate ions (HCO_3^-). If an acid is added to the system, the excess H⁺ will be buffered by the HCO_3^- and more carbonic acid is formed, which dissociates into CO_2 and water. The bicarbonate system has a pKa of 6.1; at pH 7.4, the system is more effective at buffering acids than alkalis. The ability of the lungs to excrete CO_2 and the kidneys to regulate HCO_3^- make this the main buffer system.

Haemoglobin has a large buffering capacity and has a pKa of 6.8. It is a more efficient buffer when deoxygenated (see *Section 1.3.4 – Carbon dioxide dissociation curve and Haldane effect*). Plasma proteins and the phosphate system are intracellular buffer mechanisms. Phosphate is also an important buffer in the urine.

1.7.4

Dissociation constant and pKa

$$Ka = \frac{[A^-]+[H^+]}{[HA]}$$

Ka = acid dissociation constant

HA = generic acid that dissociates into A⁻ (conjugate base) and H⁺

$$Kb = \frac{[BH^+]+[OH^-]}{[B]}$$

Kb = base dissociation constant

B = generic base that becomes BH⁺ (conjugate acid) and OH⁻ when protonated

$$pKa = -\log_{10} Ka$$

$$pKb = -\log_{10} Kb$$

The strength of an acid or base correlates with the proportion of the substance that has reacted with water to produce ions. The stronger an acid or base, the greater the proportion of it is ionized in solution. The strongest acids and bases are virtually completely ionized in solution.

A dissociation constant is an equilibrium constant that measures the readiness of a substance to reversibly dissociate. Acid dissociation constants (Ka) and base dissociation constants (Kb) are measures of the strength of an acid and base, respectively. The greater the dissociation constant, the more likely the acid or base will dissociate in solution. As with hydrogen ion activity, Ka and Kb span many orders of magnitude. A logarithmic scale is therefore used to facilitate easy application of these concepts as pH, pKa and pKb, respectively.

The pKa is the pH at which the acid is 50% dissociated, i.e. [HA] = [A⁻]. The lower the pKa the stronger the acid. Previously, the pKa was used to describe an acid and pKb a base. However, pKa is now commonly used to denote both variables. As the order of acid strength is the inverse of base strength, the weaker the acid, the stronger the conjugate base. As such, the higher the pKa, the stronger the base.

Local anaesthetic agents are drugs whose pKa influences their action. They are weak bases and all have a pKa above physiological pH (7.4), meaning that their ionized form predominates in the body (see *Section 4.14 – Local anaesthetics – properties*). However, it is their unionized form that crosses cell membranes to produce an effect. This paradox also explains the reason why they are less effective in infected tissue where the environment tends to be more acidic: the reduced pH means that even less of the drug will be in the unionized form.

1.7.5

Henderson–Hasselbalch equation

$$pH = pKa + \log_{10}\left[\frac{\text{proton acceptor}}{\text{proton donor}}\right] = pKa + \log_{10}\left[\frac{A^-}{HA}\right]$$

The Henderson–Hasselbalch equation describes the relationship between pH and pKa of a buffer solution. Derived from the acid dissociation equation, the Henderson–Hasselbalch equation may be applied as follows.

- pH calculation of a buffer solution created with known amounts of conjugate pairs. This equation indicates that buffer pH does not depend on total concentration of the buffering acid and conjugate base, but only on pKa and the ratio of concentrations of the conjugate pair. In contrast, the buffering capacity, defined as how much acid or base the buffer solution can neutralize before pH changes appreciably, is dependent on actual concentrations.
- Determination of the effect on buffer solution pH with additions of small amounts of acid or base. Adding an acid or base to a buffer leads to an equilibrium shift of the conjugate pair in an attempt to maintain constant pH.
- Calculation of the amount of acid or salt required to make a buffer solution of desired pH. This equation is used to derive blood gas bicarbonate concentration.
- Determination of optimal pH for preparation of drugs that are weak electrolytes. Weak electrolytes undergo ionization in solution. This principle may facilitate stable storage of parenteral drugs and improve drug solubility at physiological pH.
  - Weak acid: pH > pKa, ionized form predominates; pH < pKa, unionized form predominates.
  - Weak base: pH > pKa, unionized form predominates; pH < pKa, ionized form predominates.

For example, phenytoin is a weakly acidic drug with a pKa of 8.1. To ensure water solubility, the ionized form must be present, necessitating a pH > 8.1. Sodium hydroxide is therefore added to the parenteral preparation, adjusting the pH to 12. To facilitate improved solubility at physiological pH, phenytoin preparations include water-miscible solvents. Propylene glycol and ethanol may be used as co-solvents in this setting.

1.7.6

Lactic acidosis

Clinical classification

Increased lactate production

- Increased rate of glycolysis due to lack of ATP (shock, hypoxia – global and regional, anaemia, carbon monoxide poisoning)
- Increased rate of glycolysis due to pro-glycolytic stimulus (β-adrenergic agonists, catecholamine excess, malignancy)
- Unregulated substrate entry into glycolysis
- Pyruvate dehydrogenase inactivity (thiamine deficiency, inborn errors of metabolism)
- Defects in oxidative phosphorylation (cyanide, nitroprusside, salicylates, metformin, propofol, isoniazid, ethanol, methanol, ethylene glycol, anti-retrovirals)

Decreased lactate clearance

- Impaired hepatic or renal function, decreased gluconeogenesis (ethanol, methanol, ketoacidosis)

Classical Cohen and Woods classification

Type A – inadequate tissue oxygen delivery (tissue hypoxia)

- Reduced arterial oxygen content
- Decreased cardiac output
- Tissue hypoperfusion
- Regional hypoperfusion
- Abnormal vascular tone or permeability

Type B – non-hypoxic processes affecting production and elimination

- Type B1 – associated with underlying disease state
- Type B2 – associated with drugs and toxins
- Type B3 – associated with inborn errors of metabolism

Lactic acidosis is a metabolic acidosis associated with a raised plasma lactate concentration (typically >2 mmol.l^{-1}). Raised levels are associated with increased mortality and may be used for risk stratification and assessment of intervention effectiveness.

Lactate is a glycolytic by-product. In the presence of sufficient oxygen, glucose is broken down into pyruvate and is able to enter the Krebs cycle and electron transfer chain in the mitochondria (see *Section 1.8.1 – Krebs cycle*). In hypoxic conditions pyruvate is unable to enter the Krebs cycle and is metabolized to lactate by lactate dehydrogenase to maintain glycolysis and ATP production. In an aqueous solution lactic acid dissociates almost completely to lactate and H$^+$ and, consequently, the terms lactic acid and lactate are sometimes used interchangeably. Lactate is buffered in the plasma by sodium bicarbonate; the liver usually clears more than 50% of blood lactate and the kidneys and muscle metabolize the rest.

NAD$^+$ and NADH (nicotinamide adenine dinucleotide) are involved in many cellular redox reactions, serving as electron acceptors or donors, respectively. One such redox reaction is the equilibrium between pyruvic acid and lactic acid, and so the ratio of pyruvate:lactate is influenced by the ratio of NAD$^+$:NADH. In a reduced redox state, i.e. low NAD$^+$:NADH ratio, there will be a shift in pyruvate to lactate. Factors producing a reduced redox state include inadequate oxygen delivery or utilization, and rapid oxidation of certain substrates such as ethanol.

1.7.7

pH

$$pH = -\log_{10}[H^+]$$

[H⁺] = hydrogen ion concentration (nmol.l⁻¹)

The pH is a measure of the acidity or basicity of a solution. The pH was first defined in 1909 as the negative logarithm of the hydrogen ion concentration. To be absolutely accurate, the pH is a measure of hydrogen ion (H^+) activity or *effective* concentration in an aqueous solution, not H^+ concentration, because H^+ activity will vary through interaction with other ions present in the solution. The pH scale is a dimensionless quantity with a relative range of 0–14, although it is possible to exceed this range in both directions. A pH of 7 is neutral, the value for pure water, and equates to a H^+ activity of 100 nmol.l⁻¹. The pH scale is logarithmic. As a result, each whole pH unit less than 7 relates to 10 times more H^+ activity than the next higher value (e.g. pH 6 corresponds to 1000 nmol.l⁻¹ H^+ activity), indicating a more acidic solution. The converse is true for pH values greater than 7, each of which has 10 times less H^+ activity than the next lower value (e.g. pH 8 corresponds to 10 nmol.l⁻¹), indicating a more alkaline solution.

In health, the pH of whole arterial blood is tightly maintained between 7.35 and 7.45, with a pH of 7.4 corresponding to H^+ activity of 40 nmol.l⁻¹. The pH scale is roughly linear over this narrow range equating to a difference of only 10 nmol.l⁻¹ H^+ activity.

1.7.8

Strong ion difference

$$SID = ([Na^+] + [K^+] + [Mg^{2+}] + [Ca^{2+}]) - ([Cl^-] + [lactate])$$
$$SID = [Na^+] - [Cl^-]$$

An alternative to the traditional approach to acid–base disturbance is the Stewart model. In aqueous solutions, water provides an infinite supply of hydrogen ions (H^+) through dissociation. This model proposes that changes in pH are influenced by variables other than H^+ concentration. Stewart identified three independent determinants.

Strong ions: strong electrolytes dissociate completely in solution, within the pH range of interest, yielding strong ions. Similar in concept to the anion gap (see *Section 1.7.2 – Anion gap*), the strong ion difference (SID) is the difference between measured strong cations and anions (normal value 40 mmol.l^{-1}). Unlike anion gap, SID does not consider bicarbonate an independent predictor of pH. The equation may be simplified to include only dominant strong ions, Na^+ and Cl^-. The SID significantly affects H^+ concentration, and pH, through its effect on water dissociation. According to the law of electroneutrality, the sum of positive and negative ions in solution should be balanced.

$$SID + [H^+] + [OH^-] = 0$$

A reduction in SID leads to greater water dissociation, increasing H^+ concentration and resultant metabolic acidosis. Therefore, SID is an indication of the presence of unmeasured ions in solution.

Weak acids: primarily phosphate and plasma proteins (e.g. albumin) act as buffers. Weak acids only partially dissociate in solution. The *apparent* SID (SIDa) does not take into account the contribution of these buffers on plasma electrical equilibrium. The *effective* SID (SIDe) is a complex equation quantifying the effect of weak acids. The strong anion gap is the difference between SIDa and SIDe.

Carbon dioxide: in a solution of strong ions, carbon dioxide acts as a source of weak anions that buffer the effect of excess strong cations or contribute to acidosis in the presence of excess strong anions.

Clinical use of this model is limited by its complex mathematics, while dependence on accurate measurements may lead to error.

1.8.1

Krebs cycle

The Krebs cycle, also known as the citric acid or tricarboxylic acid cycle, is the final common pathway for oxidation of carbohydrates, fats and proteins. Occurring exclusively in the mitochondria, it produces adenosine triphosphate (ATP), replenishes nicotinamide adenine dinucleotide (NADH) and provides amino acid precursors. The cycle begins

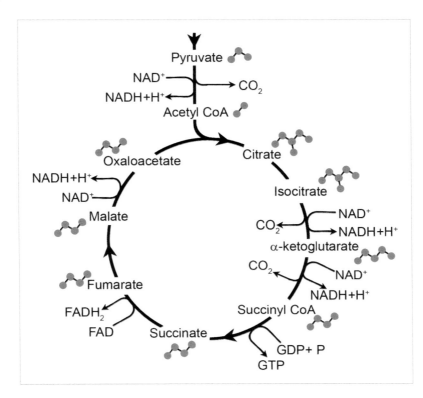

with acetyl CoA (2 carbon atoms – denoted by red dots) condensing with oxaloacetate (4 carbon) to produce citrate (6 carbon). Carbohydrate and fat metabolism produce acetyl CoA via oxidation of pyruvate and beta-oxidation of fatty acids, respectively. Protein metabolism produces several intermediates that enter the cycle as acetyl CoA, fumarate, succinyl CoA or α-ketoglutarate. As the cycle proceeds, intermediate compounds are oxidized yielding 3 molecules of NADH, 1 molecule of flavin adenine dinucleotide ($FADH_2$) and 1 molecule of high-energy phosphate in the form guanosine triphosphate (GTP). With each turn of the cycle, two decarboxylation reactions occur with carbon atoms lost as two molecules of carbon dioxide.

Oxidative phosphorylation

Energy is released as electrons are transferred from electron donors (e.g. $FADH_2$ and NADH) to electron acceptors (e.g. oxygen) via reduction–oxidation reactions. These reactions occur within the inner mitochondrial membrane in a series of protein complexes called the electron transport chain. Potential energy generated is utilized by ATP synthase to allow flow of hydrogen ions down an electrochemical gradient, catalysing ATP production. The majority of energy produced via aerobic metabolism is generated through re-oxidation of high-energy carriers ($FADH_2$ and NADH) produced in the Krebs cycle. Theoretically, one molecule of glucose will produce between 30 and 36 ATP molecules by oxidative phosphorylation, compared to only 2 ATP molecules generated by glycolysis. Dependence on oxygen to replenish NAD^+ and FADH labels the Krebs cycle aerobic. Although the Krebs cycle does not utilize oxygen directly, in an anaerobic setting, the pathway would cease as NAD^+ and FADH supplies are exhausted.

1.8.2

Liver lobule

The liver lobule describes an anatomical division of the liver at a histological level. It is a hexagonal unit with a central vein (a branch of the hepatic vein) at the centre and portal triads at the periphery. The portal triads consist of branches of the bile ducts, hepatic artery and portal vein. The lobule is made up of hepatocytes arranged in cords that are separated by sinusoids.

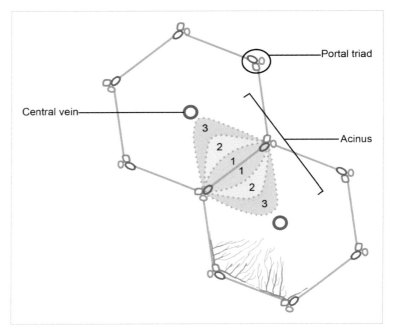

Sinusoids are vascular spaces with fenestrated endothelium that allow plasma to pass into the space of Disse. Blood from the portal venules and hepatic arterioles mixes in the sinusoids and drains into the central vein. Hepatic macrophages (Kupffer cells) are also found in the endothelium and play a role in hepatic immunity.

The functional unit of the liver is called the acinus, a diamond-shaped area in cross section that encompasses triangular portions of two adjacent lobules. It is divided into three zones depending on blood supply and metabolic function. Zone 1 is located around the portal triad with a rich blood supply from the hepatic arteries and zone 3 is located around the central vein with a poor oxygen supply. Zone 2 is morphologically and functionally intermediate between zones 1 and 3. Zone 1 hepatocytes are rich in mitochondria and perform oxidative metabolism and glycogen synthesis. The oxygen-poor cells of zone 3 have a role more in anaerobic metabolism and the biotransformation of the majority of drugs and toxins due to an abundance of endoplasmic reticulum and cytochrome P450. Zone 3 cells are more vulnerable to ischaemic injury with drug metabolism being affected early in an ischaemic process.

Nutrition and energy

Nutrient	Average normal adult daily requirement
Water	30–40 ml.kg^{-1}
Energy	30–40 cal.kg^{-1}
Protein	0.8 g.kg^{-1}
Nitrogen	0.2 g.kg^{-1}
Fat	1 g.kg^{-1}
Carbohydrate	4.3 g.kg^{-1}
Electrolytes Sodium Potassium Chloride Phosphate Calcium Magnesium	 1 mmol.kg^{-1} 1 mmol.kg^{-1} 1.5 mmol.kg^{-1} 0.2–0.5 mmol.kg^{-1} 0.1–0.2 mmol.kg^{-1} 0.1–0.2 mmol.kg^{-1}
Trace elements Iron Zinc Selenium	 0.2 mg.kg^{-1} 0.2 mg.kg^{-1} 1 μg.kg^{-1}
Vitamins	Vary from 0.1 to 20 μg.kg^{-1}

To maintain health, an adequate and balanced daily supply of nutrients is required. Nutrition may be administered via oral, enteral, parenteral or combined routes. Research has demonstrated the benefits of nutritional support in a variety of patient populations (e.g. elderly hospitalized, malnourished, major elective surgical and cancer patients) including a reduction in mortality, re-admission rates and infectious complications.

Nutritional support in the critically ill

Assessment of nutritional state should guide requirement of nutritional support. Estimated energy requirements may be calculated using the Schofield equation, estimating basal metabolic rate with adjustments for activity and physiological stress. In the critically ill, nutritional requirements are often overestimated because catabolism releases some energy from the tissues. Although still a contentious issue, some research has demonstrated mortality benefits in patients receiving 33–66% of estimated energy requirements, compared to patients receiving greater than or less than this amount. Nutritional need should be recalculated throughout the clinical course to account for varying energy demands at different stages of disease.

Internationally, guidelines recommend the use of enteral nutrition over parenteral nutrition in critically ill patients. In addition to reducing stress-related catabolism, enteral nutrition aims to minimize bacterial translocation and maintain intestinal mucosal integrity. Early enteral nutrition (within 24–48 h) is recommended as a supplement or sole nutritional technique. Enteral nutrition supplementation is often complicated by GI dysfunction leading to malabsorption. Controversy exists as to the optimal timing of parenteral nutrition to supplement insufficient enteral nutrition.

1.8.4

Vitamins – sources and function

Vitamin	Function	Sources	Daily requirement if on TPN
A (retinol)	Aids night vision, retinal pigments, growth and development of tissues, skin and mucosa	Liver, kidney, oily fish, dairy (provitamin in some fruit and vegetables)	3300 IU
D	Involved in calcium and phosphorus homeostasis	Sunlight, oily fish, egg yolk	200 IU
E	Antioxidant properties	Dark green vegetables, nuts, seeds, cereals	10 IU
K	Important role in blood coagulation	Dark green vegetables, fruit, dairy	2–4 mg/week (if not on warfarin)
B1 (thiamine)	Coenzyme – carbohydrate metabolism	Fortified cereals, milk, vegetables, fruit	3 mg
B2 (riboflavin)	Coenzyme – carbohydrate, fat, protein metabolism	Fortified cereals, milk	3.6 mg
B3 (niacin)	Coenzyme – involved in oxidation and reduction	Meat, fish, fortified cereals, pulses	40 mg
B6 (pyridoxine)	Haemoglobin production, co-enzyme	Eggs, meat, fish	4 mg
Folic acid	DNA synthesis, red blood cell production	Green leafy vegetables, fortified cereals	0.4 mg
B12	Red blood cell production, myelination of nerves	Dairy, eggs, fish, meat (absorption requires intrinsic factor)	5 mg
C (ascorbic acid)	Synthesis of collagen, bone and connective tissue, iron absorption, antioxidant	Citrus fruits, vegetables	100 mg

A vitamin is an organic compound, required in small amounts to maintain health, that cannot be synthesized by an organism and therefore has to be derived from the diet. The commonly recognized vitamins, named A to K, are classified by their activities rather than their structures.

Vitamins have diverse biochemical functions, as shown in the table. They can be divided into fat-soluble (A, D, E and K) and water-soluble (folic acid, B vitamins and vitamin C). Patients on total parenteral nutrition (TPN) require supplementation of vitamins and trace elements. The table shows the daily requirements for an average adult (70 kg) on TPN.

The word vitamin comes from the combination of 'vital' and 'amine'; suggested by the Polish scientist Funk in 1911 because he believed they were essential for life and that they were chemically amines. The 'e' was later dropped when it was found that they are not all amines. The letters were initially assigned according to order of discovery, however, vitamin 'K' was so named due to its role in 'koagulation' by a Danish scientist, Henrik Dam.

Vitamins – toxicity and deficiency

Vitamin	Deficiency	Toxicity
A (retinol)	Night blindness, increased risk of infection, poor growth	Teratogenic in high doses in pregnancy
D	Rickets/osteomalacia	Rare, can cause weight loss and diarrhoea
E	Neurological abnormalities, anaemia	Can cause muscle weakness
K	Bleeding	
B1 (thiamine)	Beriberi (dry – affecting peripheral nervous system, wet – affecting cardiovascular system), Wernicke's encephalopathy, Korsakoff's syndrome	Insomnia, headache
B2 (riboflavin)	Tongue and oral mucosal inflammation	
B3 (niacin)	Pellagra (diarrhoea, dermatitis and dementia), diarrhoea	Liver impairment, skin irritation
B6 (pyridoxine)	Rare – nervous system disorders	Peripheral nervous damage
Folic acid	Megaloblastic anaemia	
B12	Megaloblastic anaemia, neurological symptoms (subacute combined degeneration of the cord)	

Vitamin A deficiency is uncommon in developed countries but remains the leading cause of preventable blindness in children worldwide. In addition to vision, vitamin A is essential for the immune response, bone growth and maintenance of epithelial surfaces and is also important in the developing fetus. Conversely, excess vitamin A can cause problems related to bone metabolism and the metabolism of other fat-soluble vitamins, and can also be harmful to the fetus.

Vitamin D deficiency can occur due to inadequate exposure to sunlight, malabsorption or poor intake. Deficiency can lead to rickets in infants and osteomalacia in adults. Individuals with an increased risk of vitamin D deficiency are those with osteoporosis, malabsorption syndromes, conditions that alter the metabolism of vitamin D and phosphate (such as chronic kidney disease), raised BMI and Black and Hispanic populations.

Vitamin K deficiency may occur due to poor absorption or due to excessive vitamin K antagonist drugs such as warfarin. It plays an important role in coagulation and therefore deficiency can lead to bruising, petechiae or even massive haemorrhage. Infants with vitamin K deficiency are at risk of haemorrhagic disease of the newborn and therefore supplements are commonly given at birth.

Subacute combined degeneration of the cord is a manifestation of vitamin B12 deficiency and describes degeneration of the posterior and lateral columns of the spinal cord. It is often associated with pernicious anaemia. Patients may present with gradual onset of neurological symptoms; posterior column disruption will cause reduced vibratory sensation and proprioception whereas the disruption of the lateral corticospinal and dorsal spinocerebellar tracts will cause spasticity and ataxia respectively. Left untreated, this can lead to permanent neurological damage. This syndrome may be precipitated by nitrous oxide anaesthesia in individuals with subclinical vitamin B12 deficiency.

1.9.1

Adrenal gland

Adrenocortical hormone action	Glucocorticoid	Mineralocorticoid
Metabolic	Protein catabolism, hepatic gluconeogenesis	None
Immunological	Immunosuppression, delayed healing	None
Renal	Weak mineralocorticoid activity	Sodium reabsorption; potassium and hydrogen excretion
Vascular	Maintain catecholamine responsiveness	None
Regulation	Hypothalamic–pituitary–adrenal axis – negative feedback	Renin–angiotensin system, plasma electrolyte concentrations

The adrenal glands are bilateral endocrine glands located just superior to the kidneys. Each gland comprises two distinct parts: cortex and medulla.

The adrenal cortex has three histological layers, each layer synthesizing and secreting distinct classes of hormones. All of the adrenocortical hormones are steroid derivatives, synthesized from cholesterol.

Zona glomerulosa (outermost layer): produces mineralocorticoids. Aldosterone accounts for 90% of mineralocorticoid activity. Acting on the kidneys, aldosterone promotes active renal sodium reabsorption with water following passively. As such, extracellular fluid volume increases whilst plasma sodium concentration remains largely unchanged. Coupled with sodium reabsorption, potassium ions, and to a lesser extent, hydrogen ions are excreted. Many factors influence aldosterone secretion. The major regulatory mechanisms include the renin–angiotensin system (see *Section 1.5.6 – Renin–angiotensin–aldosterone system*) and changes in plasma electrolyte concentrations. An increase in plasma potassium concentration or decrease in sodium concentration stimulates aldosterone release.

Zona fasciculata (middle layer): produces glucocorticoids, primarily cortisol. Glucocorticoids impact several homeostatic mechanisms. Metabolic effects aim to stabilize plasma glucose concentrations during periods of stress. Mobilization and metabolism of proteins generates precursors for gluconeogenesis. Further actions include stimulation of gluconeogenesis, primarily within the liver, with simultaneous inhibition of peripheral glucose uptake. Glucocorticoids exert potent anti-inflammatory effects through inhibition of T-cell lymphocyte proliferation and down-regulation of pro-inflammatory proteins.

Zona reticularis (innermost layer): produces male sex hormones, primarily dehydroepiandrosterone (DHEA), with small quantities of the female sex hormones, oestrogen and progesterone. Androgen effects are largely exerted via peripheral conversion to testosterone.

The adrenal medulla is located at the core of the gland. Neuroendocrine cells, called chromaffin cells, synthesize, store and release noradrenaline and adrenaline (see *Section 1.9.3 – Catecholamine synthesis*). Catecholamine production and release is influenced by sympathetic activity. As preganglionic sympathetic fibres synapse directly on the adrenal medulla, this structure may be considered a specialized sympathetic ganglion.

Adrenergic receptor actions

Receptor	Site	Action
α-1	Blood vessels	Vasoconstriction
	Bowel	Smooth muscle relaxation
	Eye	Mydriasis
α-2	Central	Sedation, analgesia, sympatholysis
	Blood vessels • central • peripheral	Vasodilatation Vasoconstriction
β-1	Heart	Positive chronotropy and inotropy
	Kidney	Increased renin release
β-2	Lungs	Bronchodilatation
	Blood vessels	Vasodilatation
	Liver	Glycogenolysis
	Uterus	Relaxation
β-3	Adipose tissue	Lipolysis

Adrenergic receptors, or adrenoceptors, are G-protein coupled receptors that are stimulated by catecholamines producing sympathomimetic effects. They prepare the body for 'fight and flight' by causing increased ventilation (via bronchodilatation), increased cardiac output (via increased inotropy and chronotropy), diversion of blood from non-vital organs, and pupillary dilatation.

There are two main subtypes of adrenoceptors.

Alpha – divided further into subtypes 1 and 2:
- Alpha-1 adrenoceptors increase the action of phospholipase C and therefore increase intracellular calcium concentration. This leads to mainly excitatory effects such as smooth muscle contraction in the peripheral vasculature causing an increased systemic vascular resistance and diversion of blood from the peripheral tissues. Agonists include phenylephrine and metaraminol.
- Alpha-2 adrenoceptors inhibit adenylate cyclase leading to reduced cAMP formation and calcium concentration. They act presynaptically to down-regulate or reduce the sympathetic response. They can cause sedation, analgesia and hypotension. Agonists include clonidine and dexmedetomidine.

Beta – divided further into subtypes 1, 2 and 3:
- Beta-1 and -2 adrenoceptors stimulate adenylate cyclase to increase cAMP formation. Beta-1 stimulation leads to positive inotropy and chronotropy, increasing cardiac output. They also act on the juxtaglomerular apparatus to increase renin release. Beta-2 receptors cause relaxation of smooth muscle causing bronchodilatation, uterine relaxation and vasodilatation of certain vascular beds. They also have some effect on the myocardium causing a degree of chronotropy and inotropy. Agonists include isoprenaline and salbutamol.
- Beta-3 adrenoceptors act to increase lipolysis. Drugs acting at this receptor were initially targeted at weight loss therapy, however, their use has been limited due to a lack of complete understanding of this receptor and concerns over drug side-effects.

1.9.3

Catecholamine synthesis

Catecholamines are neurotransmitters composed of a catechol (benzene ring with two hydroxyl groups) and an amine group. Naturally occurring catecholamines are dopamine, noradrenaline, and adrenaline. Catecholamines are produced within chromaffin cells of the adrenal medulla and postganglionic fibres of the sympathetic nervous system. Like all monoamine neurotransmitters, catecholamines are derived from aromatic amino acids. Catecholamine synthesis begins in the cytoplasm with the amino acid tyrosine, obtained from the diet or via hydroxylation of phenylalanine in the liver. Each step in the synthetic process is dependent on a specific catalytic enzyme. Tyrosine hydroxylase is the rate-limiting enzyme, converting l-tyrosine to DOPA. In dopaminergic neurons of the CNS, this is the end product of synthesis. In noradrenergic neurons and chromaffin cells, dopamine is converted to noradrenaline. Conversion of noradrenaline to adrenaline occurs exclusively in the adrenal medulla.

Catecholamines are actively transported into synaptic storage vesicles, providing a means for release of a predetermined amount of neurotransmitter and protection of catecholamines from degradation. Catecholamine release via exocytosis is stimulated by calcium influx in response to neuronal membrane depolarization and, in the adrenal medulla, by acetylcholine release from sympathetic preganglionic neurons. A wide range of complex regulatory mechanisms modulate catecholamine release. These include control of calcium channel activity and negative feedback via presynaptic autoreceptors through which a neurotransmitter can regulate its own release (e.g. noradrenaline occupation of presynaptic α-2 adrenoceptors inhibits further noradrenaline release).

Uptake and metabolism

The primary mechanism controlling duration and spread of catecholamine activity is active uptake of these neurotransmitters into the liver or back into nerve terminals. This rapid uptake explains the short circulatory catecholamine half-life of less than 2 minutes. Metabolism occurs through a variety of pathways, including deamination by monoamine oxidase and methylation by catechol-O-methyltransferase, with the latter occurring exclusively in extraneuronal tissues.

1.9.4

Hypothalamic–pituitary–adrenal axis – anatomy

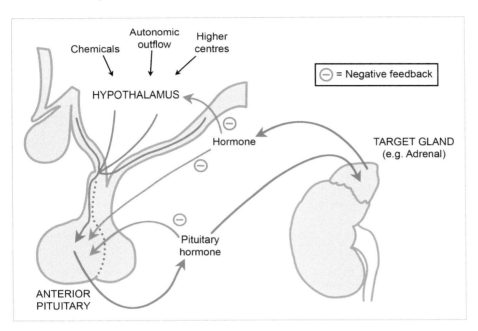

The pituitary gland is divided into two parts based on embryological origin and function:
- anterior – adenohypophysis, ectodermal origin from Rathke's pouch; secretes six peptide hormones
- posterior – neurohypophysis, from floor of third ventricle; secretes two peptide hormones.

The hypothalamus is found in the floor of the third ventricle below the thalamus. The pituitary gland sits directly below this in the middle cranial fossa in a depression of the sphenoid bone called the sella turcica (Turkish saddle). They are connected by neuronal and vascular tissue in the infundibular stalk that passes through a sheet of dura separating the optic chiasm from the anterior pituitary (the diaphragma sellae).

The blood supply to the hypothalamus is from the circle of Willis, whereas the anterior and posterior pituitary receive blood from the superior and inferior hypophyseal arteries, respectively (a branch of the internal carotid). A portal circulation connects the hypothalamus to the anterior pituitary.

Pituitary tumours may present due to their mass effect or by increased or decreased hormone secretion. The commonest pituitary hormones secreted by these tumours are prolactin (35%), growth hormone (20%) and adrenocorticotropic hormone (7%).

1.9.5

Hypothalamic–pituitary–adrenal axis – hormones

Pituitary hormone	Releasing factor	Site of action	Effect of hypersecretion	Effect of hyposecretion
Anterior				
Adrenocorticotropic hormone (ACTH)	Corticotrophin releasing hormone (CRH)	Adrenal cortex	Adrenal hyperplasia (Cushing's if pituitary tumour)	Secondary adrenocortical insufficiency
Growth hormone (GH)	Growth hormone releasing hormone (GHRH)	Multiple sites	Acromegaly (adults) Gigantism (children)	Dwarfism
Follicle-stimulating hormone (FSH)	Gonadotrophin releasing hormone (GnRH)	Testes and ovaries	Target organ hyperstimulation	Target organ failure
Luteinizing hormone (LH)	GnRH	Testes and ovaries	Target organ hyperstimulation	Target organ failure
Thyroid-stimulating hormone (TSH)	Thyrotropin releasing hormone (TRH)	Thyroid	Secondary hyperthyroidism	Secondary hypothyroidism
Prolactin (PRL)	Prolactin releasing hormone (PRLH)	Breasts	Hyperprolactinaemia	Hypoprolactinaemia
Posterior				
Antidiuretic hormone (ADH)	Reduced osmolality/ circulating volume	Kidney, blood vessels	Syndrome of inappropriate ADH secretion (SIADH)	Diabetes insipidus
Oxytocin	Suckling	Breasts	Target organ hyperstimulation	Target organ failure

The hypothalamic–pituitary–adrenal axis regulates many endocrine functions essential to body homeostasis. Inputs to the hypothalamus can stimulate production of hypothalamic factors that travel via the portal circulation, stimulating or inhibiting the release of their corresponding anterior pituitary hormones. When released into the circulation these hormones cause effects at target glands. They also exert a negative feedback effect (along with the hormones from the target gland) preventing further release from the hypothalamus and anterior pituitary.

ADH and oxytocin are synthesized in the supraoptic and paraventricular nuclei of the hypothalamus, respectively, and travel via nerves to the posterior pituitary where they are released into the circulation. Increased plasma osmolality detected by hypothalamic osmoreceptors is the main stimulus to ADH release, while negative feedback prevents further ADH release once osmolality normalizes. A baroreceptor-detected reduction in circulating volume may also stimulate ADH release. Oxytocin release is stimulated by suckling and stimulates secretion of milk from milk ducts.

1.9.6
Vitamin D synthesis

Vitamins are organic compounds necessary in limited amounts for health and growth. These essential micronutrients cannot be synthesized *in vivo* in amounts sufficient to meet demands and must therefore be obtained from diet. Vitamins are classified according to biological and chemical activity. Each vitamin comprises a number of vitamer compounds, fulfilling the same vitamin function and having similar molecular structures.

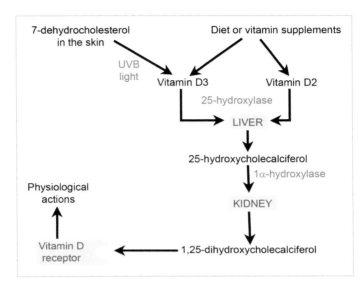

Vitamin D has two physiologically important vitamers for human health, D2 and D3. Fungi and yeasts are dietary sources of vitamin D2 (ergocalciferol), produced in response to UV irradiation. Vitamin D3 (cholecalciferol) may be obtained through dietary ingestion of fish oils or through cutaneous synthesis. In the skin, the precursor compound reacts with UV light to generate vitamin D3. Because individuals receiving sufficient UV light exposure do not require dietary supplementation, vitamin D is not a true vitamin.

Vitamin D, present as either D2 or D3, does not have significant biological activity. These compounds undergo activation to the hormonally active form, 1,25-dihydroxycholecalciferol. Activation involves a two-step process of hydroxylation, firstly in the liver, forming 25-hydroxycholecalciferol, then in the kidney forming 1,25-dihydroxycholecalciferol. Production of the active vitamin D metabolite is largely regulated via 1α-hydroxylase enzymatic activity. Production of 1,25-dihydroxycholecalciferol suppresses enzyme activity whilst upregulation occurs in response to parathyroid hormone release or reduction in serum calcium and phosphate concentrations. The active metabolite exerts its actions through binding to intracellular vitamin D receptors.

Primary physiological effects of vitamin D are as follows.
- Contributes to calcium homeostasis by facilitating intestinal absorption of calcium and stimulating bone resorption.
- Support of bone mineralization by regulating synthesis of bone matrix proteins and osteoblast/osteoclast activity.
- Other effects include antiproliferative, anti-inflammatory and immunomodulatory properties in a variety of cells and tissues. Current research is attempting to exploit these properties to develop treatments for autoimmune diseases and cancer.

1.10.1

Body fluid composition

Electrolyte (mmol.l⁻¹)	Extracellular fluid		Intracellular fluid
	Plasma	Interstitial fluid	
Cations			
Sodium (Na⁺)	153.2	145.1	12.0
Potassium (K⁺)	4.3	4.1	150.0
Calcium (Ca²⁺)	3.8	3.4	4.0
Magnesium (Mg²⁺)	1.4	1.3	34.0
Cation total	162.7	153.9	200.0
Anions			
Chloride (Cl⁻)	111.5	118.0	4.0
Bicarbonate (HCO₃⁻)	25.7	27.0	12.0
Phosphate (PO₄⁻)	2.2	2.3	40.0
Protein	17.0	0.0	54.0
Other	6.3	6.6	90.0
Anion total	162.7	153.9	200.0

Ionic composition differs between body fluid compartments. An overriding principle across compartments is the law of electroneutrality; each compartment must have the same concentration of cations and anions. Even when there is a potential difference across a cell membrane, the law of electroneutrality applies. By definition, membrane potential is the electrical potential difference between the interior and exterior of a cell. Electrical charge arises from unequal total concentrations of cations and anions across a membrane. The resulting potential difference is created exclusively at the membrane interface, with ionic balance still being maintained in the bulk solution.

Extracellular fluid (ECF): comprises plasma and interstitial fluid (see *Section 1.10.2 – Fluid compartments*). The major cation in ECF is Na⁺, and the balancing anions are Cl⁻ and HCO₃⁻. Interstitial fluid is an ultrafiltrate of plasma. As such, ionic composition between these compartments is similar. Proteins are abundant within plasma but, due to their large molecular size, movement across the small pores of capillary membranes is restricted, accounting for their absence in interstitial fluid. To maintain electroneutrality, plasma contains slightly less Cl⁻ to balance negatively charged plasma proteins.

Intracellular fluid (ICF): major cations are K⁺ and Mg²⁺, and balancing anions are proteins and phosphates.

The concentrations of Na⁺ and K⁺ in ECF and ICF are nearly opposite. This distribution of ions reflects the activity of Na⁺/K⁺-ATPase pumps (see *Section 1.12.5 – Sodium/potassium–ATPase pump*).

Electrolytes, such as organic salts, dissociate in solution and carry electrical charge. Non-electrolytes are substances that do not dissociate in solution, such as glucose, creatinine and urea, and therefore have no electrical charge. Electrolytes have greater osmotic activity because each electrolyte molecule dissociates into at least two ions. Water moves freely between the body compartments along osmotic gradients. Electrolytes, especially Na⁺, establish these gradients, influencing the movement of water between compartments.

1.10.2

Fluid compartments

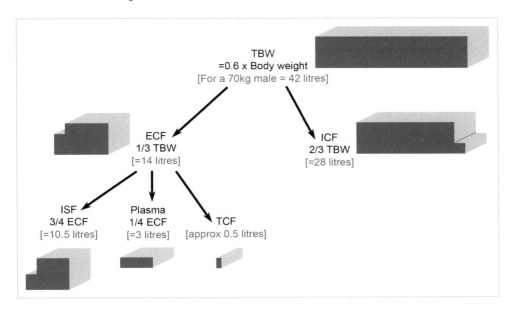

TBW
=0.6 x Body weight
[For a 70kg male = 42 litres]

ECF
1/3 TBW
[=14 litres]

ICF
2/3 TBW
[=28 litres]

ISF
3/4 ECF
[=10.5 litres]

Plasma
1/4 ECF
[=3 litres]

TCF
[approx 0.5 litres]

Total body water (TBW) is equivalent to approximately 60% of the total adult body weight. It is contained in numerous tissues that, for comparison, are grouped into larger physiologically similar collections. The main compartments are intracellular fluid (ICF) and extracellular fluid (ECF).

- ICF – approximately two-thirds of the TBW. Maintained by a metabolically active membrane. It has low sodium and high potassium/magnesium concentrations.
- ECF – approximately one-third of the TBW. Divided into interstitial fluid (ISF), plasma and transcellular fluid (TCF) compartments. These are separated by location and different kinetic characteristics. As a group, the composition is roughly opposite to ICF, with low potassium/magnesium and high sodium/chloride concentrations.
  - ISF – comprises the ECF not found in the plasma. It is approximately three-quarters of the ECF volume and is biochemically similar to plasma, but with lower protein concentrations. It provides a link between the ICF and intravascular compartment. During illness, surrounding membranes can become more permeable, allowing access for immunological mediators and the formation of oedema.
  - Plasma – makes up approximately one-quarter of the ECF volume. Functions as one discrete unit rather than a collection of smaller compartments. It transports blood cells and nutrients, assists in coagulation and has widespread immunological functions.
  - TCF – a small compartment representing all body fluids formed from the transport activities of cells, e.g. CSF, GI fluids, bladder urine, aqueous and vitreous humour and synovial fluid. Fluid composition varies depending on the type and function of the cells from which it is derived.

Variations occur due to the following factors.
- Age – TBW decreases with age. In neonates, TBW is approximately 75–80% of total body weight (with proportionally more in the ECF than ICF). This drops to approximately 50% in those over 60 years old.
- Adipose tissue – there is a lower ratio of TBW to total body weight in obese individuals.

1.10.3

Intravenous fluid composition

Content (mmol.l⁻¹ unless stated)	Plasma	0.9% Saline	5% Dextrose	Hartmann's solution	Plasma-Lyte 148	5% Human albumin solution
pH	7.35–7.45	5.0	3.5–5.5	6.5	7.4	6.9
Sodium	135–145	154	–	131	140	100–160
Chloride	95–105	154	–	111	98	100–160
Potassium	3.5–5.3	(can be added)	(can be added)	5	5	<2
Bicarbonate	24–32	–	–	29 (as lactate)	–	–
Calcium	2.2–2.6	–	–	2	–	–
Magnesium	0.8–1.2	–	–	–	1.5	–
Glucose	3.5–5.5	–	278	–	–	–
Osmolarity (mOsm.l⁻¹)	275–295	308	278	281	295	270–300
Miscellaneous	–	–	Glucose 50 g.l⁻¹	Lactate 29	Acetate 27 Gluconate 23	Albumin 50 g.l⁻¹ Citrate <15

To make appropriate fluid replacement choices it is important to understand how fluid is distributed in the body (see *Sections 1.10.1 – Body fluid composition* and *1.10.2 – Fluid compartments)*, how it moves between compartments (see *Section 1.2.7 – Starling forces in capillaries*), and the composition of replacement fluids available.

Intravenous fluids can be divided into crystalloids, colloids and blood products. The composition and characteristics of commonly used fluids can be seen in the table.

- Crystalloids are the most frequent choice of fluid replacement, usually normal (0.9%) saline or Hartmann's solution (compound sodium lactate – CSL). These are used for fluid replacement and volume expansion. Crystalloids are water-based solutions with electrolytes added in an attempt to approximate the content of plasma. They vary in their formulations: some are hypotonic to plasma while others are iso- or hypertonic. Normal saline has a high chloride concentration and can cause hyperchloraemic acidosis when large volumes are infused. For this reason a more balanced solution, such as Hartmann's, may be chosen instead. Hartmann added lactate to the solution to reduce the chloride load and potential for acidosis seen with saline. Lactate is metabolized in the liver and kidney to bicarbonate.
- Colloids have a crystalloid solution base with an added colloid substance that does not freely diffuse across a semi-permeable membrane. The presumed benefit, therefore, is their ability to raise the colloid osmotic pressure of patients requiring volume resuscitation. However, concerns about synthetic colloid safety, their increased cost and increased allergy risk compared to no demonstrable benefit have currently led to a reduction in their use. Synthetic colloids include hetastarches, dextrans (both containing polysaccharides) and gelatins.
- Human albumin solution is a colloid containing serum albumin with a molecular weight of 69 kDa and can be either iso- (5%) or hyperoncotic (20%) compared to plasma.

1.11.1

Blood groups

Blood group	A	B	AB	O
Genotype	AA or AO	BB or BO	AB	OO
Red cell antigen	A	B	A and B	None
Plasma antibody (usually IgM)	Anti-B	Anti-A	None	Anti-A and anti-B
UK incidence (%)	42	10	4	44

The ABO group antigens are the most immunogenic of all blood group antigens. The *ABO* gene encodes a protein involved in the production of A and B antigens. Inheritance is co-dominant, because both the A and B alleles are dominant (i.e. the AB genotype expresses both A and B antigens). The O allele encodes an inactive protein, resulting in a lack of antigen production.

Anti-A and anti-B antibodies are not present from birth. They are synthesized in the first year of life in response to environmental exposure to ABO-like antigens. Anti-A and anti-B antibodies bind to A and B antigens, respectively, found on the surface of the red blood cells. The complement cascade is activated, ultimately resulting in red blood cell lysis.

Acute haemolytic transfusion reaction

This immune-mediated, Type II (IgM) hypersensitivity reaction occurs secondary to ABO-incompatible blood transfusion. Antibodies in recipient plasma bind to corresponding donor red blood cell antigens, leading to intravascular haemolysis of transfused red blood cells. Activation of the complement cascade generates the production of cytokines and the release of vasoactive mediators. These substances lead to systemic symptoms of inflammation, increased vascular permeability, hypotension and platelet aggregation. Clinical effects are often immediate and, in the conscious patient, include fever, skin rash, hypotension and shortness of breath. Disseminated intravascular coagulopathy and renal failure may also occur. In the anaesthetized patient, hypotension and excessive bleeding may be the only clinical features observed.

To minimize the incidence of ABO-incompatible blood transfusions, the Serious Hazards of Transfusion (SHOT, UK) report emphasizes the necessity for confirmation of patient identity at every stage of the transfusion process.

1.11.2

Coagulation – cascade (classic) model

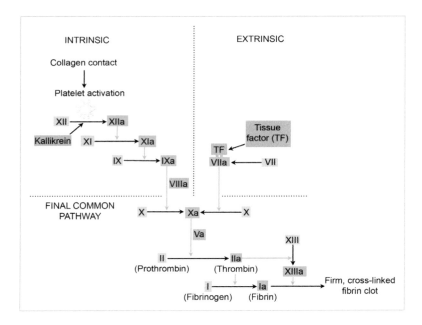

Haemostasis is a complex process that limits blood loss from damaged vessels, coordinated by vascular, platelet and plasma factors. Haemostasis involves two phases:

- Primary haemostasis begins immediately following vessel endothelial damage, characterized by temporary vascular constriction and platelet plug formation. Von Willebrand factor (vWF), produced by vascular endothelial cells, adheres to exposed collagen at the injury site. Platelets adhere to vWF and become activated by contact with collagen. Activated platelets bind circulating fibrinogen, promoting platelet aggregation and formation of an unstable platelet plug.
- Secondary haemostasis stabilizes the platelet plug with formation of a fibrin clot. Two models, classic and cell-based, describe this process. The classic model proposes sequential activation of coagulation factors by the preceding factor. Initiation of this process consists of two pathways.
  - The intrinsic pathway requires proteolytic enzymes and protein cofactors present in plasma. Circulating clotting factor (F) XII, exposed to the membrane of activated platelets, becomes activated to FXIIa. This protease amplifies its own generation through activation of kallikrein. In addition, FXIIa initiates a cascade of enzyme activation culminating in generation of FXa.
  - The extrinsic pathway requires an activator, tissue factor (TF), in addition to circulating plasma components. As TF is present in subendothelial tissue, this protein does not contact blood in the absence of injury. Endothelial damage exposes TF to circulating FVII leading to non-proteolytic activation to FVIIa. This TF–FVIIa enzyme complex converts FX to FXa.

The final common pathway begins with activation of FX via either pathway. In the presence of FVa, FXa forms a prothrombinase complex, converting prothrombin to thrombin. Thrombin generation leads to proteolysis of fibrinogen to fibrin monomers. Thrombin also activates FXIII, facilitating cross-linking of these monomers to form a stable fibrin mesh. Amplification of the final pathway, via further activation of thrombin and FVa, is mediated by thrombin.

1.11.3

Coagulation – cell-based model

The classic model of coagulation fails to fully reflect haemostatic events observed *in vivo*, nor why deficiencies of some clotting factors result in bleeding whilst others do not. The cell-based model, defined by four phases, highlights the importance of specific cell surface interactions with clotting factors (F).

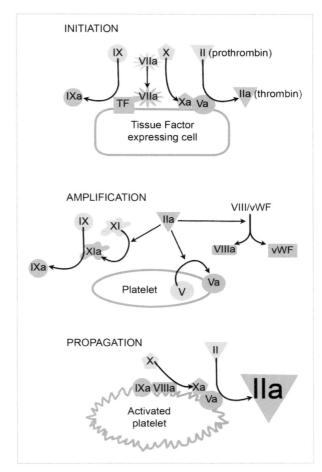

- **Initiation phase** – localized to cells expressing tissue factor (TF) (e.g. smooth muscle, vascular endothelium). As in the classic model, TF binds circulating FVIIa, forming TF–FVIIa complex that activates FX and FIX. Associated with its cofactor (FVa), FXa forms a prothrombinase complex on the surface of TF-expressing cells, generating a small amount of thrombin.
- **Amplification phase** – mediated by thrombin generated during initiation. Thrombin amplifies the procoagulant signal through platelet and plasma protein activation. Circulating FVIII forms a stable, inactive complex with von Willebrand factor (vWF) to avoid rapid degradation. Upon activation by thrombin, FVIIIa dissociates, becoming available to serve as a cofactor for FIXa.
- **Propagation phase** – activation of clotting factors on the platelet surface leading to generation of FXa. Binding with FVa, generated in the amplification phase, FXa produces large quantities of thrombin, the 'thrombin burst'. Fibrinogen cleavage and clot stabilization continues as in the classic model.
- **Termination phase** – confines coagulation to the site of vascular injury, avoiding thrombosis in areas of normal vasculature. This process is regulated by endogenous anticoagulants. Antithrombin (ATIII) inhibits the activity of thrombin and other proteases (e.g. FXa). Protein C inactivates FVa and FVIIIa, with activity enhanced by the cofactor protein S. Protein C is activated by thrombin bound to the surface of intact endothelial cells.

Haemophilia is a group of hereditary bleeding disorders. Haemophilia A and B are recessive X-linked disorders due to functional deficiencies of FVIII and FIX, respectively. Haemophilia C is a rare autosomal disorder resulting from deficiency of FXI.

1.11.4

Complement cascade

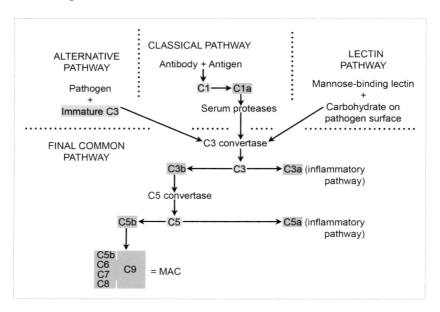

The complement cascade describes a series of over 30 serum proteins that help antibodies and phagocytic cells clear pathogens from the body. It is part of the innate immune system but can also be recruited by the acquired immune system. Complement proteins are synthesized in the liver and circulate in their inactive form in the plasma. They are activated by proteases in response to certain triggering factors. Activation occurs in a sequential manner whereby each activated component leads to activation of the next component resulting in amplification. This results in massive amplification and activation of the membrane attack complex (MAC).

Three biochemical pathways activate the complement system; the classical, the alternative and the lectin pathway. These three pathways all lead to activation of a common pathway and activation of the MAC.

- The classical pathway is activated when an antibody–antigen complex activates the C1 complement.
- The alternative pathway, part of the innate immune system, results from the combination of a pathogen with immature C3.
- The lectin pathway occurs when mannose-binding lectin (MBL, an opsonin) combines with a carbohydrate, such as glucose or mannose, found on a pathogen's surface resulting in common pathway activation.

The common pathway starts with the activation of C3 convertase that converts C3 to C3a and C3b. C3b then cleaves C5 into C5a and C5b. C5b combines with C6, C7, C8 and C9 to produce the MAC. This coats the pathogen and introduces transmembrane channels leading to cell lysis. Macrophages then phagocytose the cellular debris.

The functions of complement include opsonization (marking of the pathogen for phagocytosis), chemotaxis, cell lysis, agglutination (binding of pathogens for enhanced elimination by phagocytosis).

C3a and C5a play an important role in allergic reactions, specifically anaphylaxis, while deficiency of the MAC may lead to recurrent *Neisseria* infections.

1.11.5

Haemoglobin

Normal haemoglobin form	Globin chains	Contribution to total haemoglobin
HbF	2α, 2γ	50–95% Hb at birth, reducing to 0.5% after 6 months
HbA	2α, 2β	Most common Hb, >97% of total adult Hb
HbA2	2α, 2δ	Normal variant, 1.5–3% of total adult Hb

Haemoglobin (Hb) is the oxygen carrying component of human blood. Found within red blood cells, the Hb molecule comprises four polypeptide globin chains, each attached to a haem moiety.

- Haem is an iron-containing porphyrin compound that reversibly binds oxygen. Each Hb molecule may bind up to four oxygen molecules. Binding of oxygen to Hb is cooperative (i.e. allosteric). As each haem molecule binds oxygen, Hb undergoes a conformation change increasing affinity for further oxygen binding.
- Globins are large protein chains tightly bound to a haem compound. The globin chain structure determines the type of Hb formed (see table).

Haemoglobin functions include the following.

- Transport of diatomic gases – oxygen to tissues, carbon dioxide from tissues to lungs as carbaminohaemoglobin.
- Buffering – globin chain histidine residues act as proton acceptors. As haem releases oxygen, the electron structure of the globin chain is altered allowing increased capacity to bind hydrogen (see *Section 1.3.4 – Carbon dioxide dissociation curve and Haldane effect*).

Porphyria

Porphyrins are complex organic compounds composed of four pyrrole rings. A pyrrole is a pentagon-shaped ring of one nitrogen and four carbon atoms. Porphyrins may be characterized by the associated centrally bound metal ion (e.g. haemoproteins contain iron).

Porphyrias are a rare group of inherited and acquired disorders of enzymes that participate in the synthesis of porphyrins and haem. Acute porphyrias (e.g. acute intermittent porphyria, variegate porphyria) have the potential to develop neurovisceral crises. Precipitating factors, such as fasting, dehydration, infection and stress, lead to an accumulation of compounds synthesized before the enzyme defect (e.g. 5-ALA). Drugs commonly used in anaesthetics including thiopentone, ketamine, sevoflurane, diclofenac and ephedrine are potential triggers. Signs and symptoms of a crisis are variable and non-specific. Acute porphyria should be considered in any case of unexplained severe abdominal pain, especially in conjunction with tachycardia and neurological symptoms. Management involves trigger removal, administration of haem arginate and supportive measures.

1.11.6

Prostanoid synthesis

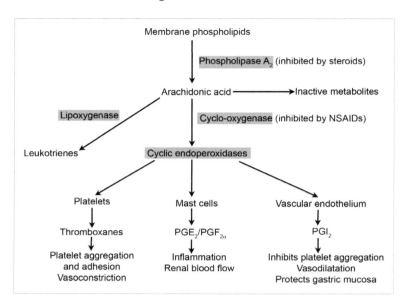

Prostaglandins, thromboxanes and prostacyclin (PGI$_2$) are prostanoids, a subclass of eicosanoids. They are a group of hormone-like compounds that produce a variety of physiological effects. They are autocrine or paracrine because they act locally to their site of secretion. They are all lipid compounds derived from fatty acids containing 20 carbon atoms, including a carbon ring. They are named with a letter (prefixed with PG) according to the type of ring structure they have, and a number indicating the number of double bonds in the hydrocarbon structure.

Prostanoids are not stored, but synthesized by cleavage of membrane phospholipids by phospholipase A$_2$ on an as required basis. This produces arachidonic acid, the rate-limiting step in prostanoid synthesis, which then enters either the cyclo-oxygenase (COX) or lipoxygenase pathways to form prostanoids or leukotrienes, respectively.

Two isoenzymes of COX exist, COX-1 and COX-2. COX-1, also known as the constitutive form, has a role in prostanoid production that controls renal blood flow, the gastric mucosal barrier and thromboxane synthesis. COX-2 is known as the inducible form because it is produced in response to tissue damage leading to an inflammatory response. Thromboxane is produced by platelets and promotes haemostasis by vasoconstriction and platelet aggregation. Conversely, prostacyclin causes vasodilatation and inhibits platelet aggregation.

Non-steroidal anti-inflammatory drugs (NSAIDs) act by inhibiting the cyclo-oxygenase enzyme and therefore prevent the production of prostanoids. They mostly produce reversible enzyme inhibition that causes the following effects.
- Anti-inflammatory – by reduced PGE$_2$ and PGF$_{2\alpha}$ synthesis.
- Antipyretic effect – by inhibition of centrally produced prostaglandins.
- Reduced platelet aggregation – by reduced thromboxane production.

Leukotrienes cause bronchospasm. In susceptible individuals (e.g. those with NSAID-sensitive asthma), inhibiting prostanoid synthesis with NSAIDs leads to an increased production of leukotrienes from arachidonic acid, and exacerbation of their asthma symptoms.

1.12.1

Cell

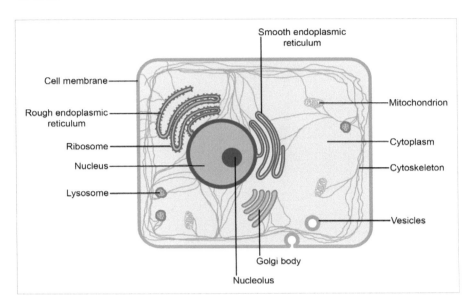

Original cell theory describes the properties of cells. Original components of this theory are:
- All organisms are composed of one or more cell.
- The cell is the basic unit of life in all living things.
- All cells are produced by division of pre-existing cells.

Modern cell theory contains four statements in addition to the original theory.
- The cell contains hereditary information (DNA) passed on from cell to cell during cell division.
- All cells are basically the same in chemical composition and metabolic activities.
- All basic chemical and physiological functions are carried out inside the cells.
- Cell activity depends on activities of subcellular structures within the cell.

Eukaryotic cell structures
- Cell membrane (see *Section 1.12.2 – Cell membrane*).
- Cytoplasm – the entire area within the cell, but outside of the nucleus, composed of organelles and cytosol.
- Cytoskeleton – protein fibre network within the cytoplasm, responsible for cell movement, cell division and organization of organelles.
- Nucleus – contains cellular genetic material. The nuclear membrane acts as an impermeable barrier, maintaining genetic integrity and regulating gene expression. The nucleolus is the site of transcription and ribosome assembly.
- Ribosomes – translation of messenger RNA into chains of amino acids.
- Endoplasmic reticulum (ER) – rough ER is studded with ribosomes, participating in protein synthesis and folding. Smooth ER, devoid of ribosomes, participates in lipid and steroid hormone synthesis and a variety of metabolic processes (e.g. drug detoxification).
- Golgi body – modification, processing and packaging of proteins synthesized by the rough ER.
- Lysosomes – store inactive hydrolytic enzymes that, when activated, contribute to degradation of biological material.
- Mitochondria – primary function is energy conversion through oxidative phosphorylation.

1.12.2

Cell membrane

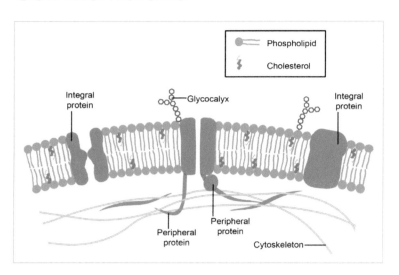

Cell membranes function to protect and organize cells. All cells (prokaryotes and eukaryotes) have a selectively permeable outer cell membrane that regulates movement of substances in and out of the cell. Eukaryotes also possess internal cell membranes that encase organelles and control exchange of cellular components.

Structure
- Lipids form the fundamental architecture of cell membranes.
  - Phospholipids possess both hydrophobic and hydrophilic regions. These molecules naturally align into a bilayer due to the sequestration of hydrophobic chains from the aqueous environment, known as the hydrophobic effect.
  - Cholesterol accounts for approximately 20% of lipids in mammalian cell membranes. Cholesterol plays a distinct role in membrane structure due to its rigid ring structure.
- Membrane proteins provide structural and functional properties.
  - Integral – one or more segments embedded within the phospholipid bilayer. Protein structure includes both hydrophilic and hydrophobic components to allow traversal of the membrane. Transmembrane proteins (e.g. G-protein-coupled receptors) completely traverse the bilayer while anchored proteins insert a hydrophobic region into one layer of the lipid membrane.
  - Peripheral – bound to cell membranes, usually by association with integral proteins. These proteins do not significantly penetrate the hydrophobic core of the bilayer.
- Carbohydrates – the glycocalyx is a carbohydrate coat on the extracellular surface of the cell. Formed by branched carbohydrates attached to lipid and integral membrane proteins, this layer is involved in cell recognition, intercellular adhesion and as hormone receptors.

The fluid mosaic model depicts biological membranes as a matrix of, predominantly, a phospholipid bilayer with randomly distributed, mobile integral membrane proteins. It has been revised to account for interactions between membrane lipids and proteins as well as membrane-associated cytoskeletal and extracellular interactions. These interactions influence non-random cooperative organization of membranes, restricting mobility of membrane structures.

Cell membrane functions include compartmentalization, transport, signal transduction, and enzymatic activity.

1.12.3

G-proteins

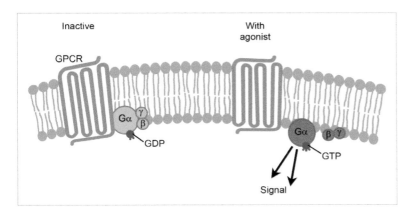

G-proteins are heterotrimeric proteins that act as transducers to bring about an intracellular change from an extracellular signal. They are called 'heterotrimeric' because they have three subunits (α, β and γ) and 'G-proteins' due to the ability of the α-subunit to bind both guanosine diphosphate (GDP) and guanosine triphosphate (GTP).

G-protein coupled receptors (GPCRs) are membrane-bound proteins with seven helical regions that traverse the membrane in a serpentine structure. The GPCR binds a ligand on the extracellular side resulting in a conformational change that activates the G-protein on the intracellular side. This causes the activation of intermediate messengers at the expense of GTP breakdown. This is a metabotropic interaction and results in signal amplification as one activated GPCR can stimulate multiple G-proteins and each G-protein can activate many intermediate messengers.

GDP is bound to the α-subunit when in its inactive form. Upon activation of the GPCR, GDP is replaced with GTP and the α-GTP dissociates from the β–γ subunits to either activate or inhibit an effector protein. This may be an enzyme, such as adenylyl cyclase or phospholipase C, or an ion channel. The α-subunit then breaks down the GTP to regenerate the α-GDP subunit and rejoins the β-γ complex.

Different types of G-proteins exist depending on their different α-subunits.
- G_s – stimulate adenylyl cyclase resulting in increased cAMP formation, e.g. β-adrenergic agonists.
- G_i – inhibit adenylyl cyclase resulting in reduced cAMP formation, e.g. opioids.
- G_q – activate phospholipase-C to form inositol triphosphate and diacylglycerol causing calcium release from the endoplasmic reticulum and activation of protein kinase C, respectively.

cAMP formed by G-proteins is broken down by phosphodiesterases, the inhibition of which leads to increased levels of intracellular cAMP. Increased cAMP leads to increased inotropy; this can therefore either be achieved with a β-adrenergic agonist or a phosphodiesterase inhibitor.

1.12.4

Ion channels

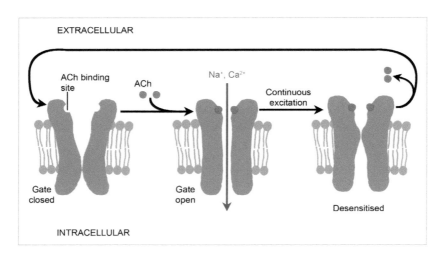

Ion channels are membrane-spanning proteins that form aqueous pores facilitating passive ion transport. Virtually all living cells have ion channels in their cell membranes. These channels are characterized in the following ways.

- Conductivity – conduct ions at very high rates with the flow of ions following the electrochemical gradient.
- Selectivity – selective for one particular ion or ion class (i.e. cation, anion).
- Gating – ion channels undergo conformational changes between 'open' and 'closed' states, as determined by an external signal. The process of opening or closing the transmembrane pore is called gating. The gate is the region of the protein that prevents ion flow in the closed state.
  - Ligand-gated – ion channels are activated by the binding of a chemical messenger (i.e. neurotransmitter) to the sensor region. Examples include nicotinic acetylcholine (ACh) receptors, glutamate receptors and GABA receptors.
  - Voltage-gated – ion channels are activated by changes in electrical membrane potential near the channel.
  - Other gating includes mechanosensitive channels (e.g. stretch, pressure activation), intracellular second messenger activation, and temperature-gated channels.

In addition to the 'open' and 'closed' states, some ion channels may adopt an 'inactivated', non-conducting state. In ligand-gated ion channels, prolonged agonist ligand exposure induces another conformational change where ion flow ceases, called desensitization. In voltage-gated channels, development of a more positive membrane potential leads to closure of an inactivation gate (e.g. ball and chain) allowing time for membrane repolarization.

Anaesthetic drug effects on ion channels

Anaesthetic agents can promote either open channel states (e.g. potentiation) or closed channel states (e.g. inhibition).

- General anaesthetics – ion channels are the most likely molecular targets with general anaesthetic agents acting as either positive or negative allosteric modulators of ligand-gated ion channels.
- Local anaesthetics – intracellular binding closes the channel inactivation gate (see *Section 4.13 – Local anaesthetics – mode of action*).

1.12.5

Sodium/potassium–ATPase pump

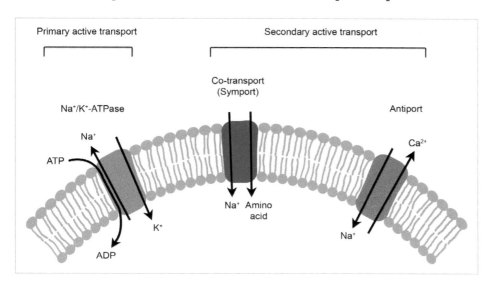

The Na$^+$/K$^+$-ATPase pump is located in the plasma membrane of cells and acts as an antiport to actively transport sodium out and potassium into cells. It is an energy-dependent pump; the high-energy phosphate bond is lost as the adenosine triphosphate (ATP) molecule is hydrolysed to adenosine diphosphate (ADP) allowing the ions to be pumped against their concentration gradients.

Under normal resting conditions sodium slowly leaks into cells and potassium leaks out. When an action potential is generated additional sodium enters and potassium leaves the cells. To maintain their concentration gradients the Na$^+$/K$^+$-ATPase pump will transport 3 sodium ions out and 2 potassium ions back into the cell, creating a negative potential within the cell.

The Na$^+$/K$^+$-ATPase pump is central to active transport in the cell, both directly and indirectly. The Na$^+$/amino acid symport in the small bowel and proximal renal tubule allows movement of amino acids when sodium is bound to the carrier protein, and moves down its concentration gradient which is generated by the Na$^+$/K$^+$-ATPase pump. A similar secondary transport mechanism can be seen in the Na$^+$/Ca^{2+} antiport where sodium ions are exchanged for calcium ions.

Digoxin is a cardiac glycoside that is used in the treatment of atrial fibrillation and flutter. It binds to and inhibits the cardiac Na$^+$/K$^+$-ATPase pump leading to increased intracellular sodium and decreased intracellular potassium concentrations. This increased sodium concentration inside the cell leads to a decrease or reversal in action of the Na$^+$/Ca^{2+} antiport and therefore an increase in intracellular calcium. This has a positive inotropic effect leading to an increase in the force of contraction and increases the refractory period of the AV node and bundle of His. Digoxin also has indirect effects; the release of acetylcholine is enhanced at cardiac muscarinic receptors further prolonging the refractory period and slowing conduction.

1.13.1

Antibody

The immune system has both innate, non-specific responses and acquired, or antibody-mediated responses to foreign material. Acquired immunity is a tailored response to specific organisms whereby certain antigens are recognized by corresponding antibodies. Acquired immunity can be either cellular or humoral; the main function of the humoral system is the production of antibodies.

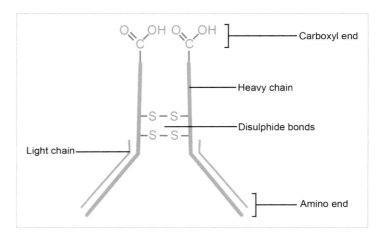

Antibodies are large (~150 kDa) 'Y' shaped glycoproteins that are produced by plasma cells (B cells) in response to antigen exposure. When an antibody binds to a specific antigen, it may:
- form an inactive complex which may be phagocytosed
- activate the complement system
- act as an opsonin and facilitate phagocytosis by macrophages and neutrophils.

Antibodies belong to the immunoglobulin superfamily. The basic structural unit consists of two heavy chains and two light chains connected by disulphide bonds. The heavy chain has a constant carboxyl end that mediates its effector functions, and a variable amino end that is the antigen-specific binding site. There are different antibody isotypes dependent on the heavy chain they possess:
- IgG – four types, forms the majority of antibody-mediated protection against pathogens; can cross the placenta providing the fetus with passive immunity.
- IgA – two types, found in mucosal areas, e.g. gut, respiratory and urogenital tract, saliva, tears and breast milk. Prevents pathogen colonization.
- IgM – can be expressed on the surface of cells or in a secreted form. Provides an early response before sufficient IgG is produced.
- IgD – part of the B cell receptor, activates basophils and mast cells.
- IgE – binds to allergens and causes histamine release from basophils and mast cells. Role in allergy and in protection against parasitic worms.

During the primary response to an antigen, memory B and T cells are formed. On repeat exposure an accelerated, or secondary, response occurs.

Hypersensitivity

	Type I	Type II	Type III	Type IV
Mediators	IgE	IgG or IgM	Immune complex	T cell
Onset time	Minutes	Hours to days	Hours to weeks	24–72 hours
Example	Anaphylaxis	Goodpasture's syndrome	Systemic lupus erythematosus	Contact dermatitis

Hypersensitivity reactions are exaggerated or inappropriate immunologic reactions occurring in response to an antigen or allergen. They can be categorized into four types using the Gell and Coombs classification, according to the type of immune response and mechanism responsible for cellular and tissue injury. Hypersensitivity reactions are implicated in the pathogenesis of several disease processes. Susceptibility to hypersensitivity reactions is, in part, genetic and often involves a triggering event (e.g. infection).

Type I – occur within minutes of antigen exposure and are mediated through pre-formed IgE antibodies bound to the surface of mast cells. On antigen exposure, mast cells rapidly degranulate releasing inflammatory mediators including histamine, platelet activating factor, leukotrienes, cytokines and prostaglandins. Widespread mast cell activation may result in an overwhelming systemic response. Examples include anaphylaxis and allergic bronchial asthma.

Type II – mediated by IgM or IgG targeting cell membrane-associated antigens. In the sensitization phase, antibodies are produced that, in the subsequent effector phase, coat the target cells (opsonization). These target cells can then be destroyed via one of three mechanisms: complement-dependent cytotoxicity, phagocytosis or antibody-dependent cell-mediated cytotoxicity. Examples include immune thrombocytopenia and Goodpasture's syndrome.

Type III – triggered by antigen exposure leading to antibody–antigen complex formation. These immune complexes precipitate in various tissues such as skin, joints, vessels or glomeruli. Complement pathway activation leads to recruitment of inflammatory cells that release cytokines and proteolytic enzymes with resultant tissue injury. Examples include systemic lupus erythematosus and rheumatoid arthritis.

Type IV – also known as delayed-type hypersensitivity reactions, they generally present 24–48 hours after exposure to soluble antigens. An antibody-independent process, reactions are mediated by antigen-specific T cells. Activated T cells release cytokines that recruit other inflammatory cells to the site of exposure. Tissue injury may also occur due to direct T cell-mediated cytotoxicity. Examples include poison ivy exposure and tuberculosis skin test.

1.13.3

Innate and adaptive immunity

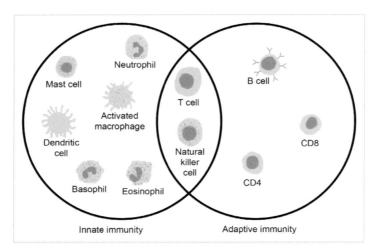

The immune response (mechanism by which a host protects against pathogens) can broadly be divided into two different types: the innate and the adaptive immune responses. There is overlap between the two in terms of the cellular response. There are four main components.

- Immediate pathogen recognition by the innate immune system.
- Consequent activation of an inflammatory response.
- Antigen presentation and consequent activation of T helper cells.
- CD4 helper T cell-coordinated targeted antigen-specific immune response involving humoral immune response (B cells) and a cell-mediated immune response (cytotoxic CD8 T cells).

The innate (non-specific) response is immediate, has no memory and consists of physical, cellular and chemical defences against pathogens.

- Physical components include skin, mucous, cilia and gut peristalsis.
- Chemical defences include stomach acidity, bile salts and lysozyme (found in tears, saliva and surfactant).
- Cellular response involves a number of cell types. The phagocyte cells (neutrophils, dendritic cells, monocytes, macrophages) identify pathogens by recognizing pathogen-associated molecular patterns (PAMPs) using pathogen recognition receptors (PRRs). Once identified these pathogens are broken down into their component proteins. These component proteins are then 'presented' to the adaptive part of the immune system via the major histocompatibility complexes (MHCs) that are now exposed. The exposure of PAMPs to PRRs also causes activation of nuclear factor kappa beta which causes cytokine release (e.g. interleukins, tumour necrosis factors and chemokine) and consequent initiation of the immune response.

Adaptive (acquired) immunity is only found in vertebrates and is specific to individual 'non-self' pathogens. It allows the development of immunological memory leading to a rapid response in the event of re-exposure. Broadly divided into humoral (controlled by B cells and antibodies) and cell-mediated response (controlled by T cells).

In autoimmune disease processes there is a specific adaptive immunity response to self-antigens. Unlike in the response to non-self-antigens, clearance of self-antigens is ineffective leading to chronic inflammatory tissue damage.

1.14.1

Actin–myosin cycle

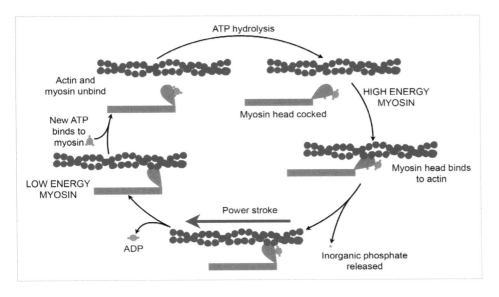

The interaction between actin and myosin filaments is responsible for many types of cell movements. Most familiar is their role in muscle contraction. However, actin and myosin have essential roles in non-muscular processes such as cell division.

Muscle contraction

The sliding filament model describes the sequence of events whereby sarcomeres shorten, achieved by sliding of actin past myosin to generate a muscle contraction. The unbound myosin head is present in the cocked state with adenosine diphosphate (ADP) and inorganic phosphate bound (products of adenosine triphosphate, ATP, hydrolysis). With exposure of the myosin binding site, myosin binds to actin and the power stroke occurs. The power stroke returns the myosin head to its low-energy conformation. In this process, the power stroke generates force, pulling the thin filament toward the centre of the sarcomere. Binding of another ATP molecule dissociates the myosin head from actin and the cycle repeats.

Excitation–contraction coupling

Excitation–contraction coupling refers to the process linking depolarization of the muscle cell membrane (sarcolemma) to muscle contraction. The cycle begins with depolarization of the muscle cell by an action potential. The action potential propagates along the sarcolemma into the muscle cell interior via the T-tubules. Voltage-gated calcium channels (VGCC) open, releasing calcium into the cytosol. Ryanodine receptors are activated leading to further calcium release from the sarcoplasmic reticulum. Calcium binds to troponin C, moving the tropomyosin/troponin complex to reveal the myosin binding site on actin. Muscle tension depends on the proportion of active actin–myosin cross-bridges. This, in turn, depends on the cytosolic concentration of calcium.

Differences between cardiac and skeletal muscle is founded in the isoforms of VGCC and ryanodine receptors present in each muscle type. In cardiac muscle, activation of the ryanodine receptor is calcium dependent. In skeletal muscle, activation is due to a direct physical interaction between the receptors.

1.14.2

Golgi tendon organ

The Golgi tendon organ (GTO) is a proprioceptor that provides the CNS with information regarding muscle and tendon tension. These sensory organs are located in series with skeletal muscle fibres at the musculotendinous junction. The GTO comprises two types of collagen fibres:

- densely packed collagen forms an external capsule
- loosely packed collagen occupies the interior.

Multiple muscle fibres insert into the collagen fibres. A single large, myelinated Ib afferent nerve innervates each GTO. This nerve bypasses the dense collagen capsule to innervate the central loosely packed collagen where it divides into smaller branches.

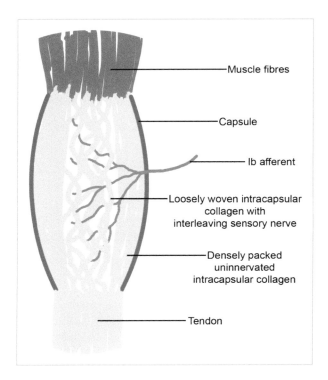

Muscle fibres

Capsule

Ib afferent

Loosely woven intracapsular collagen with interleaving sensory nerve

Densely packed uninnervated intracapsular collagen

Tendon

Golgi tendon reflex (see also Section 1.4.13 – Reflex arc)

The GTO functions as the sensory component of the reflex pathway. When a muscle contracts, the muscle body shortens, increasing tendon tension. This causes some of the loosely packed collagen fibres to straighten. The Ib afferent nerve endings become compressed between these collagen fibres leading to depolarization. With an adequate stimulus, the threshold potential is reached and an action potential is initiated. This afferent sensory signal is propagated to the dorsal root of the spinal cord where it synapses with an inhibitory interneuron. Activation of this interneuron reduces the firing rate of the α motor neuron supplying the same muscle, inhibiting further muscle contraction and force. Muscle contraction is a more effective stimulation of the GTO than muscle stretch because most of the force associated with stretch is absorbed by the muscle fibres.

This negative feedback loop, also known as autogenic inhibition reflex, serves to protect muscles from injuries due to excessive force by causing sudden muscle relaxation. In conjunction with muscle spindles (see *Section 1.14.3 – Muscle spindle*), GTOs control position and movement by providing the CNS with information regarding muscle fibre length/contraction velocity and muscle–tendon complex length, respectively.

1.14.3

Muscle spindle

Muscle spindles are proprioceptors that provide the CNS with information regarding absolute muscle length and changes in muscle length. These receptors are located deep within the muscle belly, parallel to the extrafusal muscle fibres (i.e. those responsible for muscle contraction). Muscle spindles comprise two types of sensory intrafusal fibres:

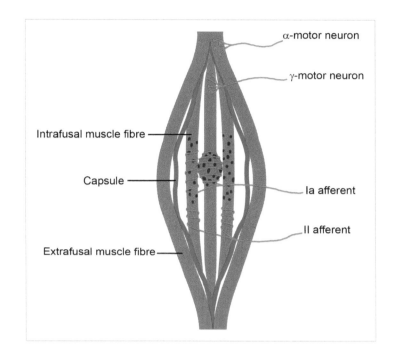

- nuclear bag which have a large number of clustered nuclei (i.e. resemble a bag) and lie within the central portion of the muscle spindle
- nuclear chain fibres which have nuclei distributed throughout the central portion.

Muscle spindles possess a non-contractile central region and contractile ends.

- The central region is innervated by Ia and II sensory afferent fibres. The Ia fibres are thick and heavily myelinated allowing fast conduction. They are rapidly adapting; when muscle length change ceases they stop discharging briefly and then begin firing at a rate appropriate for the new resting muscle length. Therefore, these Ia fibres provide dynamic information relating to the velocity of muscle length change. Type II afferents are also myelinated, but are thinner than the Ia fibres. These afferents are slowly adapting; the rate of firing increases with increased muscle length and continues at this increased rate even after the muscle stops moving. It is the dynamic response of Ia afferents that initiates the response seen with a deep tendon reflex. The tendon tap rapidly stretches muscle fibres, and muscle spindles, increasing the firing of Ia afferents. As the change in muscle length is small, little change in type II afferent firing is observed.
- The contractile end regions are innervated by efferent γ-motor neurons. Unlike α-motor neurons, these efferents are not directly involved in muscle contraction. Instead, γ-motor neurons keep the central region of the muscle spindles taut, allowing spindles to remain sensitive to muscle stretch.

1.14.4

Muscle types

Structure	Skeletal	Cardiac	Smooth
Striated	Yes	Yes	No
Sarcoplasmic reticulum	Well developed	Moderately developed	Poorly developed
Transverse tubules	Well developed	Moderately developed	No
Troponin or calmodulin	Troponin	Troponin	Calmodulin
Initiation of contraction	Nerve impulse	Pacemaker cells	Pacemaker potential
Gap junctions	No	Yes, intercalated discs	Yes

There are three types of muscle tissue originating from the mesodermal layer of embryonic germ cells.
- Skeletal – aids movement, maintains posture (unconscious control), provides joint stability and has a role in heat production. Generally contracts with conscious thought; therefore termed voluntary. Attached to bones by tendons.
- Smooth – found within walls of organs, e.g. oesophagus, stomach, intestines, bronchi, uterus, bladder, blood vessels and in hair arrector pili muscles. Contracts without conscious thought; therefore termed involuntary.
- Cardiac muscle – myocardium, found only in the heart. Involuntary muscle but structure more similar to skeletal than smooth muscle.

Striated muscle typically contracts in short bursts whereas smooth muscle has sustained, longer contractions. Skeletal and cardiac muscle are striated because they contain regularly arranged sarcomeres; smooth muscle lacks this structure. The sarcomeres of skeletal muscle are arranged in parallel bundles while those in cardiac muscle have intercalated discs with connections at more irregular angles.

Despite their differences all muscle types create contraction using the movement of actin against myosin. Skeletal muscle contraction is initiated by nerve transmission of electrical impulses whereas internal pacemaker cells initiate contraction in cardiac and smooth muscle.

Traditionally, skeletal muscle was divided into slow and fast twitch fibres depending on speed of contraction. Histochemical staining for myosin ATPase activity has superseded this, although correlations remain (the main subtypes are in bold and some texts use 'B' rather than 'X').
- Type I – slow twitch or 'red'. Two subtypes (I and IC). Contract for long periods but with little force. Has dense capillary network with multiple mitochondria and myoglobin.
- Type II – fast twitch. Five subtypes (IIC, IIA, IIAX, IIXA and IIX). Contract quickly with greater force but fatigue more quickly, sustaining only short anaerobic bursts. Type IIX is 'white' muscle and has the lowest density of mitochondria and myoglobin.

1.14.5

Neuromuscular junction

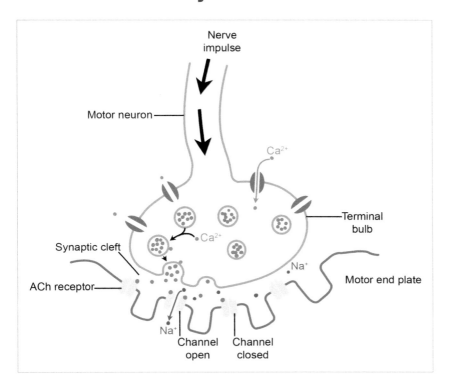

The neuromuscular junction (NMJ) is the synapse between the nervous system and a muscle fibre. Each motor neuron synapses with several muscle fibres to form a motor unit. Each muscle fibre has only one NMJ. Acetylcholine (ACh) is the neurotransmitter at the NMJ.

- As a motor neuron approaches a muscle fibre it divides into several terminal branches that lie embedded in post-junctional folds on the sarcolemma. ACh is synthesized and stored in the terminal motor neuron. Depolarization of the terminal bulb triggers fusion of ACh-containing vesicles with the pre-synaptic membrane and release of the neurotransmitter into the synaptic cleft. Pre-junctional ACh receptors present on the terminal bulb augment neurotransmitter production through a positive feedback mechanism.
- The synaptic cleft is the space between the terminal motor neuron and sarcolemma. This space is approximately 50 nm wide and is filled with interstitial fluid.
- The motor end plate is the specialized region of the sarcolemma forming the post-synaptic surface of the NMJ. Nicotinic ACh receptors are located near the cleft edge of the post-junctional folds. These receptors are ligand-gated ion channels comprising five subunits forming a ring around a central pore. The adult receptor consists of two α subunits, one β, one δ and one ε subunit. In the fetal receptor, a γ subunit replaces the ε subunit. When Ach molecules are bound to both α subunits, a conformational change opens the central non-specific cation channel. Cation movement, primarily sodium, into the cell causes depolarization. When a threshold of -50 mV is achieved, voltage-gated sodium channels open leading to rapid depolarization and generation of an action potential. Within the clefts of the post-junctional folds, acetylcholinesterase rapidly removes ACh from the synaptic cleft, thereby limiting the active period of the ACh receptor.

1.14.6

Sarcomere

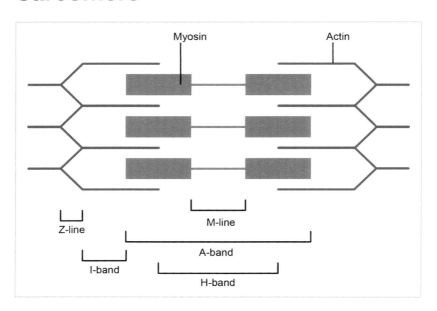

The sarcomere is the basic contractile unit of skeletal muscle. It is delineated by two Z-lines and consists of multiple thick (myosin) and thin (actin) filaments arranged in a parallel fashion.

The thick filaments consist of bundles of myosin molecules combined with myosin-binding proteins. These function to bind the myosin molecules together and potentially have a role in regulating contraction. The myosin fibres consist of a head and tail; the head possesses actin and ATP-binding sites that assist in muscle contraction. The thin filaments are formed from two actin chains helically wound together. Tropomyosin, a protein complex formed by troponin C, I and T, wraps around the actin filament and covers the binding sites for myosin.

The dark band formed by the thick filaments is called the A-band (as it is anisotropic, or directionally dependent, under a polarizing microscope). Areas of thin filaments not overlapped by the thick filaments form the I-band (from isotropic, meaning uniform in all directions). Conversely, the H-band represents the portion of the thick filaments that are not overlapped by the thin filaments (and is seen as a paler area within the A-band using polarizing microscopy). The M-line represents the cross-linkage of myosin filaments and forms the middle of the sarcomere. The dark Z-lines (also known as Z-discs or Z-bodies) form the boundaries between adjacent sarcomeres and represent the cross-linkage of actin filaments and other structural proteins. Titin is one such protein, connecting the Z-line and M-line together and providing structural stability to the sarcomere.

During skeletal muscle contraction the thick and thin filaments overlap more causing the Z-lines to move closer together and the width of the H- and I-bands to decrease. The width of the A-band remains the same because the length of the thick filament does not change.

1.14.7

Skeletal muscle structure

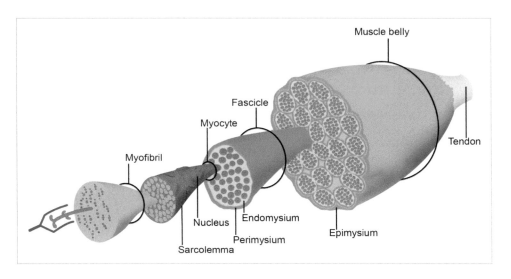

Skeletal muscles produce movement, maintain posture and stabilize joints. They are under both voluntary and involuntary control. The embryonic precursors of skeletal muscle are mononucleated myoblasts. Fusion of myoblasts gives rise to elongated, cylindrical, multinucleated myocytes (also called muscle fibres or muscle cells). Each myocyte contains hundreds to thousands of specialized contractile organelles called myofibrils. Myofibrils are cylindrical structures that extend the entire length of the myocyte. The structural components of the myofibril are the myofilaments that are organized as a series of repeating sarcomeres (see *Section 1.14.6 – Sarcomere*). The alignment of the thick and thin myofilaments within parallel myofibrils gives rise to the striated (striped) appearance of skeletal muscle when viewed under high magnification.

Skeletal muscle extracellular matrix

- Endomysium – ensheathes individual myocytes. The endomysium directly covers the sarcolemma, the cell membrane of the myocyte.
- Perimysium – binds myocytes together into fascicles. Within the fascicle, myocytes are organized in parallel.
- Epimysium – a relatively thick and tough connective tissue extending from the tendon, enveloping a number of muscle fascicles to form a distinct muscle.

Dystrophinopathies

Dystrophin, encoded on the X chromosome, is a cytoplasmic protein integral to the structural stability of the myocyte. This protein connects the myocyte cytoskeleton (proteins within the sarcoplasm such as actin and myosin) to the sarcolemma. This link is extended to the extracellular matrix via the dystroglycan complex. This link between intracellular and extracellular components is important in transmission of force generated by the sarcomeres. Duchenne and Becker muscular dystrophies are caused by mutations of the dystrophin gene resulting in functional loss of this protein. This deficiency leads to instability of the sarcolemma eventually resulting in progressive weakness and atrophy of skeletal muscle. The dystrophinopathies demonstrate an X-linked recessive inheritance pattern.

1.15.1

Fetal circulation

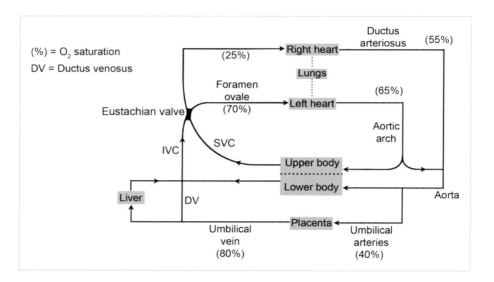

The fetal circulation demonstrates significant differences to the circulation of a baby after birth.

Site of oxygen exchange – in the fetus, oxygen exchange occurs at the fetal–placental interface. Deoxygenated blood arrives at the placenta via the umbilical arteries and oxygenated blood returns via a single umbilical vein. The fetal lungs are non-functional. A high pulmonary vascular resistance, due to the presence of fluid in the lungs, ensures only a small fraction of the right ventricular output passes through the pulmonary system (~12%).

Circulation in parallel – the fetal circulation comprises two parallel circuits (systemic/placental circulation, right/left heart) characterized by the presence of shunts and preferential streaming that aim to deliver more highly oxygenated blood to vital organs (e.g. brain, coronary circulation).
- Ductus venosus (DV) – channels half of the oxygenated blood returning from the placenta to bypass the portal system and its associated oxygen extraction. This more highly oxygenated blood is streamed along the inferior vena cava (IVC) separate from deoxygenated blood returning from the fetal lower body.
- Foramen ovale – allows flow of blood from the right atrium (RA) to the left atrium. The Eustachian valve at the junction of the IVC and RA preferentially streams highly oxygenated blood from the DV across the foramen ovale so decreasing flow through the redundant pulmonary circulation. Left ventricular output enters the proximal aorta to supply the brain and upper extremities.
- Ductus arteriosus – connects the pulmonary artery to the proximal descending aorta (distal to branches that supply the brain and upper limbs). Desaturated blood from the superior vena cava and IVC (blood from portal and systemic circulations) is ejected from the right ventricle into the pulmonary artery. The majority of this blood bypasses the lungs via the ductus arteriosus into the descending aorta and supplies the lower body and umbilical arteries with relatively desaturated blood.

1.15.2

Paediatric differences I

	Paediatric considerations	Implications for anaesthetist
Airway	Large head, short neck, prominent occiput	Neutral head positioning
	Large tongue	Can obstruct upper airway
	High anterior larynx	Can make intubation more challenging
	Obligate nasal breathers (neonates)	High nasal resistance, nasal passages can obstruct easily
Breathing	Limited respiratory reserve	Prone to desaturation
	Horizontal rib positioning	Breathing is predominantly diaphragmatic
	Low functional residual capacity (FRC)	Closing volume is greater than FRC under 6 years
	Minute ventilation is rate-dependent	
Circulation	Stiff ventricle	Cardiac output is rate-dependent
	Parasympathetically driven	Prone to bradycardia
	Increased blood volume	

Airway – neonates and infants have a relatively large head, short neck and prominent occiput making them prone to neck flexion. Their large tongue, high anterior larynx and floppy epiglottis can make mask ventilation and intubation challenging. The trachea is highly compliant, short and in line with the right main bronchus. Neonates are obligate nasal breathers and due to the small diameter of their nasal passages, have high upper airway resistance and can easily obstruct.

Breathing – chest wall is compliant and ribs are horizontal meaning that tidal volume is diaphragm-dependent. Infants are obligatory nasal breathers so if blocked, even partially, this can lead to breathing difficulties and difficulty feeding. Any obstruction to diaphragmatic movement (e.g. full stomach) restricts movement and dramatically reduces tidal volume. Closing volume is greater than functional residual capacity leading to increased airway closure. This, coupled with a high cardiac output and low respiratory reserve, leads to rapid desaturation following apnoea.

Circulation – myocardium is less compliant and stroke volume is reduced compared to adults. There is also an increased cardiac workload for the cardiovascular system due to a higher metabolic rate. There is less functional cardiac reserve in response to increased preload and afterload. Cardiac output is more rate-dependent than in adults. Children have predominant parasympathetic tone until later in infancy and are therefore prone to bradycardias. They have an increased blood volume per kg compared to adults.

1.15.3

Paediatric differences II

	Paediatric considerations	Implications for anaesthetist
Renal	High renal vascular resistance	Renal blood flow and GFR are low
	Tubular function is immature	Unable to excrete large sodium load
	Urine output 1–2 ml.kg^{-1}.h^{-1}	Dehydration is poorly tolerated; increased insensible losses
Hepatic	Decreased function liver enzymes	Liver function immature, reduced metabolism of drugs
Central nervous system	Immature descending pain pathways and blood–brain barrier	Drug dosing
	Fragility of cerebral blood vessels	Greater pain experienced
	Unpredictability of drug metabolism	Increased risk of cerebral haemorrhage

Renal and hepatic – function immature. Renal vascular resistance is high and renal blood flow and glomerular filtration rate are low. Liver enzymes are immature and drug metabolism is reduced. Hypoglycaemia is common in neonates. The bladder in children is located high above the pelvis so is easily palpated.

Haematology and temperature control – at birth, haemoglobin is predominantly HbF. The oxygen dissociation curve shifts to the right as the levels of HbA and 2,3-DPG rise. The shorter lifespan of erythrocytes in neonates is one of the factors involved in neonatal hyperbilirubinaemia. Vitamin K-dependent clotting factors and platelet function are deficient at birth. Babies have a large surface area to volume ratio and readily lose heat. Brown fat is required for non-shivering thermogenesis (a metabolically active process).

Central nervous system – the proportion of cerebral blood flow is greatest in children between 1 and 3 years, at about 40–50% of the cardiac output, thus increasing their vulnerability to cerebral ischaemia during periods of systemic hypotension. Pain pathways are intact *in utero*, however, descending pathways involved in modulation are immature; children may experience greater pain. The blood–brain barrier is immature; drugs pass more freely to their site of action. Cerebral blood vessels are thin and fragile in neonates; they are prone to intraventricular haemorrhages related to physiological stress.

1.15.4

Physiological changes in pregnancy I

System	Physiological changes
Cardiovascular	Cardiac output increases by 50% by third trimester
	Stroke volume increases by 35% due to increased blood volume
	Peripheral vascular resistance reduced due to vasodilatation
	Heart rate increases by 15–25%
Respiratory	Increased risk of difficult airway secondary to upper airway oedema and vascular engorgement, enlarged breasts and increasing obesity
	Diaphragmatic displacement, increased chest diameter and rib flaring
	Expiratory reserve volume, residual volume and functional residual capacity reduced as pregnancy progresses, by approximately 20–30% at term
	Inspiratory reserve volume is increased
	Vital capacity, total lung volume and FEV_1 unchanged
	Reduced airways resistance secondary to bronchodilatation (progesterone effect)
	Respiratory rate increased by 15%, tidal volume increased by 40%, both increasing minute ventilation
	Alveolar ventilation 70% higher by end of pregnancy

Cardiovascular – progesterone levels increase throughout pregnancy. This leads to a decrease in systemic vascular resistance causing a decrease in diastolic blood pressure during the first and second trimesters in particular. In response, cardiac output increases up to 50%. LV hypertrophy and dilatation help facilitate this increased cardiac output; contractility remains the same. An increase in sodium and water retention, due to activation of the renin–angiotensin system, leads to an increase in total blood volume. The upward displacement of the diaphragm shifts the position of the heart apex resulting in ECG changes. Aortocaval compression occurs as pregnancy progresses and causes reduced venous return and therefore preload and cardiac output. This may lead to reduced uteroplacental and renal blood flow and potentially fetal compromise.

Respiratory – a progesterone-associated chronic respiratory alkalosis develops in pregnancy (related to increased sensitivity to carbon dioxide levels). Anatomically, fetal growth causes upward diaphragmatic displacement compensated for by increases in both the transverse and anteroposterior diameters of the thoracic cavity. Reduced FRC leads to closure of the airways when supine in 50% of parturients at term. Increase in metabolic rate leads to an increase in both tidal volume (30–50%) and ventilation rates, resulting in an increase in minute volume of up to 50% by the third trimester. Due to increased airway diameter later in pregnancy, anatomical headspace increases significantly (up to 45%).

Preoxygenation is less effective and, coupled with the increased oxygen consumption, leads to rapid desaturation following apnoea.

1.15.5

Physiological changes in pregnancy II

System	Physiological changes
Haematology	Blood volume increased
	Plasma volume increased by 45% due to renin–angiotensin–aldosterone system activation
	Total body water increased secondary to renal sodium retention
	Red cell mass increased by 20–30% secondary to increased erythropoietin production
	Physiological anaemia of pregnancy
	Hypercoagulable state
Renal	Renal blood flow increases by 50%
	Increased GFR from 100 to 150 ml.min^{-1}
Endocrine	Increase in size of thyroid gland and total T_3 and T_4 levels
	Relative insulin resistance
	Progressive increase in oestrogen and progesterone levels
	Increased lipolysis
Hepatic	Increased cholesterol synthesis
	Change in liver biochemical profile
Gastrointestinal	Raised intragastric pressure and reduced lower oesophageal sphincter tone

Haematology – blood volume increase is proportionally higher than that of red cell mass leading to physiological anaemia. This reduces the impact of maternal blood loss at delivery. Plasma concentrations of clotting factors and fibrinogen increase, except factor XI and XIII. Platelet production is increased but actual count falls due to dilution and consumption. Risk of venous thromboembolic disease increases 10-fold in pregnancy and 25-fold post-partum.

Renal – increased clearance of urea, creatinine and drugs due to increased renal blood flow and GFR. Increased GFR (by up to 50% as early as end of first trimester) exceeds reabsorption capacity leading to increased urine glucose and protein. Increased progesterone and relaxin cause smooth muscle relaxation leading to dilatation of the collecting system, increasing the chance of urinary stasis and UTIs.

Endocrine – increase in size of thyroid gland and total T_3 and T_4 levels. However, free T_3 and T_4 levels remain static due to increased production of thyroid-binding globulin. Increased hCG levels stimulate TSH receptors in anterior pituitary leading to transient hyperthyroidism and hyperemesis gravidarum. A diabetogenic state occurs with relative insulin resistance and compensatory increased insulin synthesis and secretion.

Hepatic – ALP may be physiologically elevated due to placental production, with other LFTs generally lower. Pregnancy-specific liver diseases can occur, including HELLP syndrome (haemolysis, elevated liver enzymes and low platelets) and acute fatty liver of pregnancy. Reduced activity of butyryl (plasma) cholinesterase.

Gastrointestinal – increased risk of gastric aspiration due to raised intragastric pressure and reduced lower oesophageal sphincter tone; treat as a full stomach from 16 weeks of gestation until 48 hours post-partum.

Abdominal wall

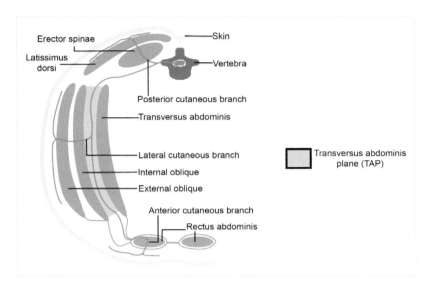

The anterolateral abdominal wall comprises five paired muscles.

Flat, layered muscles
- The external oblique is the most superficial, originating from the inferior 8 ribs. Following an inferiomedial path, some fibres insert onto the iliac crest whilst other fibres end in a thick aponeurosis. Anteriorly, the aponeurosis joins those of the internal oblique and transversus abdominis to form the rectus sheath. Inferiorly, the external oblique aponeurosis forms the inguinal canal.
- The internal oblique is the intermediate layer originating from the iliac crest, the inguinal ligament and the thoracolumbar fascia. The muscle fibres follow a superiomedial course to insert on the inferior ribs and linea alba.
- The transverse abdominis is the innermost layer originating from the inguinal ligament, the iliac crest, the inferior 6 ribs and the thoracolumbar fascia. This muscle runs in a transverse direction ending in a broad aponeurosis.

Central, vertical muscles
- The rectus abdominis and pyramidalis lie within the rectus sheath. They are separated from parallel, mirrored muscles by the linea alba, a midline band of connective tissue.

Sensory supply of the abdominal wall

Innervation arises from the anterior rami of spinal nerves T7 to L1 and includes the intercostal nerves (T7 to T11), the subcostal nerve (T12) and the iliohypogastric and ilioinguinal nerves (L1). The anterior divisions of T7 to T11 continue from the intercostal space into the abdominal wall travelling between the internal oblique and the transversus abdominis muscles (site of local anaesthetic deposition in 'transversus abdominis plane' block). The nerves continue anteriorly where they pierce the rectus abdominis to end as the anterior cutaneous branch, supplying skin of the anterior abdomen. The anterior branch of T12 contributes a communicating branch to L1 as part of the lumbar plexus. The iliohypogastric and ilioinguinal nerves supply sensation to skin overlying the hypogastrium, upper gluteal region and genitalia.

2.1.2
Antecubital fossa

The antecubital fossa is an anterior triangular depression found between the anatomical arm and forearm at the elbow joint. It has the following borders.

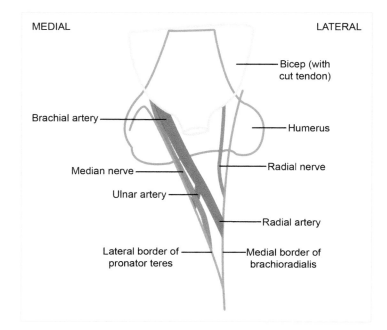

- Superior – an imaginary line connecting the medial and lateral epicondyles of the humerus.
- Medial – lateral border of the pronator teres muscle.
- Lateral – medial border of the brachioradialis muscle.
- Floor – formed proximally by the brachialis and distally by the supinator muscles overlying the capsule of the elbow joint.
- Roof – formed from skin and fascia (including the bicipital aponeurosis). The medial cubital vein runs in the superficial fascia joining the cephalic and basilic veins.

The contents from medial to lateral are as follows.
- The median nerve.
- Brachial artery bifurcating at the apex of the fossa into its terminal branches: the radial and ulnar arteries.
- Biceps tendon and bicipital aponeurosis.
- Radial and posterior interosseous nerves (overlapped by brachioradialis). The radial nerve divides into its deep and superficial branches as it passes underneath brachioradialis.

Clinical relevance
- Venepuncture – the basilic, median cubital and cephalic veins are easily seen within the antecubital fossa (from medial to lateral).
- Blood pressure measurement – the brachial artery is palpated or auscultated at this point. It can also be cannulated for invasive measurement, although caution is advised because it is an end artery.
- Nerve blocks – although rarely performed, the median nerve can be anaesthetized by injecting local anaesthetic between the biceps tendon and the medial epicondyle.
- Supracondylar fractures – a transverse fracture running between the two epicondyles of the humerus. Fragment deplacement can damage contents of the antecubital fossa. Untreated damage to the brachial artery can lead to ischaemic contracture, a permanent flexion contracture of the hand and wrist resulting in a claw-like deformity of the hand and fingers.

2.1.3

Autonomic nervous system

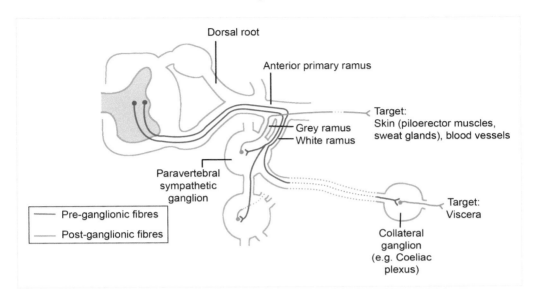

Dorsal root
Anterior primary ramus
Grey ramus
White ramus
Target:
Skin (piloerector muscles, sweat glands), blood vessels
Paravertebral sympathetic ganglion
Pre-ganglionic fibres
Post-ganglionic fibres
Target:
Viscera
Collateral ganglion (e.g. Coeliac plexus)

The autonomic nervous system (ANS) is a complex system of neurons that regulates involuntary visceral functions. Two complementary components, the sympathetic and parasympathetic nervous systems, employ the hypothalamus and brainstem as their central points of integration.

Sympathetic nervous system (SNS) activates the 'fight or flight' response but is also essential for maintaining basal homeostasis. Cell bodies, located in the lateral horn of the spinal cord from T1 to L2 (thoracolumbar outflow), leave the spinal cord to form the white rami communicantes: myelinated, preganglionic sympathetic outflow. These fibres enter the sympathetic chain that extends from the base of skull to the coccyx. Lying in close proximity to the vertebral column bilaterally, the sympathetic chain comprises 23–24 paravertebral ganglia; 3 cervical, 12 thoracic, 4 lumbar and 4–5 sacral. On entering the sympathetic chain, a preganglionic axon may take one or more of the following paths.

- Synapse in the nearest ganglion, the postganglionic nerve joining the spinal nerve at that vertebral level (T1 to L2) via the grey rami communicantes; unmyelinated, postganglionic sympathetic outflow.
- Ascend or descend to synapse in another paravertebral ganglion, joining the spinal nerve at that level; each spinal nerve receives a grey rami communicantes from the sympathetic chain.
- Pass through the paravertebral ganglion to synapse in a collateral ganglion; sympathetic ganglia separate from the sympathetic chain targeting deeper visceral organs.
- Pass through the paravertebral ganglion to synapse in the adrenal medulla.

Parasympathetic nervous system promotes 'rest and digest' response. Outflow is craniosacral with nerve fibres arising from cranial nerves III, VII, IX and X and sacral spinal nerves S2 to S4. In contrast to the SNS, parasympathetic ganglia lie on, or adjacent to, their target tissue. Therefore, myelinated preganglionic fibres possess long axons to synapse with postganglionic neurons near the end organ.

2.1.4

Base of skull

The base of the skull forms the floor of the cranial cavity. It is a complex anatomical region made up of the ethmoid, sphenoid, occipital, paired frontal and paired temporal bones and through which many important structures pass.

It is divided into three regions: the anterior, middle and posterior cranial fossae. The middle cranial fossa is further subdivided by the petro-occipital fissure into a central and two lateral components.

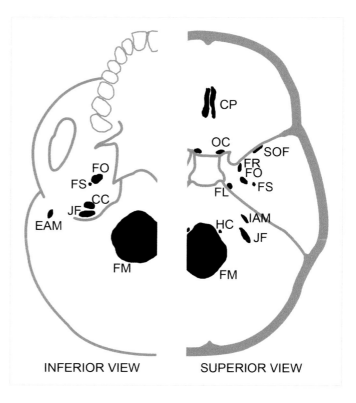

INFERIOR VIEW   SUPERIOR VIEW

Foramina	Structures passing through foramina
Anterior cranial fossa	
Cribriform plate (CP)	Olfactory nerves (CN I)
Middle cranial fossa	
Optic canal (OC)	Optic nerve (CN II)
Superior orbital fissure (SOF)	Ophthalmic nerve (CN V1), occulomotor nerve (CN III), trochlear nerve (CN IV), abducent nerve (CN VI)
Foramen rotundum (FR)	Maxillary nerve (CN V2)
Foramen lacerum (FL)/ carotid canal (CC)	Internal carotid artery
Foramen ovale (FO)	Mandibular nerve (CN V3)
Foramen spinosum (FS)	Middle meningeal artery
Internal acoustic meatus (IAM)	Facial nerve (CN VII)
Posterior cranial fossa	
Foramen magnum (FM)	Medulla, accessory nerve (CN XI), vertebral arteries, spinal arteries
Jugular foramen (JF)	Glossopharyngeal nerve (CN IX), vagus nerve (CN X) and spinal accessory nerve (CN XI), sigmoid sinus (to become internal jugular vein)
Hypoglossal canal (HC)	Hypoglossal nerve (CN XII)

Brachial plexus

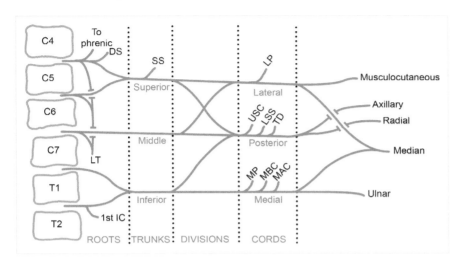

The brachial plexus is a network of nerves providing sensory and motor innervation to the upper limb. Subdivision is as follows.

- **Roots** – five roots arise from the anterior rami of spinal nerves C5 to T1 and lie in the interscalene groove. An interscalene approach may be performed to anaesthetize roots C5 to C7.
- **Trunks** – the roots merge to form three trunks that pass between the anterior and middle scalene muscles. The trunks may be anaesthetized via a supraclavicular approach.
- **Divisions** – as the trunks pass behind the clavicle, each splits into an anterior and posterior division. There are no nerve branches at this level.
- **Cords** – three cords lie in the axilla, named according to their relationship with the axillary artery. The posterior cord is formed from the three posterior divisions (C5–T1). The lateral cord is the anterior divisions from the upper and middle trunks (C5–C7). The medial cord is a continuation of the anterior division of the lower trunk (C8, T1).
- **Branches** – the terminal branches are the musculocutaneous, axillary, radial, median and ulnar nerves. These branches all contain both motor and sensory fibres. Located in the axilla, the radial, median and ulnar nerves may be anaesthetized via an axillary approach.

The brachial plexus can be injured during the perioperative period. Mechanisms include the excessive stretching of the plexus from poor patient positioning (especially arm abduction with external rotation), compression and direct trauma related to surgery or regional anaesthetic techniques.

Other nerves arising from the brachial plexus are:

LT – long thoracic
1st IC – first intercostal
DS – dorsal scapular
SS – suprascapular
LP – lateral pectoral
USS – upper subscapular
LSS – lower subscapular

TD – thoracodorsal
MP – medial pectoral
MBC – medial brachial cutaneous
    (aka medial cutaneous nerve of arm)
MAC – medial antebrachial cutaneous
    (aka medial cutaneous nerve of forearm)

2.1.6

Bronchial tree

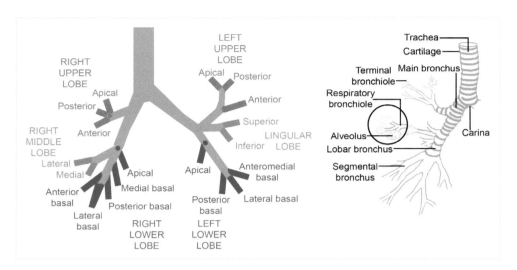

The trachea overlies the C6 to T4 vertebral bodies, bifurcating at the T5 level (carina). It is about 10 cm long in adults and 'D' shaped, being reinforced by 'C' shaped cartilages anteriorly. The trachealis muscle runs down the posterior border and is useful for orientation during bronchoscopy.

The right main bronchus is wider and shorter than the left, measuring about 3 cm in adults. It enters the right lung at approximately T5 and splits into three secondary, or lobar, bronchi which communicate with the three lobes of the right lung. The right upper lobe branch comes off after about 2 cm; again, a useful landmark during bronchoscopy. The left main bronchus is smaller, longer and more horizontal than the right, measuring about 5 cm in adults. It enters the left lung at the level of approximately T6 and divides into two lobar bronchi communicating with the two lobes of the left lung (the lingular 'lobe', is a tongue-like projection from the upper lobe and may be the evolutionary remnant of the middle lobe).

The lobar bronchi further subdivide into tertiary, or segmental, bronchi which supply the bronchopulmonary segments. These are divisions that are separated from the rest of the lung by septa, allowing surgical removal without affecting other segments. The segmental bronchi divide into bronchioles, then terminal bronchioles that become respiratory bronchioles, alveolar ducts and sacs. Hyaline cartilage is present in the bronchi, with the amount decreasing until it disappears at the bronchiole level. Smooth muscle is present continuously around the bronchi, increasing in amount as the cartilage decreases.

Sympathetic and parasympathetic nerve supply comes from the cardiac plexus (T2–4) and vagus nerve, respectively. Blood supply to the bronchi comes from bronchial arteries (from the aorta) and intercostal arteries. They contribute to true, or anatomical, shunt along with the Thebesian veins of the heart.

Cardiac vessels – cardiac veins

Venous drainage from the myocardium is via the coronary veins. Blood is collected in venules that join together to form the coronary veins which roughly follow the path of the coronary arteries. They eventually join to form the coronary sinus located on the posterior aspect of the heart. This drains into the right atrium between the opening of the inferior vena cava and the tricuspid valve. The opening has a protective endothelial fold called the semilunar valve of the coronary sinus.

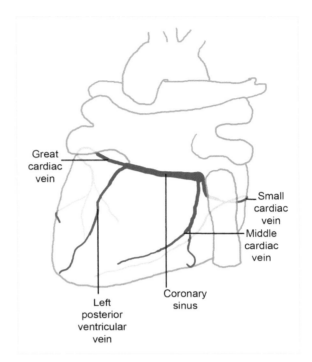

Tributaries of the coronary sinus include the:

- **great cardiac vein** – runs from the apex of the myocardium in the anterior interventricular septum with the LAD artery and drains the areas of the heart supplied by the left coronary artery
- **middle cardiac vein** – runs with the posterior descending artery in the posterior interventricular groove and drains the area of the myocardium supplied by the posterior descending artery
- **small cardiac vein** – runs in the posterior atrioventricular groove and drains blood from the posterior part of the right atrium and ventricle
- **oblique vein** – descends across and drains blood from the left atrium.

There are other veins that drain directly into the right atrium, independent of the coronary sinus. The anterior cardiac veins of the right ventricle are small veins that arise on the anterior surface of the right ventricle, cross the coronary sulcus and enter the anterior wall of the right atrium.

The Thebesian veins are the smallest of the cardiac veins. They drain the myocardium and pass through the endocardial layer to empty directly into the cardiac chambers and contribute to true, or anatomical, shunt.

2.1.8

Cardiac vessels – coronary arteries

The right and left coronary arteries supply blood to the myocardium and originate at the base of the aorta from openings located behind the aortic valve leaflets; the coronary ostia. Conversely, the innermost endocardium receives its blood supply directly from the blood within the chambers.

The right coronary artery arises from the anterior, or right, aortic sinus and runs between the pulmonary trunk and auricle of the right atrium. It descends in the right atrioventricular groove and then interventricular groove on the posterior aspect of the heart. It divides into the right marginal and posterior descending, or interventricular, arteries. It supplies the:

- sinoatrial node in 60% of people
- atrioventricular node in 80% of people
- right atrium, most of the right ventricle and the diaphragmatic surface of the left ventricle
- posterior third of the septum.

The left coronary artery arises from the left posterior aortic sinus and runs in the coronary groove between the pulmonary trunk and auricle of the left atrium. It branches into the left circumflex and left anterior descending (LAD), or interventricular, arteries. The LAD artery anastomoses with the posterior descending branches of the right coronary artery. It supplies the:

- left atrium
- majority of the left ventricle
- anterior two-thirds of the septum
- sinoatrial node in 40% of people (from the circumflex artery).

Coronary artery	Anatomical region supplied	ECG pattern
Left anterior descending	Anteroseptal	V1–V4
Left circumflex	Anterolateral	I, aVL, V5–V6
Left anterior descending	Septal	V1–V2
Left circumflex	Lateral	V5–V6, aVL
Right posterior descending	Inferior	II, III, aVF
Right coronary	Posterior	V1–V4 (reciprocal changes)

Although there are anatomical variations, the table indicates the regions of the heart that are supplied by the coronary arteries and therefore the ECG patterns that may be seen with disease in these vessels.

Circle of Willis

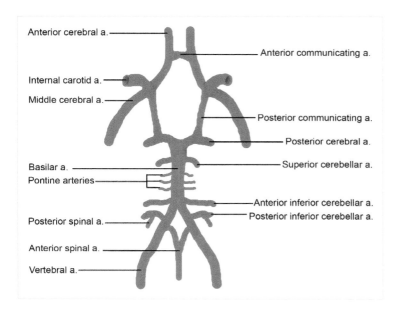

The circle of Willis is a circulatory anastomosis delivering arterial blood to the brain. Two-thirds of the cerebral arterial blood is provided via the internal carotid artery (ICA), with the remaining one-third via the vertebral arteries. The circle of Willis creates collateral circulation between these vascular structures in an attempt to preserve cerebral perfusion, even in the setting of vascular occlusion. The following vessels comprise the arterial circle.

- Internal carotid artery (paired) – arising from the common carotid arteries, the ICAs enter the cranium via the carotid canal.
- Anterior cerebral artery (ACA; paired) – one of the terminal branches of the ICA. Supply blood to the superior/medial portions of the parietal lobe and the medial portion of the frontal lobe.
- Anterior communicating artery (ACOM; unpaired) – this small artery joins the right and left ACAs.
- Posterior cerebral artery (PCA; paired) – these vessels arise from bifurcation of the basilar artery which, in turn, is formed by the union of the two vertebral arteries. The PCAs provide blood supply to the occipital lobes and medial temporal lobes.
- Posterior communicating artery (PCOM; paired) – a branch of the ICA, these vessels join the PCAs to the ICAs.

The middle cerebral arteries (MCAs), also terminal branches of the ICA, are technically not part of the circle of Willis. These bilateral vessels supply most of the lateral cerebral cortex.

Rupture of an intracranial aneurysm is the most common aetiology of non-traumatic subarachnoid haemorrhage. Aneurysms frequently develop at vascular bifurcations within the circle of Willis. Approximately 70% of lesions arise in the anterior circulation:

- junction of ACA and ACOM – 30–40%
- junction of ICA and PCOM – 30%.

Other sites of intracranial aneurysm development include:

- MCA – 20–30%
- posterior circulation (basilar tip, superior and posterior inferior cerebellar arteries) – 10%.

2.1.10

Cranial nerves

Cranial nerve	Fibres	Structures innervated	Functions
I. Olfactory	Sensory	Olfactory mucosa	Olfaction
II. Optic	Sensory	Retina	Vision
III. Oculomotor	Motor	Superior/middle/inferior rectus, inferior oblique, levator palpebrae	Eye movement
	PNS	Pupillary constrictor, ciliary muscle	Pupillary constriction and accommodation
IV. Trochlear	Motor	Superior oblique	Movement of eye
V. Trigeminal	Sensory	Face, scalp, cornea, nasal and orbital cavities, anterior dura mater	General sensation
V1 - Ophthalmic	Motor	Mastication muscles	Opening, closing mouth
V2 - Maxillary		Tensor tympani muscle	Tension tympanic membrane
V3 - Mandibular			
VI. Abducens	Motor	Lateral rectus	Eye movement
VII. Facial	Sensory	Anterior 2/3 tongue	Taste
	Motor	Muscles of facial expression	Facial movement
		Stapedius muscle	Tension of ossicles
	PNS	Salivary and lacrimal glands	Salivation, lacrimation
VIII. Vestibulo-cochlear	Sensory	Cochlea	Hearing
		Vestibular apparatus	Head proprioception, balance
IX. Glosso-pharyngeal	Sensory	Eustachian tube, middle ear	General sensation
		Carotid body and sinus	Chemo/baroreceptors
		Pharynx, posterior 1/3 tongue	Taste
	Motor	Stylopharyngeus	Swallowing
	PNS	Salivary glands	Salivation
X. Vagus	Sensory	Pharynx, larynx, oesophagus, external ear	General sensation
		Aortic bodies and arch	Chemo/baroreceptors
		Thoracic and abdominal viscera	Visceral sensation
	Motor	Soft palate, larynx, pharynx, upper oesophagus	Speech, swallowing
	PNS	CV, respiratory and GI systems	Control of these systems
XI. Accessory	Motor	Sternomastoid, trapezius	Movement of head and shoulders
XII. Hypoglossal	Motor	Muscles of tongue	Movement of tongue

PNS – parasympathetic nervous system, CV – cardiovascular, GI – gastrointestinal.

The cranial nerves are 12 paired nerves numbered according to their attachments to the brain in a rostral–caudal direction. All, with the exception of the optic nerve, comprise part of the PNS. The optic nerve is considered part of the CNS due to its embryonic development. The olfactory and optic nerves emerge directly from the brain with the remaining 10 pairs originating from the brainstem. All cranial nerves innervate structures within the head and neck with the exception of the vagus nerve, which also supplies structures in the thorax and abdomen. The cranial nerves may be classified as motor (efferent), sensory (afferent) or mixed, with some containing parasympathetic axons (see table above).

Cross-section of neck at C6

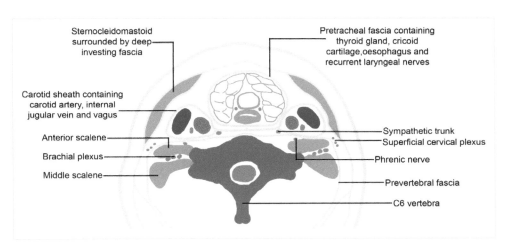

The cross-section demonstrates the relationship of many of the important structures that are found in the neck at this level. Areas of interest to anaesthetists include the following.

- Cricoid cartilage – signet ring shaped, with the narrow portion at the front. It slopes posteriorly and seats the arytenoid cartilages.
- Carotid sheath – a tube of neck fascia running from the base of the skull to the root of the neck. It contains the carotid artery, internal jugular vein and vagus nerve.
- Scalene muscles and brachial plexus – the anterior scalene originates from C3–5 and inserts onto the first rib. The phrenic nerve runs over it and the subclavian vein lies anterior to it. The interscalene groove, between the anterior and middle scalenes, contains the subclavian artery and brachial plexus.
- Cervical plexus – originates from the anterior rami of C2–4 and emerges from the posterior border of sternocleidomastoid. Supplies sensation to the front and sides of the neck.
- Sympathetic trunk/chain – the cervical chain ganglia lie between the prevertebral fascia and carotid sheath. The middle cervical ganglion lies at the level of the C6 vertebral body.

The stellate ganglion is a fusion of the inferior cervical and T1 ganglion providing sympathetic supply to the head, neck and upper limb. It lies anterior to the neck of the first rib at the level of C7. A stellate ganglion block can be performed for pain syndromes (such as complex regional pain syndromes I and II, refractory angina and herpes zoster) or for vascular insufficiency (such as Raynaud's syndrome, scleroderma, obliterative vascular disease and trauma). It is usually performed at the C6 tubercle (Chassaignac's), avoiding the vertebral artery at C7 and the dome of the pleura. Successful blockade will produce a picture similar to Horner's syndrome (pupillary constriction, partial ptosis and anhydrosis).

2.1.12

Cross-section of spinal cord

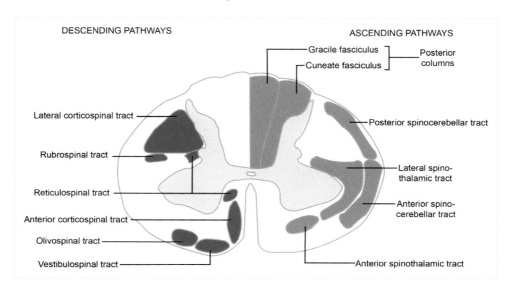

The spinal cord extends from the foramen magnum to terminate, in adults, at the level of the first or second lumbar vertebrae as the conus medullaris. Below this level the filum terminale continues to attach to the coccyx, providing longitudinal support to the cord.

A cross-section of the spinal cord demonstrates butterfly-shaped grey matter (nerve cell bodies) surrounded by white matter (nerve fibres) peripherally. A small central canal runs the length of the cord, continuous with the fourth ventricle of the brain. Although similar structures are present at all spinal cord levels, regional differences exist; grey matter contour varies and white matter volume reduces distally through the cord. The spinal cord contains ascending sensory tracts and descending motor tracts.

Ascending

- Cuneate and gracile fasciculus lie in the posterior white column and transmit fine touch and proprioceptive information to the sensory cortex on the opposite side of the body. The crossover occurs in the medulla after synapsing with the cuneate and gracile nuclei.
- Two spinothalamic tracts, anterior and lateral, transmit sensory information to the contralateral thalamus with crossover occurring in the cord at the level of entry. The anterior tract conveys crude touch and pressure, the lateral tract conveys pain and temperature sensation.
- Two spinocerebellar tracts, anterior and posterior, transmit proprioceptive sensation to the ipsilateral cerebellum without crossover.

Descending

- Two corticospinal tracts, anterior and lateral, facilitate conscious control of skeletal muscle. The lateral tract, the major motor pathway, arises in the pyramidal cells of the motor cortex to cross in the medulla and descend in the contralateral pyramidal tract. The anterior tract, lying near the anterior median fissure, descends from the motor cortex with fibres crossing at each segmental level.
- The remaining motor tracts facilitate subconscious regulation of balance, position and muscle tone.

2.1.13

Dermatomes

A dermatome is an area of skin that is innervated by sensory fibres from a single spinal nerve. There are 31 paired dermatomal segments consisting of 8 cervical, 12 thoracic, 5 lumbar, 5 sacral and 1 coccygeal. The sensory nerve fibres to the spinal nerve root of a specific vertebra transmit sensory information from each dermatome.

The dermatomes are stacked like discs along the thorax and abdomen and then run longitudinally along the arms and legs. There may be significant overlap between dermatomes and individuals display variable anatomy.

Important dermatomes and anatomical landmarks are as follows.

- C6 – dorsal surface of proximal phalanx of thumb.
- C7 – dorsal surface of proximal phalanx of middle finger.
- T4 – level of the nipples.
- T6 – level of the xiphoid process.
- T10 – level of the umbilicus.
- L4 – anterior aspect of knee (L3 in some texts).
- L5 – heel (S1 in some texts).
- S1 – lateral aspect of the foot.
- S4/5 – perineum.

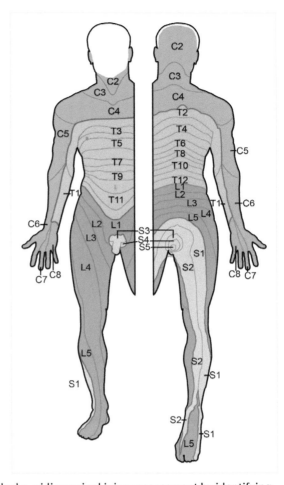

Dermatomes are useful in assessing nerve blocks, aiding spinal injury assessment by identifying neurological sensory levels and in referred pain.

2.1.14

Diaphragm

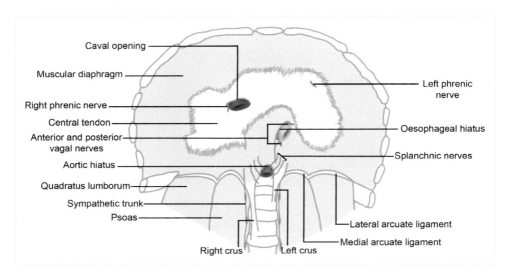

Caval opening

Muscular diaphragm

Right phrenic nerve

Central tendon

Anterior and posterior vagal nerves

Aortic hiatus

Quadratus lumborum

Sympathetic trunk

Psoas

Left phrenic nerve

Oesophageal hiatus

Splanchnic nerves

Lateral arcuate ligament

Medial arcuate ligament

Right crus   Left crus

The diaphragm is a dome-shaped musculotendinous septum located between the thorax and abdomen.

Peripheral muscle – radial muscle fibres originate anteriorly from the xiphoid process, laterally from the inferior six ribs and posteriorly from the arcuate ligaments and lumbar vertebrae. The medial and lateral arcuate ligaments are tendinous structures that fuse with fascia of the psoas and quadratus lumborum muscles, respectively. The diaphragm is attached to the vertebral column via the right and left crura. The crura are musculotendinous bundles arising from the anterior surfaces of the lumbar vertebrae (right crus from L1 to L3, left crus from L1 to L2). The crura unite centrally to form the median arcuate ligament.

Central tendon – this thin but strong aponeurosis has a trefoil leaf shape, functioning as an insertion point for the muscular portion of the diaphragm.

A number of diaphragmatic openings permit passage of structures between the thorax and abdomen. The caval opening (level of T8), in the central tendon, transmits the inferior vena cava and right phrenic nerve. The oesophageal hiatus (level of T10) conveys the oesophagus, vagus nerves and left gastric vessel. Located within the muscle of the right crus, this aperture forms an anatomical sphincter preventing reflux of gastric contents when intra-abdominal pressure increases during inspiration. Through the aortic hiatus (level of T12) pass the aorta, azygos vein and thoracic duct. This opening is located behind the arch formed by the union of the crura. As such, blood flow through the aorta is not affected by muscular diaphragmatic contractions.

Motor innervation of the diaphragm is exclusively via the right and left phrenic nerves, formed from the anterior rami of spinal nerves C3–5. Sensory innervation is largely via the phrenic nerves with input to peripheral portions of intercostal nerves T5–12.

2.1.15

Epidural space

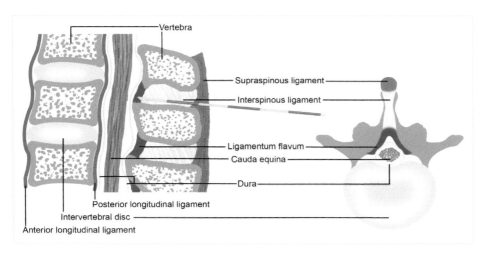

The epidural space extends from the foramen magnum to the sacral hiatus. It surrounds the dural sac (i.e. is the extradural space) within the vertebral canal and contains:
- spinal nerve roots
- venous plexus (of Batson)
- connective tissue
- lymphatics
- fat.

The veins drain into the azygous system and then into the inferior vena cava. Being valveless they distend with increased intra-abdominal pressure, e.g. pregnancy and prone position; the risk of inadvertent intravascular injection of epidural solution is therefore increased.

When performing an epidural, the needle passes through (in order) skin, subcutaneous tissue, supraspinous ligament, interspinous ligament and ligamentum flavum. The ligaments have no sensory supply and can be pierced painlessly during insertion. The epidural space is a potential space and a loss of resistance technique is used to identify the correct position.

The space is widest posteriorly and can have divided folds of dura mater creating compartments that do not always communicate. This can lead to a patchy or unpredictable block. The subdural space is a thin potential space between the dura and arachnoid mater and can be inadvertently entered when attempting epidural placement; local anaesthetic injected into this space can cause an unexpectedly extensive block. Although the epidural space ends superiorly at the foramen magnum, this cannot be relied upon. Inadvertent passage of drugs into the cranial cavity causing a 'total spinal' block is possible.

An effective epidural after surgery requires knowledge of how the surface anatomy relates to the vertebral canal and the arrangement of the dermatomes supplied by the nerves. Useful surface anatomy for identifying corresponding levels of the vertebral bodies include:
- inferior angle of the scapula (T7)
- lower rib margin (T10)
- intercristal (Touffier's) line at the highest points of the iliac crests (L3/4)
- posterior superior iliac spines (S2).

2.1.16
Femoral triangle

Borders
- Superior: inguinal ligament – extends from the anterior superior iliac spine (ASIS) to the pubic tubercle.
- Medial: medial border of adductor longus.
- Lateral: medial border of sartorius.
- Floor: adductor longus, pectineus, psoas and iliacus muscles.
- Roof: fat, fascia lata, subcutaneous tissue and skin.

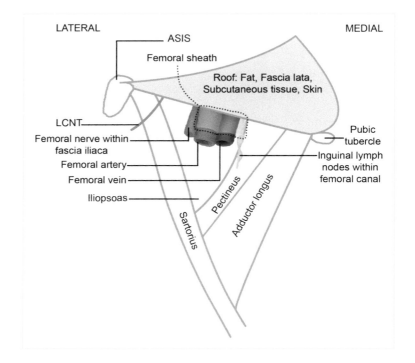

Contents
- Femoral sheath: continuation of extraperitoneal fascia; contains the femoral artery, femoral vein and inguinal lymph nodes.
- Femoral nerve: lies within fascia iliaca.
- Lateral cutaneous nerve of the thigh (LCNT).

Femoral nerve blockade
Research has demonstrated a reduction in systemic opioid requirements in patients receiving femoral nerve blockade (FNB) as adjuvant analgesia. The femoral nerve may be blocked by performing a lumbar plexus block, '3 in 1' technique or fascia iliaca compartment block (FICB).
- **Indications**: peri-operative analgesia for patients with hip fracture, post-operative analgesia for hip and knee surgery, surgical anaesthesia (often in combination with sciatic nerve blockade).
- **Lumbar plexus blockade**: blocks the femoral nerve, obturator nerve and LCNT as they run within the psoas muscle. This block is performed using a landmark approach. It has the potential for serious complications such as fatal haemorrhage, epidural/spinal spread of local anaesthesia and local anaesthetic toxicity (as plexus lies within a large muscle bed).
- **'3 in 1' and FICB**: in principle, both techniques block the femoral nerve, obturator nerve and LCNT, although the LCNT may be missed using the '3 in 1' approach. Landmark and ultrasound techniques may be employed for either technique. The point of injection for the FICB is more lateral to ensure injection into this potential space. Both approaches are easy to perform and associated with infrequent and relatively minor complications.

Intercostal space

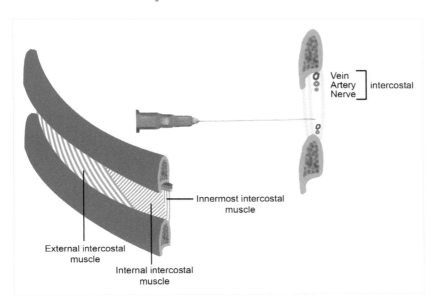

There are 11 intercostal spaces, each named by the rib above, containing:
- muscles – external, internal and innermost
- intercostal arteries and veins
- intercostal nerves
- lymph nodes.

The muscles run between the ribs and are involved in the mechanics of ventilation:
- **External intercostals** – originate on ribs 1–11 and insert onto 2–12, passing forwards and downwards. Elevate the ribs and expand the transverse dimension of the chest. Aid quiet and forced inhalation.
- **Internal intercostals** – originate on ribs 2–12 and insert onto 1–11. Run in the opposite direction to the externals, i.e. forward and upwards. Pull the ribs inwards and reduce the diameter of the chest. Aid forced expiration (quiet expiration is passive).
- **Innermost intercostals** – a layer of muscles, comprising the transversus thoracis anteriorly, lateral muscle slips laterally and subcostalis posteriorly.

The neurovascular bundle (from above, downward; vein, artery, nerve – VAN) runs high in the space between the internal and innermost muscles, protected by the rib above in the costal groove. A collateral bundle may also be found just superior to the rib below. The nerves arise from the anterior rami of T1–T11 and have various branches. The T12 nerve runs forward in the abdominal wall as the subcostal nerve, communicating with either the 1st lumbar or iliohypogastric nerve.

An intercostal nerve block can provide anaesthesia and analgesia for thoracic and high abdominal procedures, chest drain insertion and fractured ribs. The needle insertion point is at the angle of the rib (about 6–8 cm lateral to the midline of the back) at the desired level. It is inserted directly above the lower rib, avoiding the neurovascular bundle, and 'walked off' the edge of the rib, then advanced another 2–5 mm with aspiration; 2–5 ml of local anaesthetic is injected per space. Risks include pneumothorax and local anaesthetic toxicity.

2.1.18

Internal jugular vein

The internal jugular vein originates as a continuation of the sigmoid sinus as it exits the skull at the jugular foramen. It takes a straight course in the neck before joining the subclavian vein behind the sternoclavicular joint.

It is found in the carotid sheath alongside the internal carotid artery and vagus nerve, initially being superficial in the upper part of the neck and then running deep to the sternocleidomastoid (SCM) muscle. Within the sheath, the relationship of the vein to artery changes

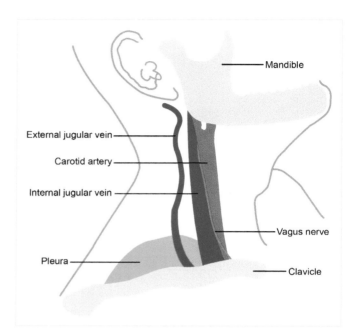

as it travels down the neck; the vein initially being posterior to the artery, moving lateral and then anterolateral in the lower part of the neck. However, there exists a degree of inter-patient variability.

The internal jugular vein is a common site for central venous cannulation due to its accessibility and safety profile. Important relations to be aware of are:
- anterior – internal carotid artery, external jugular vein, vagus nerve, SCM and platysma muscles
- posterior – sympathetic chain, dome of the pleura, thoracic duct (left)
- medial – carotid arteries, cranial nerves IX–XII.

An ultrasound-guided technique is advised when performing central venous cannulation, however, awareness of the landmark technique is important. One approach is to insert the needle in the centre of a triangle formed by the two lower heads of the SCM muscle and clavicle at approximately the level of the thyroid cartilage (C4). The carotid artery should be palpated and the needle guided lateral to this, aiming caudally and towards the ipsilateral nipple. Complications include:
- pneumothorax/haemothorax
- air embolism
- carotid artery cannulation
- infection
- arrhythmias (from the guidewire irritating the right atrium)
- chylothorax (left only as the thoracic duct that drains lymph from the majority of the body empties into the junction of the left subclavian and jugular veins).

Laryngeal innervation

Recurrent laryngeal nerve injury	Phonation	Vocal cord position
Unilateral nerve damage	Hoarseness	Ipsilateral vocal cord paralysis, affected vocal cord drawn inwards
Bilateral nerve damage	Airway closure	Vocal cords overlap due to unopposed adduction
Nerve transection – unilateral/bilateral	Whisper	Cadaveric position of vocal cord(s) – partially abducted (open)

Motor and sensory innervation to the larynx is via two paired branches of the vagus nerve.
- **Superficial laryngeal nerves** (SLNs) – descend lateral to the pharynx and divide into internal and external branches at the level of the hyoid bone. The external laryngeal nerve provides motor innervation to the cricothyroid muscle. The internal laryngeal nerve provides sensory innervation to the laryngeal cavity above the vocal cords and to the inferior epiglottic surface.
- **Recurrent laryngeal nerves** (RLN) – supply motor innervation to all the intrinsic muscles of the larynx, with the exception of cricothyroid, as well as sensation to the larynx below the vocal cords. The right RLN originates in the root of the neck, enters the thorax and loops beneath the subclavian artery. The left RLN originates in the thorax and passes beneath the aorta. Both nerves ascend in the tracheo-oesophageal groove and enter the larynx posteriorly.

Injuries to laryngeal nerves

Laryngeal nerve damage may be caused by inadvertent injury during surgery (e.g. thyroidectomy or thoracic surgery), tumours of the skull base, neck and chest, viral infections or following endotracheal intubation.

Injury to the SLN results in hoarseness due to paralysis of the cricothyroid muscle. If injury is unilateral, the functioning cricothyroid muscle will compensate returning the voice quality to normal with time. Bilateral injury results in permanent hoarseness.

Injury to the RLN is more complex because this nerve innervates the muscles responsible for opening and closing the laryngeal inlet. Partial paralysis affects the abductor muscles more than the adductors. As a result, the corresponding vocal cord is drawn inwards due to unopposed adduction. This has significant clinical implications with bilateral nerve injury because the airway may become completely obstructed.

2.1.20

Larynx

The larynx is a functional sphincter of the respiratory tract with a primary function of protecting the tracheobronchial tree and lungs from foreign bodies. Other functions include sound production (phonation), coughing, straining and modification of respiration. The larynx is located in the anterior neck, extending from the base of tongue to the cricoid cartilage.

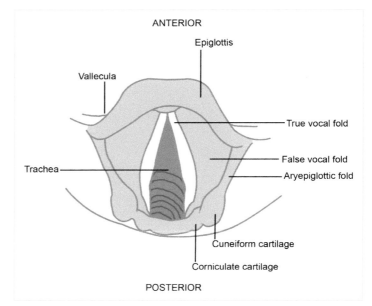

ANTERIOR

Epiglottis

Vallecula

True vocal fold

False vocal fold

Trachea

Aryepiglottic fold

Cuneiform cartilage

Corniculate cartilage

POSTERIOR

Cartilages – the larynx comprises three large, unpaired cartilages (thyroid, epiglottic and cricoid) and three small, paired cartilages (arytenoid, corniculate and cuneiform). The hyoid bone is, technically, not part of the larynx but provides muscular attachments to aid laryngeal movement.

Ligaments – intrinsic ligaments serve to connect cartilages within the larynx to each other.
- The cricothyroid ligament attaches the cricoid cartilage to the anterior thyroid cartilage and ends, superiorly, as a free upper margin. This free upper margin thickens, joining the thyroid and arytenoid cartilages, to form the vocal ligament (within the true vocal cord).
- The upper border of the quadrangular membrane joins the lateral epiglottis with the arytenoid and corniculate cartilages, forming the aryepiglottic fold. The free lower margin of this ligament thickens to form the vestibular ligament (within the false vocal cord).
- Extrinsic ligaments serve to connect laryngeal cartilages with surrounding structures and include the thyrohyoid, hyoepiglottic and cricotracheal ligaments.

Muscles – intrinsic muscles adjust the tension, length, shape and spatial positioning of the vocal folds. There are two tensor muscles, the cricothyroid and vocalis. Contraction of the cricothyroid muscle results in elongation and increased tension of the vocal cords, producing higher pitch phonation. The posterior cricoarytenoid muscle is the vocal fold adductor. There are three abductor muscles, the lateral cricoarytenoids, thyroarytenoid and interarytenoid muscles. The thyroarytenoid muscle consists of two parts: the vocalis, which acts as an antagonist to the cricothyroid muscle, and a lateral portion which adducts and lengthens the vocal cord.

2.1.21
Limb muscle innervation (myotomes)

Spinal level	Myotome
C5	Shoulder abductors (deltoid) and elbow flexors (mainly biceps)
C6	Wrist extensors (extensor carpi radialis longus and brevis)
C7	Elbow extensors (triceps)
C8	Finger flexors (flexor digitorum profundus)
T1	Hand intrinsic (interossei)
L2	Hip flexors (iliopsoas)
L3	Knee extensors (quadriceps)
L4	Ankle dorsiflexors (tibialis anterior)
L5	Long toe extensors (extensor hallucis longus)
S1	Ankle plantar flexors (gastrocnemius, soleus)
S2	Knee flexors (hamstrings)
S4	Perianal reflex (anal wink – external anal sphincter)

A myotome is a group of muscles that are innervated by the motor fibres of a single spinal nerve root and could be thought of as the motor equivalent of a dermatome (see *Section 2.1.13 – Dermatomes*). Like dermatomes, there is a degree of anatomical variability. In embryology, it is the portion of the somite (bilateral paired segments of paraxial mesoderm) that develops into muscle tissue.

During neurological testing, the passive and resistive strength in various myotomes can indicate the spinal level of pathology. Muscle strength can be graded using the Medical Research Council Scale for Muscle Strength. It is graded from 0 to 5:
  0 – no muscle contraction is visible
  1 – muscle contraction is visible but there is no movement of the joint
  2 – active joint movement is possible with gravity eliminated
  3 – movement can overcome gravity but not added resistance
  4 – movement can overcome gravity and some added resistance
  5 – full and normal power against resistance.

2.1.22

Lumbar plexus

The lumbar plexus comprises intersecting nerves originating from the anterior rami of spinal nerve roots L1–4 with a variable contribution from T12. The plexus forms within the psoas muscle.

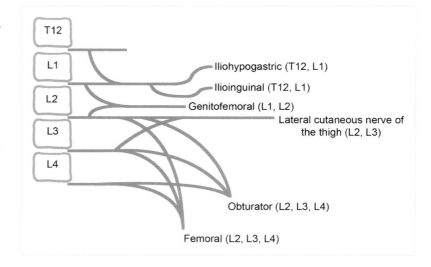

T12

L1 — Iliohypogastric (T12, L1)

L2 — Ilioinguinal (T12, L1)

Genitofemoral (L1, L2)

L3 — Lateral cutaneous nerve of the thigh (L2, L3)

L4

Obturator (L2, L3, L4)

Femoral (L2, L3, L4)

Iliohypogastric nerve – emerges from the lateral psoas border and perforates the transversus abdominis muscle near the iliac crest to lie within the transversus abdominis plane. Sensory branches supply the suprapubic skin and posterolateral gluteal region.

Ilioinguinal nerve – emerges from the psoas just below the iliohypogastric nerve, following the same course to the transversus abdominis plane. The nerve pierces the internal oblique muscle to accompany the spermatic cord through the superficial inguinal ring to provide sensation to the superomedial thigh and genitals.

Genitofemoral nerve – emerges medially and divides into genital and femoral branches. The genital branch enters the inguinal canal via the deep ring. Accompanying the spermatic cord to the scrotum, this branch supplies motor innervation to the cremaster muscle and sensation to scrotal skin (this branch is lost upon the round ligament in females). The femoral branch provides sensation to skin overlying the femoral triangle.

Lateral cutaneous nerve of the thigh – emerges laterally to lie on the iliacus muscle. Passing deep to the inguinal ligament, this branch provides sensation to the skin of the lateral thigh.

Obturator nerve – emerges from the medial border of psoas near the pelvic brim. It enters the thigh via the obturator foramen, supplying a motor branch to obturator externus (hip stabilizer and lateral rotator). Further branches supply motor innervation to the thigh adductors and sensation to skin of the medial thigh.

Femoral nerve – the largest terminal branch, emerging laterally to lie between the psoas and iliacus. Travelling beneath the inguinal ligament, the nerve divides into numerous sensory (anterior thigh, medial lower leg) and motor (quadriceps) branches.

Nose

The nose consists of the external nose and pyramidal nasal cavity that extends from the anterior nares to the choanae at the posterior septum. Squamous epithelium line the cavity anteriorly, becoming columnar ciliated epithelium with abundant seromucinous glands as you move

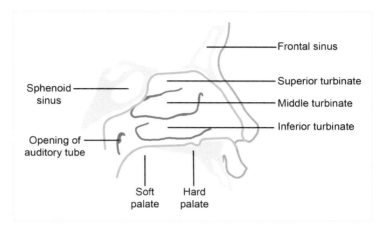

posteriorly. Superior, middle and inferior turbinates or concha exist on the lateral walls of the nostrils with corresponding passages, the superior, middle and inferior meatus, through which various sinuses and ducts drain.

Nasal cavity boundaries
- Floor – hard palate (anterior – maxilla, posterior – palatine).
- Roof – sphenoid and ethmoid (cribriform plate).
- Medial wall – septum (paired nasal, maxillary and palatine bones, unpaired ethmoid and vomer bones, septal and greater alar cartilages).
- Lateral wall – medial orbit, ethmoid air cells, maxillary sinus.

Superiorly, the external skeleton is formed by the nasal and maxillary bones. Inferiorly it consists mainly of cartilages: the lateral, major and minor alar and the cartilaginous septum.

Nasal cavity blood supply
- Predominantly from branches of the maxillary artery (from the external carotid).
- Sphenopalatine artery being the most important.
- Anastomoses with the superior labial branch of the facial artery; a common site of epistaxis.
- Veins principally follow the arterial pattern, draining into the cavernous sinus. There is potential risk for intracranial spread of infection.

Nasal cavity nerve supply
- Branches of the ophthalmic and maxillary divisions of the trigeminal nerve.
- Anteriorly supplied by the anterior ethmoid nerve (branch of ophthalmic).
- Posteriorly supplied by the nasal, nasopalatine and palatine branches of the pterygopalatine ganglion (branch of maxillary).
- Parasympathetic supply to the lacrimal gland and glands of the nose and palate come from the pterygopalatine ganglion.
- Olfactory nerves arise from the olfactory mucus membrane that lines the superior turbinate and spheno-ethmoidal recess. They pass through the cribriform plate to the olfactory bulb.

2.1.24

Orbit

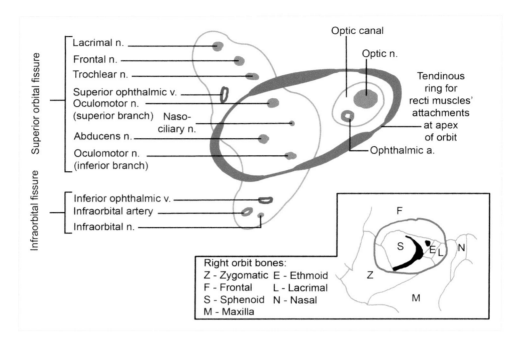

The orbits are bony cavities occupied by the eyes and associated structures. Each orbit is roughly shaped as a quadrilateral pyramid, the apex contains the optic canal and the base lies in plane with the orbital rim. The orbit is composed of seven main bones.
- Roof: frontal bone and lesser wing of the sphenoid.
- Medial wall: ethmoid bone, lacrimal bone, maxillary bone and lesser wing of the sphenoid.
- Floor: sphenoid and maxillary bones. A minute orbital process of palatine bone lies between the maxillary and ethmoid bones, although this is of little importance to the structure of the orbit (and not shown in diagram).
- Lateral wall: zygoma and greater wing of the sphenoid.

The nerves and blood vessels to the orbit and globe enter via three posterior openings:
- **Superior orbital fissure** – a bony cleft bound by the greater and lesser wings of the sphenoid. This fissure serves as a conduit for cranial nerves (CN) III, IV, V and VI. The oculomotor nerve (CN III) divides into superior and inferior branches prior to entering the orbit. These branches innervate the majority of extraocular muscles (see *Section 2.1.10 – Cranial nerves*). The trochlear nerve (CN IV) supplies the superior oblique extraocular muscle. The ophthalmic division of the trigeminal nerve (CN V_1) divides into three small sensory branches: the lacrimal, frontal and nasocillary nerves which supply the lacrimal gland, conjunctiva, upper eyelid, forehead, globe and lateral nose. The abducens nerve (CN VI) innervates the lateral rectus extraocular muscle. The superior ophthalmic vein is the only vascular structure to pass through the superior orbital fissure.
- **Inferior orbital fissure** – separates the lateral wall from the floor of the orbit. Through this cleft pass two branches of the maxillary nerve (CN V_2), the zygomatic and infraorbital nerves. The infraorbital artery and inferior ophthalmic vein also pass through this fissure.
- **Optic canal** – lies at the apex of the orbit within the sphenoid bone, transmitting the optic nerve and ophthalmic artery.

Rib

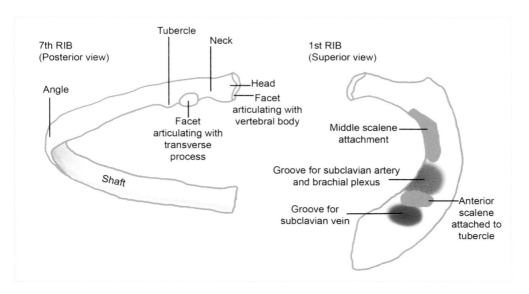

The human body has 12 pairs of ribs. They are long curved bones that serve to protect the vital organs of the thoracic and upper abdominal cavities and have an important role in the mechanics of breathing. The first 7 ribs (1–7) are known as 'true ribs' because they attach directly to the sternum. The following five sets are sometimes known as 'false ribs': ribs 8–10 have a common cartilaginous attachment to the sternum and the last two (11–12) are floating.

The main structures of a typical rib are as follows.
- Head – articulates with corresponding vertebral body.
- Neck – between the tubercle and the head.
- Angle – beginning of the anterior curve.
- Shaft – contains an inferior costal groove in which the neurovascular bundle runs (see *Section 2.1.17 – Intercostal space*).

The first rib is unique in its structure because it is shorter, flatter and more C-shaped than the others. It forms the lateral boundary of the thoracic inlet (see *Section 2.1.29 – Thoracic inlet and first rib*) and attaches to the T1 vertebra posteriorly and the sternum anteriorly.

The ribs tend to increase in length from rib 1 to 7 and then decrease again through to rib 12. Their angles change so that ribs 1–9 become progressively more oblique and then become less so by rib 12. Rib movement contributes to respiration by increasing the diameter and volume of the thoracic cavity. The lateral diameter of the chest is increased due to movement of the posterior ends of the ribs on the transverse processes of the vertebrae. The anteroposterior diameter is increased due to movement of the anterior ends of the ribs moving up and out (often described as a bucket handle movement). Rib movement contributes approximately 25% to the increase in thoracic volume during respiration while diaphragmatic movement contributes approximately 75%.

2.1.26

Sacral plexus

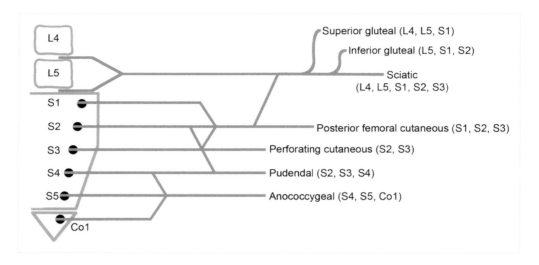

The sacral plexus, lying between the pelvic fascia and piriformis, is derived from the lumbosacral trunk (L4–5) and anterior rami of spinal nerves S1–4. These nerves unite, forming a flattened band near the greater sciatic foramen. All branches of the sacral plexus exit the pelvis via this foramen.

- Superior gluteal nerve – supplies motor function to gluteus medius, gluteus minimus and tensor fasciae latae muscles.
- Inferior gluteal nerve – innervates the gluteus maximus muscle.
- Sciatic nerve – supplies nearly the whole of the skin of the leg and muscles of the lower leg, foot and posterior thigh. Descending between the femoral greater trochanter and ischial tuberosity, the sciatic nerve continues within the posterior compartment of the thigh to divide into two large branches; the tibial and common fibula (peroneal) nerves. Division occurs approximately 6–7 cm proximal to the posterior knee crease, although anatomic variability is common.
  - o The tibial nerve and its branches provide motor innervation to flexor muscles of the lower leg and foot. A cutaneous branch joins the fibula anastomotic branch, forming the sural nerve. Distal to the medial malleolus, the tibial nerve divides into medial and lateral plantar nerves, supplying sensation to the sole of the foot.
  - o The common fibula nerve travels around the fibular neck, dividing into superficial and deep branches. The superficial branch supplies skin over the majority of the dorsum of the foot and innervates muscles in the lateral compartment of the lower leg. The deep branch supplies sensation to the webbing between the greater and second toes and motor innervation to the extensors of the foot and toes.
- Posterior cutaneous nerve of the thigh – descends in the posterior thigh, supplying sensation to the gluteal region, perineum and posterior thigh and leg.
- Branches to the pudendal plexus may arise from the sacral plexus.

Sacrum

The sacrum is a large, triangular bone composed of five fused sacral vertebrae. Located at the base of the vertebral column, the sacrum articulates with the L5 vertebra above, coccyx below and ilia laterally. The sacral canal is continuous cranially with the lumbar epidural space. The canal contains sacral nerves, cauda equina, epidural venous plexus, lymphatics and fat.

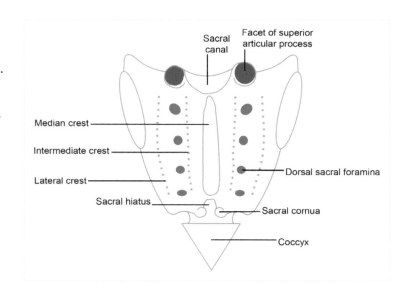

Present on the dorsal surface are several longitudinal crests.
- Median crest – forms through fusion of the rudimentary spinous processes of the upper sacral vertebrae, with laminae on either side forming sacral grooves. Failure of the fifth sacral lamina to fuse results in an opening of the posterior canal wall, termed the sacral hiatus, which is covered by the sacrococcygeal membrane.
- Intermediate crests – present lateral to the sacral grooves, formed through fusion of the articular processes. The articular processes of the fifth sacral vertebrae form osseous protuberances; the sacral cornua.

Lateral to the intermediate crests are eight paired dorsal sacral foramina, through which pass the posterior divisions of the sacral nerves.

Caudal blockade involves injection of local anaesthetic into the sacral canal via the sacral hiatus. It is performed to facilitate perioperative analgesia in children and as a component of chronic pain management in adults. Important differences relevant to the technique exist between these populations.
- Anatomical – at birth, the dura ends at S4, ascending to S2 by the age of 2 years. Accidental intrathecal injections are therefore more common in children less than 2 years of age.
- Physiological – in children less than 8 years of age, negligible cardiovascular instability accompanies injection due to a lower circulatory volume of the legs and splanchnic system and a relatively vasodilated systemic vasculature. Spread of local anaesthetic in those aged over 12 years is unpredictable, in part, secondary to a lower density of epidural fat in children.

2.1.28

Spinal nerve

A spinal nerve is a mixed motor, sensory and autonomic nerve that carries information between the spinal cord and the rest of the body. There are 31 pairs of spinal nerves that emerge from the cord. As the cord is shorter than the vertebral canal they exit at increasingly oblique angles and lengths to reach the corresponding vertebral foramina through which they exit. There are 8 pairs of cervical nerves,

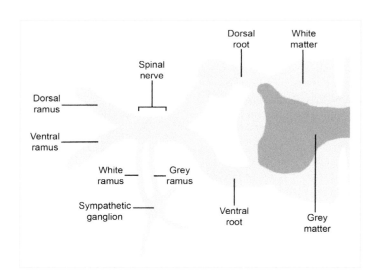

12 thoracic, 5 lumbar, 5 sacral and 1 pair of coccygeal nerves. The cervical nerves are numbered by the vertebra below, except C8, which exits above T1 (as there are only 7 cervical vertebrae). The C1 nerve emerges between the occipital bone and the atlas (C1). Conversely, the thoracic, lumbar and sacral nerves are numbered by the vertebra above.

Each spinal nerve is formed from the combination of the ventral and dorsal nerve fibres from the spinal cord. The ventral root is efferent, carrying motor fibres away from the brain, and the dorsal root is afferent, carrying sensory information to the brain.

Once outside the vertebral column each spinal nerve branches as follows.
- Dorsal ramus – visceral motor, somatic motor and somatic sensory to the skin and muscles of the back.
- Ventral ramus – visceral motor, somatic motor and sensory information to and from the anterolateral body and limbs.
- Meningeal branches – re-enter the intervertebral foramen to supply the ligaments, dura, intervertebral discs, blood vessels, joints and periosteum of the vertebrae.
- Rami communicantes – grey and white. Supply sympathetic nerve fibres to the sympathetic ganglion.

The dorsal and ventral rami may merge to form an interconnecting network of nerves called a plexus, including the cervical, brachial, lumbar and sacral plexuses.

The terms dorsal and ventral are synonymous with the terms posterior and anterior (respectively) in this setting.

Thoracic inlet and first rib

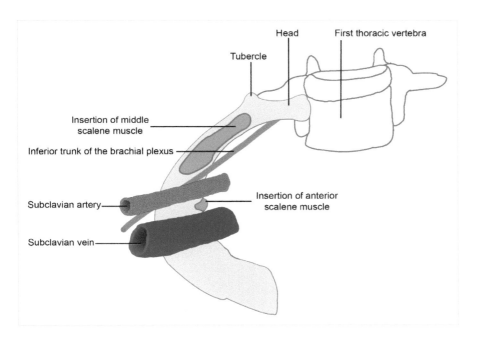

The thoracic inlet is the superior opening of the thorax. It is bound by the manubrium anteriorly, the bony ring of the first ribs curving laterally, and the first thoracic vertebra (T1) posteriorly. The plane of the inlet is oblique as determined by the first rib sloping anteriorly and inferiorly from articulation with T1 to the manubrium. Structures passing through the inlet may be categorized as either midline or those passing on either side.

Midline structures – behind the manubrium pass the strap muscles and inferior thyroid veins. Posteriorly, the trachea and oesophagus travel in close proximity to the recurrent laryngeal nerves. Posterior to the left oesophageal margin lies the thoracic duct.

On either side – the lung apices, covered by cervical pleura, extend upwards. The sympathetic trunk and superior intercostal artery travel posterior to the lung. Medial to the lung pass the internal thoracic artery, vagus nerve and phrenic nerve. The subclavian vessels pass anteriorly.
- Additional structures present on the right are the brachiocephalic artery (unilateral) and vein.
- Additional structures on the left are left common carotid artery and left brachiocephalic vein.

First rib

The first rib is short, broad and flattened in the horizontal plane. The small head has a single facet joint for articulation with the T1 body. The thick tubercle possesses an articular surface for articulation with the T1 transverse process. Two shallow grooves are present on the superior surface of the shaft, separated by the scalene tubercle. The subclavian vein lies in the anterior groove, whilst the subclavian artery and lowest (inferior) trunk of the brachial plexus lie in the posterior groove. The phrenic nerve lies on the anterior surface of the anterior scalene muscle, which inserts onto the scalene tubercle. Behind the posterior groove is the insertion site of the middle scalene muscle.

2.1.30

Vertebra

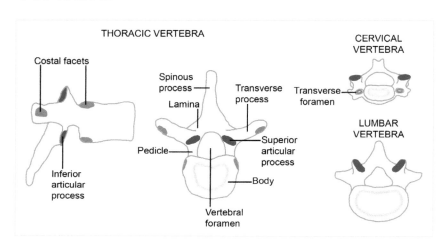

Structure	Cervical	Thoracic	Lumbar
Vertebral foramen	Large and triangular Largest at C2–3	Small and circular	Large and triangular
Spinous process	Short, bifid	Long, slopes postero-inferiorly	Shorter, broader and more horizontal
Articular processes	Fused to form articular pillars	Nearly vertical facets facing posteriorly (superior) and anteriorly (inferior)	Directed posteromedial (superior) and anterolateral (inferior)
Transverse processes	Foramen transversarium C1–6 with vertebral artery and vein	Long and strong	Long and slender
Vertebral body	Small, broad, concave superiorly, convex inferiorly	Heart shaped, one or two facets for articulation with the head of the rib	Large, kidney shaped

The vertebral column consists of 7 cervical, 12 thoracic and 5 lumbar vertebrae, articulating with the base of the skull above and sacrum below. With a similar basic structure, anatomical variations exist appropriate for their location and function.

The cervical spine has two specialized vertebrae, C1 (atlas) and C2 (axis), providing enhanced mobility. C1 serves as a ring that the skull sits upon (atlanto-occipital joint, allowing flexion) and articulates in a pivot joint with the odontoid process (or peg) of C2 (atlanto-axial joint, allowing rotation). It is stabilized by the transverse ligament that holds the odontoid peg close to the posterior aspect of the anterior arch of C1. The C7 vertebra (vertebra prominens) has a distinctive, long spinous process.

Thick intervertebral shock absorbing discs, with a central nucleus pulposus and outer fibrous annulus, join adjacent vertebral bodies. Two synovial joints also exist between the articular processes of adjacent vertebrae. The anterior and posterior longitudinal ligaments are continuous bands that run down the vertebral bodies and discs providing support to the vertebral column. The supraspinous, interspinous, intertransverse ligaments and ligamentum flavum provide further support.

2.2.1

Axillary

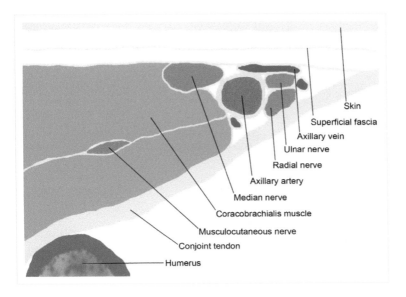

Skin
Superficial fascia
Axillary vein
Ulnar nerve
Radial nerve
Axillary artery
Median nerve
Coracobrachialis muscle
Musculocutaneous nerve
Conjoint tendon
Humerus

The nerves at the axilla are the terminal branches of the brachial plexus cords (see *Section 2.1.5 – Brachial plexus*). The medial cord divides into five nerves: the medial origin of the median nerve, ulnar, medial pectoral, medial brachial cutaneous (aka medial cutaneous nerve of the arm), and medial antebrachial cutaneous (aka medial cutaneous nerve of the forearm). The lateral cord divides into three nerves: the lateral origin of the median nerve, the musculocutaneous and lateral pectoral nerve. The posterior cord divides into five nerves: the radial, axillary, thoracodorsal, lower subscapular and upper subscapular.

The muscles surrounding the brachial plexus at this location are:
- Biceps – anterior and superficial
- Coracobrachialis – anterior and deep
- Conjoint tendon of teres major and latissimus dorsi – medial and posterior.

The median, ulnar and radial nerves are contained within the brachial plexus sheath, while the medial brachial cutaneous nerve and medial antebrachial cutaneous nerve may travel either inside or outside the plexus. The musculocutaneous nerve is usually found outside of the plexus, between the biceps and coracobrachialis muscles, or in the body of coracobrachialis itself.

The axillary approach to the brachial plexus (including the musculocutaneous nerve) results in anaesthesia of the upper limb from the mid arm distally, including the hand. The skin over the deltoid muscle and medial skin of the upper arm are not covered (supplied by the axillary and intercostobrachial nerves).

The axillary approach to the brachial plexus is best performed where the plexus sits on the conjoint tendon. The veins are easily compressed with pressure from the ultrasound probe and therefore must be identified by varying pressure and colour Doppler. The nerves are found in close proximity to the axillary artery; the median on the biceps side superior to the artery, the ulnar on the triceps side, often beneath the main axillary vein and the radial nerve deep to the artery usually on the conjoint tendon.

2.2.2

Femoral

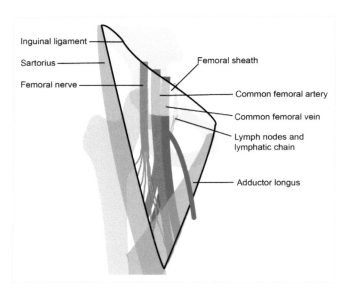

Inguinal ligament
Sartorius
Femoral nerve
Femoral sheath
Common femoral artery
Common femoral vein
Lymph nodes and lymphatic chain
Adductor longus

The femoral triangle (see *Section 2.1.16 – Femoral triangle*) has the following borders:
- superior – inguinal ligament
- lateral – medial border of sartorius
- medial – medial border of adductor longus.

The floor is formed from the adductor longus, pectineus, psoas major and iliacus muscles, and roof from the fascia lata. The femoral triangle acts as a conduit for structures entering and leaving the anterior thigh.

The contents of the femoral triangle, from lateral to medial:
- femoral nerve – innervates the anterior compartment of the thigh and sensory supply to the medial side of the leg and foot
- femoral artery – gives off the deep profunda branch in the triangle
- femoral vein – great saphenous vein joins femoral vein in the triangle
- femoral canal – contains lymph nodes and some vessels.

The mnemonic NAVEL helps recall of the contents, from lateral to medial: Nerve, Artery, Vein, Empty space (allows veins and lymph vessels to distend), and Lymph nodes.

The femoral nerve originates from the L2–L4 lumbar nerves and is the largest branch of the lumbar plexus. At the level of L5, it exits the psoas muscle deep to the fascia iliaca and continues caudally, entering the anterior compartment of the thigh under the inguinal ligament, anterior to iliopsoas and lateral to the blood vessels. It gives off multiple branches in the triangle; the most medial part, the saphenous nerve, descends alongside the femoral artery to provide innervation to the patella, superficial structures of the knee and medial aspect of the leg.

The femoral nerve block provides analgesia for femoral and knee surgery, and in combination with a sciatic and obturator block, can provide anaesthesia for knee and lower limb surgery. The saphenous nerve can be blocked in the adductor canal, in the medial aspect of the mid-thigh, and can provide analgesia for knee surgery with a reduction in motor weakness compared with the femoral block.

2.2.3

Interscalene

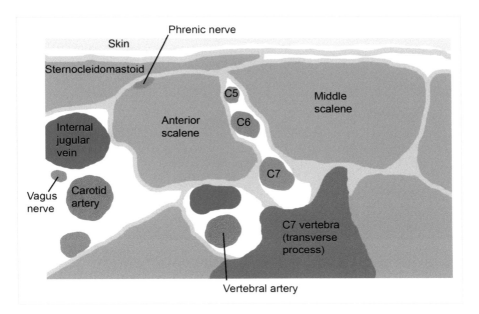

The interscalene groove is located between the anterior and middle scalene muscles and posterior to the sternocleidomastoid muscle (SCM) at the level of the cricoid cartilage (C6). It contains the C5, C6 and C7 roots of the brachial plexus (see *Section 2.1.5 – Brachial plexus*), which then continue to form the superior (C5 and C6), middle (C7) and inferior trunks (C8 and T1) before descending below the clavicle. There can be marked anatomical variation within the groove.

The ultrasound appearance can be identified by either tracking back the anatomy from the supraclavicular fossa or by scanning laterally at the level of the cricoid. The nerve roots are hypoechoic, due to the high density of conducting axons compared to connective tissue, and must be differentiated from vascular structures. The roots are often arranged vertically in a 'traffic light' orientation between the two scalene muscles, the C5 root being cephalad and the C7 root caudad. The way to differentiate these roots is to trace the anatomy back to the transverse processes of the corresponding vertebra and to identify the prominent anterior tubercle of the C6 vertebra (Chassaignac's tubercle).

The phrenic nerve also passes through the interscalene groove before traversing over the anterior surface of the anterior scalene muscle and into the thoracic cavity. The interscalene block consistently produces an ipsilateral phrenic nerve block (incidence of up to 100% depending on the volume of local anaesthetic used) and hemi-diaphragmatic paralysis. Patient selection is therefore particularly important; respiratory compromise or contralateral paresis of the phrenic or recurrent laryngeal nerves being relative contraindications.

An interscalene nerve block provides anaesthesia for shoulder, clavicle and proximal arm surgery because it consistently blocks the C5 and C6 nerve roots, but is unsuitable for hand and forearm surgery due to sparing of the C8 and T1 nerve roots.

2.2.4

Popliteal

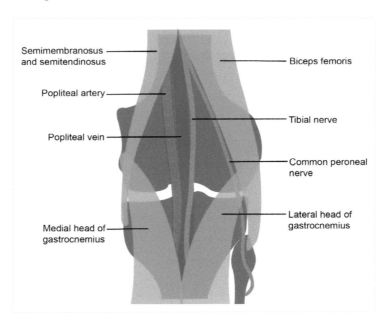

Semimembranosus and semitendinosus

Popliteal artery

Popliteal vein

Medial head of gastrocnemius

Biceps femoris

Tibial nerve

Common peroneal nerve

Lateral head of gastrocnemius

The popliteal fossa has four borders:
- superomedial – semimembranosus
- superolateral – biceps femoris
- inferomedial – medial head of gastrocnemius
- inferolateral – lateral head of gastrocnemius and plantaris.

The floor is formed by the posterior surface of the capsule of the knee joint, the popliteus muscle and the femur. The roof is derived from the popliteal fascia, which is continuous with the fascia lata of the leg.

The sciatic nerve is made up of the tibial nerve (TN) and the common peroneal nerve (CPN) which travel from the pelvis down the posterior aspect of the leg in a common fascia (Vloka's sheath). The point at which they diverge compared to the popliteal crease varies between individuals; they then continue below the knee in separate sheaths. The TN is larger than the CPN and gives rise to medial and lateral plantar nerves and collateral branches to form the cutaneous sural nerve. The CPN gives rise to the superficial and deep peroneal nerves, which innervate the muscles of the lateral and anterior compartments of the leg.

The popliteal sciatic nerve block is ideal for surgeries on the lower leg, particularly the foot and ankle. The medial side of the leg will not be covered with this block and therefore a saphenous or femoral nerve block may be required. The patient can be positioned supine, lateral or prone, with the lateral approach being most common. The ultrasound probe is placed in the popliteal crease to identify the popliteal artery with the TN more superficial to it; caudal angulation may be required to clearly identify the nerve. Once the TN is identified, scanning more proximally will usually identify the smaller, more superficial CPN on the lateral side. The block is usually performed at the point at which the nerves diverge but are still in their common sheath.

2.2.5

Sciatic

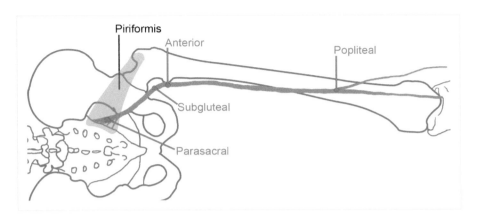

The sciatic nerve is the largest in the body. It is derived from L4–S3 and innervates the muscles of the posterior thigh and the hamstring portion of the adductor magnus (remaining portion innervated by the obturator nerve). Its terminal branches, the tibial and common peroneal nerve, innervate all the muscles of the leg and foot and the skin of the lateral leg, heel, and the dorsal and plantar surfaces of the foot.

It is derived from the lumbosacral plexus and enters the gluteal region via the greater sciatic foramen of the pelvis. It travels inferiorly to the piriformis muscle and then descends in the posterior compartment of the thigh. As it approaches the popliteal fossa, it divides into the tibial and common peroneal nerves.

The sciatic nerve can be targeted with ultrasound at any point along its course with consideration to the structures involved in the relevant surgery. The sciatic nerve is anisotropic and therefore small changes in transducer angle can change the appearance of the nerve. There are four common cited approaches with ultrasound.

- **Parasacral** – block performed at a point distal to lateral edge of the sacrum and caudal to the sacroiliac joint. More accurately described as a sacral plexus block at the level of the greater sciatic foramen. This approach can be used for pelvic and hip surgery, above-knee amputation and lower leg surgery.
- **Subgluteal** – block performed between the ischial tuberosity and the greater trochanter as the nerve traverses the subgluteal space. Caution because of vascular structures in close proximity. Can be used for analgesia for above-knee amputation, knee surgery and lower leg surgery.
- **Anterior** – block performed in the proximal thigh with the patient supine. Can be challenging due to the depth of the nerve with this approach. Can be used for surgery at or below the knee.
- **Popliteal** – see *Section 2.2.4 – Popliteal*.

2.2.6
Supraclavicular

Around the level of the clavicle, the brachial plexus (see *Section 2.1.5 – Brachial plexus*) consists of superior (C5, C6), middle (C7) and inferior trunks (C8, T1) which then separate into anterior and posterior divisions. A fascial sheath surrounds the neurovascular bundle and extends from the deep cervical fascia to the border of the axilla.

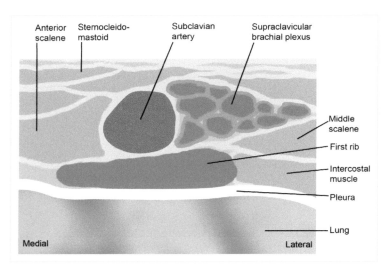

Anterior scalene | Sternocleido-mastoid | Subclavian artery | Supraclavicular brachial plexus | Middle scalene | First rib | Intercostal muscle | Pleura | Lung | Medial | Lateral

Key landmarks along the first rib from lateral to medial are:
• middle scalene muscle
• brachial plexus
• subclavian artery
• anterior scalene muscle
• subclavian vein.

The subclavian artery is the main landmark for the supraclavicular block. It crosses over the rib between the insertions of the anterior and middle scalene muscles, posterior to the midpoint of the clavicle. The brachial plexus is found lateral and superficial to the subclavian artery. The landmark approach to this block carries a high risk of pneumothorax due to the proximity to the dome of the pleura; with ultrasound this risk can be greatly reduced. It is important to identify the following structures on ultrasound.
• **Subclavian artery** – anechoic round structure.
• **Pleura** – hyperechoic bright linear structure below and on both sides of the artery, with lung markings seen below (comet tail sign).
• **First rib** – hyperechoic bright linear structure with acoustic shadow, deep to the subclavian artery.
• **Brachial plexus** – triangular bundle of hypoechoic round nodules posterior and superficial to the artery. Identifying the plexus where it sits on the rib reduces the risk of pneumothorax on needling.

The supraclavicular approach to the brachial plexus provides reliable anaesthesia to the arm from the level of the mid humerus. The plexus is tightly packed at this level, resulting in a reliable and high quality block, and is often known as the 'spinal of the arm'. The medial skin of the arm (intercostobrachial nerve, T2) may not be covered by the block and may require subcutaneous infiltration distal to the axilla.

3.1

Clearance

$$Cl = k_e \times V_d$$

$$Cl_{organ} = Q \times \frac{(C_{in} - C_{out})}{C_{in}}$$

$$Cl_{organ} = Q \times ER$$

Cl = clearance (ml.min⁻¹)

k_e = elimination rate constant (min⁻¹)

V_d = volume of distribution (ml)

Q = cardiac output (ml·min⁻¹)

C = concentration (g·L⁻¹)

ER = extraction ratio

Clearance is the theoretical volume of plasma completely cleared of drug per unit time. It is a measure of drug elimination from the body via excretion and/or metabolism. Once a drug has undergone biotransformation it is deemed eliminated, although its metabolite may still remain. Distribution of a drug to organs and tissues is not considered clearance if the unchanged drug is subsequently released back into the plasma. Total body clearance is the sum of all clearance pathways for a specific compound.

The drug clearance of an organ is determined by its blood flow and extraction ratio (ER). The ER describes the efficiency with which an organ eliminates a drug, with those efficient at drug removal having a ratio approaching 1 (i.e. 100% extraction). Propranolol undergoes exclusive hepatic metabolism with a high ER (0.9). Clearance is therefore dependent on the rate of drug delivery to the liver (i.e. hepatic blood flow); as flow increases, clearance increases. In contrast, hepatic metabolism of phenytoin demonstrates a low ER; even with an increase in hepatic blood flow, clearance will remain low.

Clearance is a proportionality factor used to determine rate of elimination (see *Section 3.5 – Elimination*). To maintain a steady-state plasma concentration, the rate of drug elimination must equal the rate of administration. Clearance may therefore be used to calculate the rate of drug administration.

Implications in the critically ill

Metabolism – hepatic metabolism is often altered as a result of disease processes affecting enzymatic activity, plasma protein concentrations and/or hepatic blood flow. Additionally, drugs can induce or inhibit hepatic enzymes.

Excretion – acute kidney injury leads to a variable reduction in drug clearance, while renal replacement therapy may provide a dramatic increase in renal drug elimination. Augmented renal clearance may be observed in situations of increased cardiac output (e.g. burn injury, sepsis and inotropic administration).

3.2

Compartment model – one and two compartments

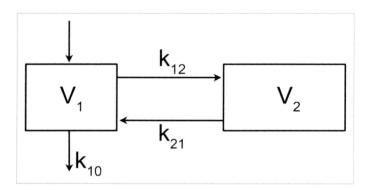

Compartment models can predict the distribution of a drug after administration. They assume the presence of a single central compartment, into which a drug will initially distribute, and one or more peripheral compartments into which a drug can move. A drug must move from peripheral compartments back into the central compartment to be cleared from the body. Although a simplification, these models can help predict plasma concentrations of drugs.

$$C = C_0 e^{-kt}$$

C = concentration

C_0 = concentration at time zero

k = rate constant for elimination

t = time

The simplest is the one compartment model. On administration, the drug distributes evenly into a single compartment, the volume of which is the volume of distribution (V_d). The drug will be removed from this compartment in an exponential manner with a single rate constant for elimination (k). This describes the proportion of plasma from which the drug is removed per unit time. The drug concentration will therefore show a monophasic decline over time, described using a single exponential term (see equation above). The one compartment model can be used to calculate aminoglycoside concentrations accurately.

The two compartment model adds a second compartment, which connects with the central compartment. A drug will initially distribute into the central compartment, with a volume V_1, before redistributing into (and out of) the second peripheral compartment, with a volume V_2; the V_d is the sum of V_1 and V_2. The drug can now leave the central compartment in two ways: by distribution into the peripheral compartment and by elimination. Its concentration over time will therefore show a biphasic pattern. The rate of transfer between the compartments is dependent on the concentration gradient between them and is assumed to be exponential. The rate constant for transfer between compartments can be described in both directions (k_{12} and k_{21}), and the rate constant for elimination from the central compartment as k_{10}. The two compartment model can be used to calculate thiopentone and vancomycin concentrations.

3.3

Compartment model – three compartments

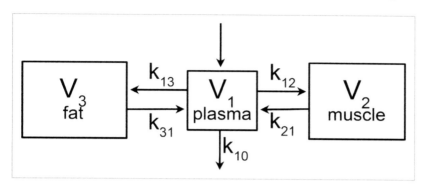

Compartment models are used to predict the distribution of a drug after administration. Multiple compartments are used to describe the different tissues into which a drug will move according to its rate of distribution into those tissues. The three compartment model is convenient to depict vessel-rich and vessel-poor compartments, although multiple compartments may be described.

As explained in the one compartment model (see *Section 3.2 – Compartment model – one and two compartments*), a drug can only enter and leave the body via the central compartment, but will distribute into and out of the other compartments at varying rates. In the three compartment model this creates a triphasic pattern for plasma concentration explained using three exponential functions. In a clinical model the central compartment represents the plasma, with the second compartment typically representing a well perfused tissue (e.g. muscle) and the third compartment a poorly perfused tissue (e.g. fat). Again, the volume of distribution (V_d) will represent the sum of the three compartment volumes. This provides a good model for distribution of many anaesthetic agents.

A single exponential function describes the elimination of the drug from the body via the central compartment. The terminal elimination half-life reflects elimination from the body once pseudo-equilibrium has taken place with the other compartments.

A three compartment model is the basis behind some target-controlled infusion (TCI) algorithms for total intravenous anaesthesia (TIVA), e.g. for propofol. It provides an initial bolus in order to fill the central compartment and then an infusion at a reducing rate to match the exponential redistribution of the drug into the peripheral compartments. If a higher plasma concentration is required a bolus is given, whereas if a lower concentration is needed the infusion will stop to allow a multi-exponential fall to the new target, before the infusion restarts at the new desired rate.

3.4

Dose–response curves

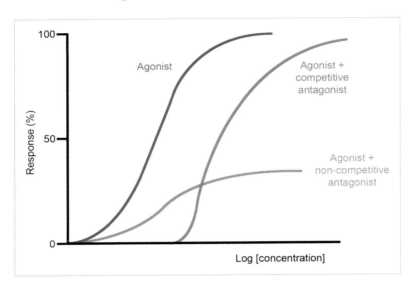

A dose–response curve depicts the pharmacological response when a drug is given. It may bind to a receptor and produce a response (agonist) or bind and produce no response but, by doing so, prevent an endogenous agonist eliciting its effect (antagonist). This response may also vary in magnitude. Affinity describes how well a drug binds to its receptor and intrinsic activity (IA), or efficacy, describes the magnitude of response that it will cause once bound.

An agonist will demonstrate high receptor affinity and full IA (IA = 1), whereas an antagonist will have a high affinity but low IA (IA = 0). A partial agonist demonstrates a similar response to an agonist but with only limited IA (0 < IA < 1). It will produce a submaximal response when bound to its receptor and therefore can act as an antagonist at high doses as it prevents the endogenous agonist from binding. An inverse agonist will produce the opposite effect to the endogenous agonist; this is different from competitive antagonism because it is exerting its own pharmacological effect rather than simply preventing the endogenous agonist from binding to the receptor.

Competitive antagonists compete for the same receptor as the endogenous agonist, e.g. non-depolarizing muscle relaxants competing with acetylcholine at the neuromuscular junction (nicotinic receptors). Conversely, non-competitive antagonists do not bind to the same receptor as the endogenous agonist, but instead cause their antagonism through conformational distortion preventing receptor activation. An example is ketamine competing with glutamate at the NMDA receptors.

The dose–response curve is often plotted with a logarithmic scale for dose (concentration), producing the classical sigmoid shape shown in the diagram. The response seen when either a competitive or non-competitive antagonist is added to a full agonist is also shown.

3.5

Elimination

$$\text{Rate of elimination} = Cl \times C_{ss}$$

$$\text{Maintenance} = Cl \times \left(\frac{C_{pl}}{BA} \right)$$

Cl = clearance (ml.min⁻¹)

C_{ss} = plasma concentration at steady state (mg.ml⁻¹)

C_{pl} = target plasma concentration (mg.ml⁻¹)

BA = bioavailability

Drug elimination is defined as the irreversible removal of drug from the body. Elimination processes encompass biotransformation and excretion.

Biotransformation/drug metabolism – the process of chemical modification of a drug to a metabolite, usually via an enzyme. Biotransformation is achieved by two successive reactions.
- Phase I reactions – unmask functional groups, e.g. hydroxyl (-OH), amino (-NH₂) and thiol (-SH), through oxidation, reduction and/or hydrolysis. This reaction produces metabolites that are more polar. Their degree of activity may also be modified. The hepatic cytochrome P450 isozyme family facilitates the majority of Phase I reactions.
- Phase II reactions – convert compounds/metabolites into more hydrophilic and excretable forms through conjugation. The liver is the primary site of drug metabolism with the kidneys, lungs, small intestine and skin also containing metabolic enzymes.

Excretion – the removal of waste substances from the body. The predominant route of excretion is the urine, however, other pathways include bile, sweat, saliva, faeces, breast milk and exhaled air. Most drugs undergo metabolism prior to excretion.

Rate of elimination

The rate of elimination (mg.min⁻¹) reflects the amount of drug removed per unit time. As most drugs are eliminated by a first-order process, the amount of drug removed is proportional to the plasma concentration of the drug. The proportionality constant relating the rate of elimination to plasma concentration is clearance.

To maintain a desired plasma concentration of a drug at steady state, the rate of elimination must equal the rate of administration. As such, the rate of administration may be calculated using the target plasma concentration and drug clearance. If the drug is administered by any route other than intravenously, the bioavailability (BA) is likely to be less than 100%. Therefore, the maintenance dose would need to be proportionally increased.

3.6

Elimination kinetics

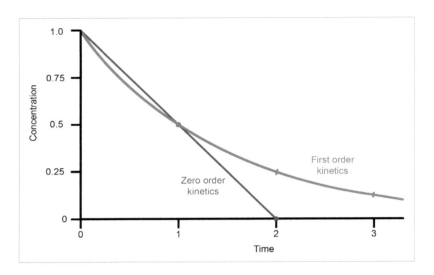

Elimination kinetics describe the relationship between plasma drug concentration and rate of drug elimination. Elimination mechanisms often exhibit excess capacity allowing effective drug elimination at therapeutic doses. However, saturation of enzyme and carrier-mediated processes alter kinetics of drug elimination. Elimination kinetics may be classified based on this principle as zero- and first-order.

Zero-order elimination – the elimination system is saturated at clinical levels as processes are functioning at maximum capacity. If plasma drug concentration increases, no further enzymatic/carrier capacity is available. Therefore, rate of elimination occurs at a constant rate, independent of plasma drug concentration. As a fixed mass of drug is eliminated per unit time, half-life decreases as plasma drug concentration decreases. The elimination processes that are most commonly saturated are enzymatic metabolism and active renal tubular secretion. Clinically, zero-order drug elimination is a concern because drugs may accumulate, leading to toxicity. Drugs demonstrating this at/near therapeutic doses include aspirin, phenytoin and ethanol.

First-order elimination – the elimination system demonstrates excess capacity. If plasma drug concentration increases, the rate of drug elimination increases. Therefore, rate of elimination is not fixed but is dependent on concentration. As a constant fraction of drug is eliminated per unit time, half-life and clearance remain constant. However, the amount of drug eliminated decreases exponentially as plasma concentration decreases. The vast majority of drugs in therapeutic doses demonstrate first-order kinetics.

Elimination kinetic equations (see Section 3.5 – Elimination)

Derivation of these equations is complex. For both zero- and first-order processes, the plasma drug concentration may be calculated for any time (C_{pt}) if concentration at time zero (C_0) and rate constant (k) are known.
- Zero-order – as rate is independent of drug concentration, reduction in plasma drug concentration is linear. This is evident numerically from the slope–intercept form of equation.
- First-order – plasma drug concentration declines exponentially with time as evidenced by the exponential function (e).

Half-lives and time constants

A half-life, $t_{1/2}$, describes the time taken for the plasma concentration of a substance to fall by 50% of its original value. When considering elimination of a drug, after one half-life there will be 50% of the drug remaining and after two half-lives 25% will remain

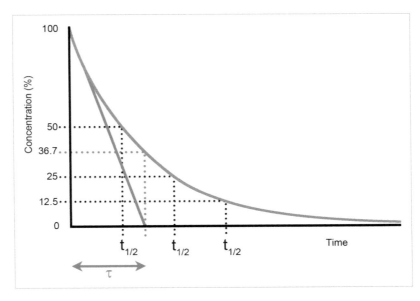

(50 divided by 2). Following this principle, after 5 half-lives only 3.125% will remain, i.e. the process will be 96.875% complete. Similarly, when administering a drug infusion it will take approximately 5 half-lives to reach steady state.

The time constant, however, describes the time it would have taken for the plasma concentration of a substance (C) to fall to zero, had the initial rate of elimination continued (i.e. the semi-log plot of the negative exponential curve $C = C_0 - e^{-kt}$ giving $\ln C = \ln C_0 - kt$; see *Section 5.8 – Exponential function*). It is represented by the symbol tau, τ, and is measured in minutes. The time constant is the inverse of the rate constant for elimination $(1/k)$, and therefore also represents the time it would take for the plasma concentration to fall by a factor of $1/e$ ($e = 2.718...$). In one time constant the plasma concentration will have fallen to approximately 36.7% of its original value. The half-life is shorter than the time constant by a factor of 0.693, so $t_{1/2} = 0.693\tau$. This is derived from the fact that C must equal $C_0/2$ at $t_{1/2}$ therefore giving:

$$\ln(C_0/2) = \ln C_0 - kt_{1/2}$$

and ultimately:

$$t_{1/2} = \ln 2/k = \ln 2\tau = 0.693\tau$$

Alternatively, one could state that the time constant is 44% longer than the half-life.

The context-sensitive half-time is used in relation to an infusion, where the context refers to the duration of the infusion. It is defined as the time taken for the plasma concentration of a substance to fall by 50% of the value at the time of stopping the infusion. The longest context-sensitive half-time will be seen after the infusion has been allowed to reach steady state (and will then equal the terminal elimination half-life). The term half-time is used rather than half-life because a half-life is constant whereas a half-time is not.

3.8

Meyer–Overton hypothesis

The Meyer–Overton hypothesis, now an outdated concept, sought to explain the mechanism of action of general anaesthetic agents. Cell structure was known to include a hydrophobic lipid cell membrane. Meyer proposed that anaesthetic agents were hydrophobic and attracted to other hydrophobic molecules. This mutual hydrophobia

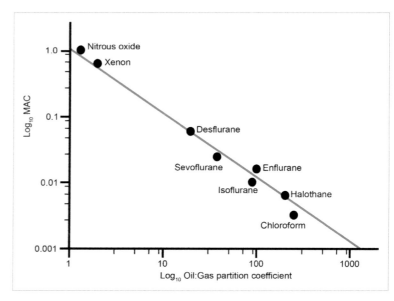

was believed to allow anaesthetic agents to dissolve within the lipid molecules of brain cells.

Meyer and Overton demonstrated a positive correlation between anaesthetic lipid solubility and potency. Lipid solubility was represented by partitioning anaesthetic agents between olive oil (lipid membrane model) and water (plasma model). Correlation was plotted on a log–log scale to accommodate the range of potencies and partition coefficients. It was proposed that anaesthesia was achieved once a certain concentration of anaesthetic molecules dissolved in the lipid membrane of brain cells, thereby changing their normal relationship to other cellular structures.

More than 50 years after Meyer and Overton proposed their hypothesis, minimum alveolar concentration (MAC) was published as a method for determining equipotency. The Meyer–Overton hypothesis was modified, using this more objective measure of potency. The original research utilized the oil:water partition coefficient. When potency became represented by MAC, the partition coefficient was changed, relating lipid membrane solubility to the alveolar gas phase. There is an equivalent correlation between the oil:gas partition coefficient of an anaesthetic agent and its potency.

Hypothesis limitation
- Some drugs with a high oil:gas partition coefficient do not produce anaesthesia.
- Drugs with similar oil:gas partition coefficients demonstrate different potencies
  (e.g. the structural isomers enflurane and isoflurane).

These exceptions to the hypothesis rendered it outdated. Several other lipid-based theories evolved, including cell membrane volume expansion and changes in surface tension. These have also since been disproved and, while the mechanism of action of general anaesthetics is still not fully understood, it is now believed likely to be receptor-mediated.

Target-controlled infusions

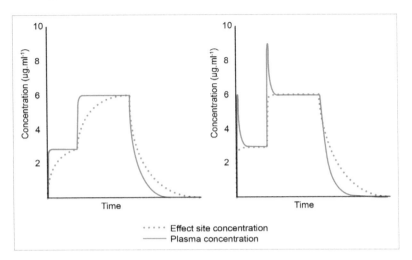

..... Effect site concentration
——— Plasma concentration

A target-controlled infusion (TCI) is an infusion controlled in a manner that achieves a user-defined drug concentration in a body compartment/organ of interest (e.g. brain). TCI systems enable improved precision and more rapid control of drug concentration compared to manual infusions.

TCI systems use pharmacokinetic models derived from drug-specific population studies, with most anaesthetic drugs conforming to a three-compartment model (see *Section 3.3 – Compartment model – three compartments*).

TCI systems are based on the original bolus elimination transfer model. The general method of use is as follows (graph on left).
- With a selected increase in target plasma concentration, the system administers a rapid bolus/infusion to quickly fill the central compartment (V_1) resulting in a stepwise increase in plasma concentration. The amount of drug infused is calculated according to estimated V_1 volume and the difference between current and new target blood concentrations. When the system calculates that target concentration has been achieved, the rapid infusion stops. A lower rate infusion begins, accounting for drug distribution to peripheral compartments and rate of elimination. Effect-site concentration (e.g. brain) increases until it reaches equilibrium with the plasma.
- With a selected decrease in target concentration, the TCI system stops the infusion until the new calculated target concentration is achieved.

TCI systems can target either plasma or effect-site concentration.
- **Plasma targeting** (graph on left) – desired plasma concentration is selected. Effect-site concentration follows passively with a temporal delay.
- **Effect-site targeting** (graph on right) – desired effect-site concentration is selected. The TCI system manipulates the delivered dose to achieve a plasma concentration higher than the targeted effect-site concentration. This generates a greater concentration gradient between plasma and effect-site, resulting in more rapid achievement of target concentration.

For most anaesthetic agents in common use, there are multiple published TCI models. Different models utilize different variables to calculate clearance rates and volumes of distribution.

3.10

Volume of distribution

$$V_d = \frac{\text{Amount of drug in body at } t_0}{C_0}$$

$$V_d = \frac{\text{Dose}}{C_0}$$

V_d = volume of distribution (l)

t_0 = time zero

C_0 = plasma concentration at time zero

The volume of distribution (V_d) describes the relationship between drug concentration and the amount of drug in the body. It is defined as the theoretical volume of fluid into which the total amount of drug administered must be diluted to achieve the measured plasma concentration.

Depending on the timing of plasma drug concentration measurement, V_d varies in accordance with the degree of drug distribution.
- Initial V_d (V_c) – immediately following intravenous administration, plasma drug concentration is maximal. The V_c is estimated by extrapolation of the drug concentration–time curve to time zero (see *Section 3.6 – Elimination kinetics*). In practice, V_c is seldom used but may be helpful in predicting initial maximal plasma concentration.
- Steady-state V_d (V_{ss}) – at equilibrium (i.e. during intravenous infusion), V_{ss} is the apparent volume of fluid into which the total amount of drug present in the body must be diluted to achieve equilibrium concentration. The V_{ss} may be used to calculate loading dose.

The V_d does not necessarily correspond to an anatomical/physiological volume and may exceed total body water volume due to drug tissue binding or sequestration in fat. Highly ionized drugs have a small V_d (e.g. atracurium, V_{ss} 0.16 l.kg^{-1}). In contrast, lipid soluble drugs, which widely distribute throughout body tissues, have a large V_d (e.g. fentanyl, V_{ss} 4 l.kg^{-1}).

Implications in the critically ill

Increased V_d reduces plasma drug concentration.
- Hydrophilic drugs (e.g. gentamicin) – increased capillary membrane permeability results in fluid shift.
- Acidic drugs (e.g. phenytoin, warfarin) – hypoalbuminaemia increases the unbound drug fraction leading to enhanced distribution.

Reduced V_d increases plasma drug concentration.
- Basic drugs (e.g. lidocaine) – bound to α-1-acid glycoprotein (AAG). Synthesis of this acute phase protein increases in critical illness, reducing the unbound drug fraction and limiting distribution.
- Clinical effect needs to be considered in conjunction with other pharmacokinetic processes (e.g. active drug plasma concentration, metabolism, elimination).

Wash-in curves for volatile agents

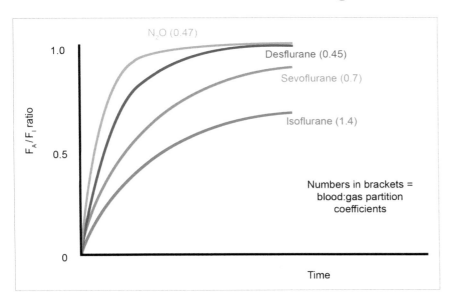

Speed of onset of a volatile agent depends on various factors. The effects of volatile anaesthetics depend on concentration at their effect sites, which parallels alveolar concentration (F_A). During the wash-in period, partial pressure of inhaled anaesthetic gas in the alveoli increases exponentially, approaching inspired fresh gas concentration (F_I). An alveolar to inspired concentration ratio (F_A/F_I) of 1 represents equilibrium. At equilibrium, the anaesthetic partial pressure in the alveoli (P_A) equals arterial (P_a) and brain partial pressures (P_B). P_A can, therefore, be used as a surrogate measure of P_B. As the brain is the effector site for anaesthetic agents, an increase in P_A will lead to a faster onset of action.

A high inspired volatile concentration and increased alveolar ventilation will produce a rapid rise in P_A and speed the onset of action. Conversely, an increase in FRC will effectively dilute the anaesthetic, lowering the P_A and slowing onset.

A high cardiac output increases the rate of removal of anaesthetic from the alveoli, preventing equilibrium between alveoli, blood, and brain. This results in a slower onset of action. A lower cardiac output has the opposite effect.

There is an inverse relationship between blood:gas partition coefficient and onset of anaesthesia. Agents with lower blood:gas partition coefficients (i.e. lower solubility in blood) exert a higher partial pressure, resulting in faster onset and offset of action.

The use of nitrous oxide (N_2O) will speed the onset of action due to concentration and second gas effects. When N_2O is used in high concentrations it is readily absorbed into the capillaries, with gas present in the conducting airways being drawn into the alveoli to maintain their volume. This leads to an increase in gas concentrations and P_A. A volatile anaesthetic, used alongside N_2O, will be concentrated by this mechanism causing a high P_A, speeding the onset of action.

4.1

Alpha-2 adrenoceptor agonists

	Clonidine	Dexmedetomidine
Structure	Aniline derivative	Imidazole derivative
Presentation	Clear, colourless solution Concentration 0.15 mg.ml⁻¹	Clear, colourless solution Concentration 100 mcg.ml⁻¹
Route	Oral, intravenous, epidural	Intravenous
Dose	IV: 0.15–0.3 mg 8-hourly Oral: 0.05–0.6 mg 8-hourly	Maintenance infusion: 0.2–1.4 mcg.kg⁻¹.h⁻¹
Uses	Antihypertensive, sedation, anxiolysis and analgesia	Sedation, anxiolysis and analgesia
Kinetics	100% oral bioavailability 20% protein-bound VD: 1.7–2.5 l.kg⁻¹ <50% hepatically metabolized 65% renally excreted unchanged Elimination half-life: 6–23 h	94% protein-bound VD: 1.33 l.kg⁻¹ Hepatically metabolized 95% of metabolites excreted in urine Elimination half-life: 2 h
Effects	*CVS*: initial transient BP increase (when given IV, due to alpha-1 stimulation) followed by sustained decrease *CNS*: decreases cerebral blood flow; depression of spontaneous sympathetic outflow & somatosympathetic reflexes *GI*: decreased gastric and small bowel motility; antisialogogue *Metabolic*: decreased catecholamine concentrations and plasma renin activity; increased blood sugar concentration *Side-effects*: drowsiness and dry mouth; rapid withdrawal can cause rebound hypertension and tachycardia	*CVS*: dose-dependent decrease in heart rate and mean arterial pressure *CNS*: sedation and anxiolysis *Metabolic*: decrease in plasma catecholamine concentrations *Side-effects*: hypotension, bradycardia, nausea and dry mouth

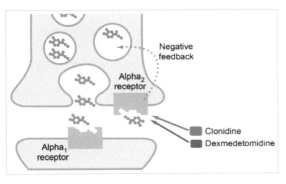

Clonidine is an alpha adrenoceptor agonist, with a 200:1 affinity for alpha-2 to alpha-1, respectively. Dexmedetomidine has similar clinical effects, but a greater affinity for the alpha-2 adrenoceptors (1600:1).

Stimulation of the presynaptic alpha-2 adrenoceptor decreases noradrenaline release from sympathetic nerve terminals, decreasing sympathetic and vagal tone. Analgesic effects are mediated via alpha-2 adrenoceptor activation in the dorsal horn of the spinal cord.

4.2

Anaesthetic agents – etomidate

Etomidate is the only imidazole intravenous hypnotic drug and demonstrates minimal impact on the cardiovascular and respiratory systems. However, use is largely limited due to potent inhibition of adrenal steroid synthesis (ketamine has now gained popularity for use in the cardiovascularly unstable patient). When given in clinical doses, etomidate enhances agonist activation of $GABA_A$ receptors. In supra-clinical concentrations, direct activation of the $GABA_A$ receptor is observed.

Red = The imidazole ring

Chemical structure – carboxylated imidazole derivative.

Presentation – presented as an enantiopure, R(+), formulation in a concentration of $2\,mg.ml^{-1}$. It is a weak base with a pKa of 4.2. Hydrophobic at physiological pH. To improve solubility, formulations contain 35% propylene glycol (associated with pain on injection) or fat emulsion.

Route of administration – intravenous (IV).

Dose – induction IV $0.3\,mg.kg^{-1}$.

Uses – induction of anaesthesia, especially in the setting of cardiovascular instability. For rapid control of hypercortisolaemia in ACTH-dependent Cushing's syndrome.

Kinetics
- Volume of distribution $4.5\,l.kg^{-1}$.
- Protein binding 76% in plasma.
- Onset of action 10–60 seconds.
- Duration of action 6–10 minutes due to rapid drug redistribution.
- Rapid metabolism by hepatic and plasma esterases.
- Inactive metabolites, majority (85%) excreted renally, remainder excreted in bile.
- Clearance $870–1700\,ml.min^{-1}$.
- Elimination half-life 1–4.5 hours.

Effects
- Respiratory – transient apnoea, reduction in tidal volume offset by compensatory increases in respiratory rate.
- Cardiovascular – relative cardiovascular stability, may induce mild reduction in mean arterial blood pressure, minimal effect on myocardial contractility.
- CNS – potent direct cerebral vasoconstrictor, decreasing cerebral blood flow and oxygen consumption, myoclonic movements common, may activate seizure foci.
- Gastrointestinal – increased incidence of post-operative nausea and vomiting.
- Metabolic – potent inhibitor of adrenal cortisol and aldosterone synthesis for 24–48 hours, even after a single dose.
- Haematological – significant antiplatelet activity.

Anaesthetic agents – ketamine

Ketamine is the only intravenous anaesthetic agent available that has analgesic, amnesic, hypnotic and local anaesthetic properties. It is a non-competitive antagonist at the N-methyl-D-aspartate (NMDA) receptor. It is commonly referred to as a dissociative anaesthetic, i.e. causes catalepsy, catatonia and amnesia, without necessarily involving complete unconsciousness, through incoming signal blockade to the cerebral cortex. It may also have some action at opioid receptors, however, its effects are not reversed by naloxone.

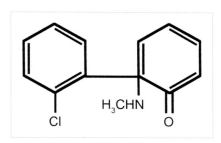

Chemical structure – phencyclidine derivative.

Presentation – presented as a racemic mixture or as the single S(+) enantiomer (more potent and less psychoactive). It is a colourless solution and available in three concentrations; 10, 50 and 100 mg.ml^{-1}. Solution has a pH of 3.5–5.5 and a pKa of 7.5. Generally contains a preservative.

Route of administration – it can be given intravenously (IV) or intramuscularly (IM). Oral, rectal, nasal and epidural (preservative-free preparation only) routes can also be used.

Dose – induction IV 1–2 mg.kg^{-1}, IM 5–10 mg.kg^{-1}; maintenance IV 0.5 mg.kg^{-1}, IM 3–5 mg.kg^{-1} approximately every 15 mins; analgesia and sedation IV 0.1–0.5 mg.kg^{-1}, IM 1–5 mg.kg^{-1}.

Uses – anaesthesia, sedation and analgesia. Useful in the shocked patient, when oxygen/ventilation equipment is not available, acute severe asthma, field anaesthesia. Safe in porphyria.

Kinetics
- Volume of distribution 3 l.kg^{-1}.
- Onset of action (IV) 30 seconds.
- Hepatic metabolism (hydroxylation or N-demethylation, conjugation).
- Active metabolite norketamine (20% potency).
- Excreted in urine.
- Clearance 18 ml.kg^{-1}.min^{-1}.
- Half-life 10 minutes.
- Elimination half-life 2.5 hours.

Effects
- Respiratory – laryngeal reflexes preserved, minimal effect on central respiratory drive, bronchodilator.
- Cardiovascular – increased blood pressure and heart rate, increased cardiac output.
- CNS – dissociative anaesthesia, analgesic, can cause hallucinations (emergence phenomenon), raised intracranial pressure.
- Gastrointestinal – increased secretions.
- Musculoskeletal – increased tone.

4.4

Anaesthetic agents – propofol

Propofol is a short-acting hypnotic agent with favourable characteristics including rapid emergence, with minimal residual drowsiness, and anti-emetic effect. Propofol enhances the inhibitory function of GABA at the $GABA_A$ receptor. In addition, it inhibits the NMDA glutamate receptor through sodium channel gating. Animal models suggest enhancement of GABA activity on $5HT_3$ receptors in the chemoreceptor trigger zone as the mechanism of anti-emetic action.

Chemical structure – a phenol derivative, 2,6-diisopropylphenol. A weak acid with a pKa of 11.

Presentation – presented as a white oil-in-water emulsion containing soybean oil (oil phase), egg lecithin (emulsifier stabilizing emulsion), glycerol (renders the preparation isotonic) and sodium hydroxide (adjusts the pH). Some preparations contain an antimicrobial agent such as metabisulfite or benzyl alcohol.

Route of administration – intravenous (IV).

Dose – induction IV 1.5–2.5 mg.kg^{-1}; increased dose in children, reduced dose in elderly or haemodynamically unstable. TCI: maintenance 2–6 mcg.ml^{-1}, sedation 0.5–1.5 mcg.ml^{-1}. Sedation in intensive care is achieved with manually controlled infusions because infusions are continued over sufficient time to achieve a steady-state concentration.

Uses – induction and maintenance of anaesthesia, sedation and management of refractory status epilepticus.

Kinetics
- Volume of distribution 60 l.kg^{-1}.
- Protein binding 95–99% in plasma.
- Onset of action less than 60 seconds.
- Duration of action 3–5 minutes after single bolus.
- Liver conjugation produces inactive metabolites. Some degree of extrahepatic metabolism.
- Clearance 23–50 ml.kg^{-1}.min^{-1}.
- Elimination half-life 0.5–1.5 hours.

Effects
- Respiratory – bolus dose causes short period of apnoea and suppression of laryngeal reflexes. Propofol infusion reduces tidal volume, increases respiratory rate and blunts response to hypercarbia and hypoxia.
- Cardiovascular – reduction in arterial blood pressure and systemic vascular resistance without compensatory increase in heart rate.
- CNS – reduction in intracranial pressure and cerebral oxygen consumption.
- Gastrointestinal – demonstrates intrinsic anti-emetic effects.

Anaesthetic agents – thiopentone

Barbiturates exhibit tautomerism, in that they transform between the keto and enol forms, depending on the surrounding pH. There are two categories depending on the functional group at the C2 position (by convention C1 is in the

Red = The barbiturate ring

12 o'clock position with further carbon atoms numbered sequentially clockwise): oxybarbiturates have oxygen and the thiobarbiturates have sulphur. Thiopentone is a thiobarbiturate and is more lipid soluble than the oxybarbiturates and therefore has a faster onset of action. Barbiturates depress the reticular activating system by inhibiting the dissociation of GABA from its receptors.

Chemical structure – thiobarbiturate.

Presentation – presented as the sodium salt of the enol form in a hygroscopic pale yellow powder containing 500 mg sodium thiopental with 6% sodium carbonate in an inert atmosphere of nitrogen. Prepared with 20 ml water or saline to create a solution containing 25 mg.ml^{-1} with a pH of 10.8 and a pKa of 7.6. Bacteriostatic solution.

Route of administration – intravenous (IV).

Dose – induction IV 4–5 mg.kg^{-1} (cerebral protection 5 mg.kg^{-1} then 5 mg.kg^{-1}.h^{-1}).

Uses – induction of general anaesthesia, cerebral protection. Contraindications – allergy, porphyria, no IV access.

Kinetics
- Volume of distribution 2.5 l.kg^{-1}.
- Onset of action within 30 seconds (rapid redistribution leads to short duration of action).
- Highly protein bound 65–85%.
- Hepatic metabolism (slow) by oxidation and desulphuration, easily saturated in infusion leading to zero order kinetics.
- Inactive metabolite phenobarbitone.
- Excreted in urine.
- Clearance 3 ml.min^{-1}.kg^{-1}.
- Half-life 8 minutes.
- Elimination half-life 11 hours.

Effects
- Respiratory – depression and apnoea, airway reflexes relatively well preserved (therefore not suitable for use with laryngeal mask airway).
- Cardiovascular – reduced cardiac output (direct depressant effect on myocardium) and blood pressure, decreased venous tone.
- CNS – reduced cerebral blood flow, cerebral metabolic rate and oxygen demand, anticonvulsant. Can be used in traumatic brain injury to lower intracranial pressure.
- Intra-arterial injection can cause vasospasm due to endogenous vasoconstrictor release.

4.6

Anticoagulants

	Unfractionated heparin	Low molecular weight heparins (e.g. dalteparin & enoxaparin)	Fondaparinux	Warfarin
Structure	Mucopolysaccharide mixture Average molecular weight 15 000–18 000 Daltons (Da)	Short polysaccharide chains Average molecular weight <8000 Da	Synthetic, specific activated Factor Xa inhibitor	Synthetic coumarin derivative
Mechanism of action	Binds reversibly to antithrombin III (AT III) causing inhibition of Factors IX–XIII, plasmin and thrombin Also inhibits platelet activation by fibrin	Interaction with AT III to cause inhibition of Factor Xa No effect on thrombin	Binds to AT III potentiating the neutralization of Factor Xa Doesn't inactivate thrombin and has no effect on platelet function or fibrinolysis	Prevents synthesis of vitamin K dependent clotting factors (II, VII, IX and X)
Dose	Intravenous bolus of 100 units.kg^{-1} followed by approximately 1000 units.h^{-1} to achieve an aPTT ratio of 1.5–2 (target ratio dependent on indication)	Once or twice daily subcutaneous injection No aPTT monitoring needed	Subcutaneous injection of 2.5–10 mg depending on patient weight	Oral 3–9 mg OD Response measured by PT/INR Maximum effect occurs 18–72 h after loading dose
Kinetics	Desulphated and depolymerized by heparinases in the liver, kidneys and endothelium Elimination half-life 0.5–2.5 h		Excreted unchanged in the urine Elimination half-life 17–21 h	
Other	Antagonized by protamine Heparin-induced thrombocytopenia: prevalence 5%; caused by formation of abnormal antibodies (IgG) which activate platelets	May be partially reversed by protamine (maximum effect <60%)		Effects antagonized by vitamin K or prothrombin complex in life-threatening haemorrhage

Anticoagulant drugs inhibit different stages of coagulation to prevent blood clotting. They are used in the prevention and treatment of venous and arterial thrombosis, acute coronary syndromes, disseminated intravascular coagulation and for priming haemodialysis and cardiopulmonary bypass machines.

Antiemetics

Post-operative nausea and vomiting (PONV) is a significant problem (incidence potentially 30%). It may cause distress and pain, and interfere with oral intake of medications, fluid and food. PONV may result in prolonged post-anaesthesia care unit stay and is a main reason for unanticipated hospital admission after day-case procedures.

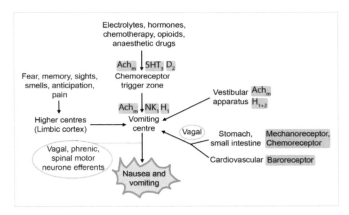

Two areas of the brain are involved.
- The vomit centre – an ill-defined region of brainstem nuclei (including the nucleus tractus solitarius) with afferents from the limbic, vestibular, gastrointestinal and cardiovascular systems.
- The chemoreceptor trigger zone (CTZ) – located outside the blood–brain barrier in the area postrema on the floor of the 4th ventricle. Efferents coordinate vomiting.

Most antiemetics antagonize the receptors of the CTZ and vomit centre afferent supply. They can be classified according to their target receptor.

Dopamine antagonists – CTZ main site of action (abundant D_2 receptors).
- Phenothiazines. Prochlorperazine is an antipsychotic and can be used for vertigo. Chlorpromazine (another antipsychotic) use is limited by its side-effects, including sedation, extrapyramidal effects and neuroleptic malignant syndrome (NMS). It can be used for intractable hiccups.
- Butyrophenones. Droperidol use has declined due to its association with prolonged QT. Intravenous domperidone is no longer available due to its association with serious arrhythmias.
- Benzamides. Metoclopramide also acts a prokinetic and has weak $5HT_3$ (5-hydroxytryptamine 3 receptor) antagonist properties. Side-effects include extrapyramidal reactions and NMS.

Anticholinergics – antagonize the muscarinic ACh receptors with minimal effect on nicotinic receptors. Hyoscine (scopolamine) is also useful in motion sickness.

Antihistamines – cyclizine is an H_1 antagonist and has anticholinergic properties. It is also useful in motion sickness and Ménière's disease.

$5HT_3$ antagonists – ondansetron and granisetron act on central and peripheral (gut) $5HT_3$ receptors. Undergo significant first pass metabolism.

Others – dexamethasone's mechanism is unclear but may include reduced release of arachidonic acid, reduced turnover of 5-hydroxytryptamine and decreased permeability of the blood–brain barrier. Total intravenous anaesthesia with propofol reduces PONV, as does acupuncture if performed prior to anaesthesia.

4.8

Antiplatelets

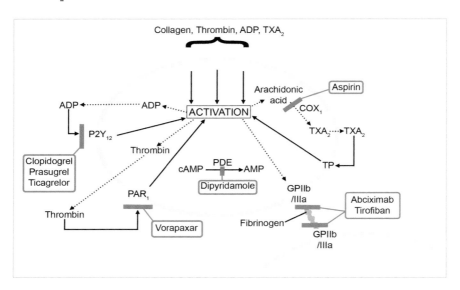

Platelets are essential for haemostasis but are also integral in thrombotic and atherosclerotic disease processes. Antiplatelets are used for both primary and secondary disease prevention. The decision to stop medication prior to surgery will depend on the nature of surgery, bleeding risk and the underlying reasons for taking the medication.

Platelet activation and aggregation occurs via several receptors found on their surface. Antiplatelets work by antagonizing these receptors or by blocking enzymes that produce messenger compounds. These target sites can be used for classification.

Cyclo-oxygenase inhibitors – aspirin is the most used antiplatelet. In low doses it irreversibly inhibits COX_1 preventing the synthesis of thromboxane A_2 (TXA_2) for the platelet's lifespan (7–10 days). At high doses COX_1 and COX_2 are inhibited. It is contraindicated in those <16 years due to the risk of developing Reye's syndrome (encephalopathy and liver dysfunction secondary to mitochondrial damage).

Adenosine diphosphate (ADP) receptor antagonists – 1st generation (e.g. ticlopidine), 2nd generation (e.g. clopidogrel) and 3rd generation (e.g. prasugrel) thienopyridine agents irreversibly bind to the $P2Y_{12}$ ADP receptor, preventing aggregation for the platelet's lifespan. Clopidogrel and prasugrel are prodrugs that require conversion in the liver to become active. Ticagrelor (a cyclopentyl-triazolopyrimidine compound) is a reversible antagonist at the same site.

Glycoprotein IIb/IIIa receptor antagonists – block fibrinogen and von Willebrand factor binding to the activated receptor, preventing cross-bridging and aggregation. Abciximab is a monoclonal antibody given as an infusion – platelets recover 48 hours following cessation. Tirofiban is a non-peptide antagonist given as an infusion – platelets recover 8 hours following cessation.

Phosphodiesterase inhibitors – dipyridamole prevents the degradation of cAMP, causing levels to increase and preventing platelet activation.

Protease-activated receptor (PAR) antagonists – vorapaxar is a PAR_1 reversible antagonist preventing thrombin-mediated platelet aggregation. However, inhibition can remain at 50% weeks after stopping the drug due to its long half-life.

4.9
Benzodiazepines

Benzodiazepines (BDZs) produce hypnosis, sedation, anxiolysis, anterograde amnesia and muscular relaxation, and are anticonvulsant.

BDZs potentiate the effects of gamma-aminobutyric acid (GABA) at $GABA_A$ receptors. $GABA_A$ is a ligand-gated chloride ion channel consisting of 5 subunits. Activation of $GABA_A$ results in augmented chloride ion conductance and membrane hyperpolarization. BDZs bind to the alpha subunit of the activated receptor.

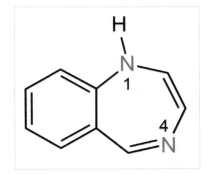

All BDZs have a common heterocyclic two-ring structure: a benzene ring and a 5 carbon, 2 nitrogen diazepine ring. Differences are due to the attachment of different side groups to the central structure.

Midazolam

Midazolam is unique among BDZs because its molecular structure is dependent on the surrounding pH. At pH 3.5, the diazepine ring structure opens resulting in an ionized molecule which is water soluble. At pH >4, the ring structure closes, is no longer ionized and becomes lipid soluble. The pKa of midazolam is 6.5, so 89% of the drug is unionized at physiological pH and therefore able to cross lipid membranes.

Midazolam is highly protein-bound, with an elimination half-life of 1–4 hours. It can be given orally (40% bioavailable), intranasally, intramuscularly or intravenously. Midazolam has a short duration of action and is hydroxylated and conjugated with glucuronic acid before being renally excreted.

Diazepam

Diazepam is rapidly absorbed orally with an oral bioavailability of 86–100%. Oral doses range between 2 and 60 mg.day^{-1}, whereas initial IV doses begin at 10–20 mg, titrated to effect.

Diazepam is approximately 95% protein-bound and oxidized by the liver to active metabolites such as desmethyldiazepam. The elimination half-life is 20–45 hours.

Flumazenil

Flumazenil is an imidazobenzodiazepine, used to reverse the effects of BDZs by competitive antagonism. Given by IV injection in 100 mcg increments, flumazenil acts within 2 minutes and has a half-life of approximately 1 hour. Seizure activity can result from administration, particularly in BDZ overdose.

4.10

Blood products

	Red blood cells	Fresh frozen plasma (FFP)	Cryoprecipitate	Platelets
Indication	Improve oxygen-carrying capacity in anaemia and blood loss	Replace coagulation factors in major haemorrhage Contains all soluble coagulation factors 2 g fibrinogen in 4 units FFP	Treatment of hypofibrinogenaemia Contains concentrated Factor VIII, XIII, vWF, fibrinogen and fibronectin	Treatment or prevention of haemorrhage in thrombocytopenia
Presentation	ABO/Rh D specific ~300 ml Hb content >40 g.unit^{-1} In saline, adenine, glucose & mannitol	Obtained from single male donor plasma via apheresis (limits transfusion-related acute lung injury – TRALI)	Available as single unit (20–40 ml) or pools of 5 units (100–200 ml) Each unit contains 400–450 mg fibrin	Either pool of 4 donations (of buffy coats in plasma of male donor) or from single donor via apheresis
Storage	2–6°C for 35 days after donation	Kept at −25°C to preserve factor activity Once thawed can be stored for 1–5 days at 4°C depending on type of thawer used	Kept at −25°C Once thawed, must be used within 4 hours	5–7 days at 22°C on an agitator
Dose	Hb transfusion trigger = 70–80 g.l^{-1} 1 unit increases Hb concentration by ~10 g.l^{-1}	12–15 ml.kg^{-1} Must be ABO compatible	Adult: 2 pools (5 units each)	1 pool Doesn't need to be ABO compatible, although care in paeds/pregnancy
Comment	Irradiated and CMV −ve RBCs available	If born after 1996, FFP sourced outside of UK & virally inactivated with methylene blue/solvent detergent		Should be transfused through a 200 μm filter which hasn't previously been used for RBC transfusion

Blood product transfusion can be a life-saving intervention. In the UK, blood donations are currently split into component parts, rather than being transfused as whole blood.

Other products:

- **Prothrombin complex** – a four-factor concentrate containing factors II, VII, IX and X with Protein C, Protein S and heparin. Indications include urgent reversal of warfarin or acquired factor deficiency.
- **Fibrinogen concentrate** – a pasteurized concentrate made from virally inactivated pooled human plasma. Available in vials containing 900–1300 mg fibrinogen concentrate for reconstitution.

Direct-acting oral anticoagulants

Direct acting oral anticoagulants (DOACs) are used for venous thromboembolism (VTE) prophylaxis in the context of elective arthroplasty, stroke prophylaxis in non-valvular atrial fibrillation, and the secondary prevention and management of deep venous thrombosis or pulmonary embolus.

Unlike warfarin's indirect mechanism of action, DOACs act directly: dabigatran inhibits thrombin (Factor II) while rivaroxaban, apixaban and edoxaban directly inhibit Factor Xa.

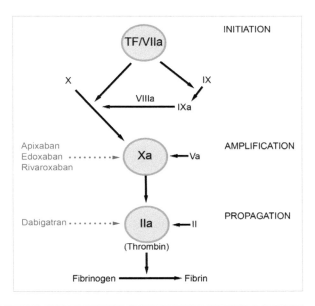

	Dabigatran	Rivaroxaban	Warfarin (for comparison)
Mechanism of action	Direct thrombin inhibitor	Direct Factor Xa inhibitor	Vitamin K epoxide reductase inhibitor
Oral bioavailability (%)	6.5	80–100	79–100
Half-life (hours)	12–17	5–13	45
Hepatic elimination (%)	20	65	~100
Renal elimination (%)	80	35	0
Time to maximal inhibition (h)	0.5–2	1–4	69

Dabigatran

A benzamidine-based, competitive, reversible direct thrombin inhibitor. Tablets contain the prodrug dabigatran etexilate that undergoes plasma and hepatic esterase hydrolysis to dabigatran. By inhibiting thrombin, it prevents the cleavage of fibrinogen into fibrin. It also inhibits platelet aggregation.

Idarucizumab, a monoclonal antibody, binds dabigatran resulting in anticoagulant reversal.

Rivaroxaban

An oxazolidinone derivative. It acts to directly inhibit Factor Xa, interrupting the amplification phase of blood coagulation. It exerts no effect on platelet aggregation.

The effects of rivaroxaban can be reversed by administration of recombinant human Factor Xa (andexanet alfa).

4.12

Intralipid

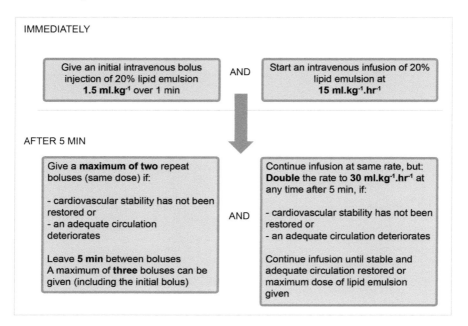

IMMEDIATELY

| Give an initial intravenous bolus injection of 20% lipid emulsion **1.5 ml.kg⁻¹ over 1 min** | AND | Start an intravenous infusion of 20% lipid emulsion at **15 ml.kg⁻¹.hr⁻¹** |

AFTER 5 MIN

| Give a **maximum of two** repeat boluses (same dose) if:

- cardiovascular stability has not been restored or
- an adequate circulation deteriorates

Leave **5 min** between boluses
A maximum of **three** boluses can be given (including the initial bolus) | AND | Continue infusion at same rate, but:
Double the rate to **30 ml.kg⁻¹.hr⁻¹** at any time after 5 min, if:

- cardiovascular stability has not been restored or
- an adequate circulation deteriorates

Continue infusion until stable and adequate circulation restored or maximum dose of lipid emulsion given |

Intralipid 20% is used in the treatment of local anaesthetic toxicity with or without circulatory arrest. It is also used in the preparation of total parenteral nutrition mixtures.

Chemical structure – a fat emulsion.

Presentation – a white, oil–water emulsion. Contains 20% soybean oil, 1.2% egg yolk phospholipids, 2.25% glycerin, sodium hydroxide and water.

Route of administration – intravenous either as a bolus or infusion.

Dose – in local anaesthetic toxicity, bolus of 1.5 ml.kg⁻¹ over 1 minute followed by infusion of 15 ml.kg⁻¹h⁻¹.

Kinetics
- Data for Intralipid is incomplete.
- Hypothesized that Intralipid is metabolized on the endothelium surface of capillaries by lipoprotein lipase.

Effects
- The exact mechanism of action in treatment of local anaesthetic toxicity remains unclear, but may involve the establishment of a concentration gradient away from primary site of local anaesthetic activity.
- Intralipid acts as an energy substrate containing 2 kcal.ml⁻¹, resulting in increased heat production and oxygen consumption.

Side-effects include pancreatitis secondary to hyperlipidaemia. Hepatic dysfunction has also been described after prolonged use. Following treatment for local anaesthetic toxicity, patients should have serial serum amylase or lipase measurements to check for pancreatitis.

Local anaesthetics – mode of action

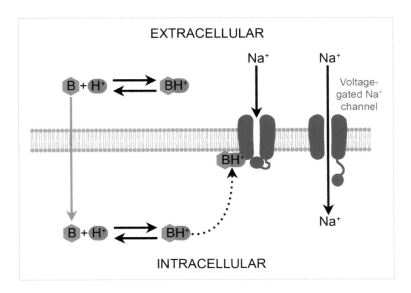

Local anaesthetic agents reversibly inhibit neuronal conduction by inhibition of voltage-gated sodium channels.

Chemical structure consists of an aromatic ring (lipophilic) linked to a basic amine side chain (hydrophilic) by either an ester or amide bond. The form of amine side chain determines, in part, molecular solubility. In the tertiary form the molecule is relatively lipid soluble whilst the quaternary form is water soluble.

Preparation – local anaesthetics are weak bases with pKa >7.4. At physiological pH these molecules are largely ionized rendering them water insoluble. To be stable in solution, local anaesthetics are formulated in the water soluble quaternary state as hydrochloride salts.

Mode of action – once injected, ionized local anaesthetics are unable to diffuse across the axonal membrane. The proportion of local anaesthetic converted to the tertiary form is dependent on pKa. This lipophilic, unionized molecule diffuses easily across the axonal membrane. Within the axon, lower intracellular pH converts local anaesthetics back to the ionized form. It is this ionized molecule that binds to, and closes, the intracellular channel inactivation gate. This occurs more readily whilst the channel is in the open or inactivated (rather than resting) states. Threshold potential is not reached because sodium influx is reduced and impulse conduction halts.

Neuronal sensitivity to local anaesthetic correlates with fibre diameter. Small diameter nerve fibres (e.g. Aδ and C) are more susceptible to local anaesthetic blockade than large fibres (e.g. Aα). As such, pain sensation is readily blocked whilst motor function is relatively resistant.

Absorption of local anaesthetic may lead to systemic toxicity. Associated factors include:
- method of administration – greatest systemic absorption with intravenous injection
- site of administration – after intravenous injection, highest peak plasma levels associated with intercostal and caudal injections
- vasoconstrictor use reduces absorption and prolongs local anaesthetic blockade.

4.14

Local anaesthetics – properties

Local anaesthetic	pKa	Protein binding (%)	Maximum safe dose (mg.kg⁻¹)
Esters			
Amethocaine	8.5	76	1.5
Cocaine	8.7	–	3
Procaine	8.9	6	12
Amides			
Lidocaine	7.9	64	3–7
Prilocaine	7.9	55	5–8
Bupivacaine	8.1	96	2
Levobupivacaine	8.1	>97	2
Ropivacaine	8.1	94	3.5

Linking bond – local anaesthetics are classified according to the type of linking bond: ester and amide. A general difference between these groups is the mechanism of drug metabolism. Esters are rapidly inactivated by non-specific plasma and liver cholinesterases. Amides are more stable in blood compared to ester local anaesthetics, accounting for their longer half-life. Amide local anaesthetics undergo hepatic biotransformation.

Time of onset – determined by the proportion of molecules that convert to the tertiary form at physiological pH as predicted by the pKa (see *Section 1.7.4 – Dissociation constant and pKa*). As all local anaesthetics are weak bases with a pKa greater than physiological pH, the quaternary form predominates in tissues with a normal pH (7.4). This process is amplified in infected, acidic tissue. The greater the pKa, the slower time to onset.

Potency – a measure of drug activity expressed in terms of the amount required to produce an effect of given intensity. For local anaesthetics, potency correlates with lipid solubility. Lipid solubility may be enhanced through substitution of carbon side chains to the aromatic ring. Greater lipid solubility facilitates diffusion through the axonal membrane increasing drug availability at the site of action.

Duration of action – local anaesthetics bind to plasma proteins (predominantly α-1-acid glycoprotein) in varying degrees. The plasma protein binding affinity correlates with the affinity of the molecule to bind to protein within sodium channels. As such, a molecule that is highly bound to circulating plasma proteins will have a relatively longer duration of action.

Stereochemistry – local anaesthetics demonstrating stereoisomerism include prilocaine, bupivacaine and ropivacaine. Although physiochemical properties of the stereoisomers are the same, biological effects may differ dramatically. Use of enantiopure formulations of bupivacaine and ropivacaine may be favoured due to their associated relative safety profiles.

Neuromuscular blockers – mode of action

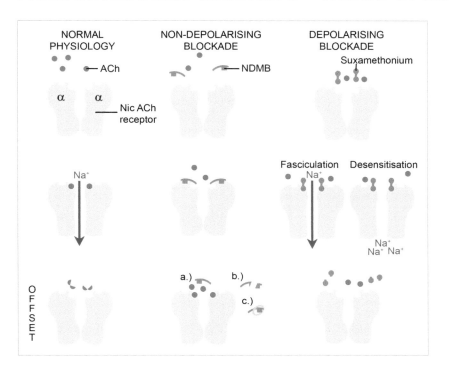

Neuromuscular blocking drugs (NMBDs) act at the neuromuscular junction (NMJ – see *Section 1.14.5 – Neuromuscular junction*). Each of the two alpha subunits of the nicotinic cholinergic receptor must be separately occupied by an acetylcholine (ACh) molecule to allow flux of sodium through the channel. Most modern NMBDs work by blocking these receptors, preventing the ACh molecules from binding. The commonly used NMBDs are divided into groups according to their mechanism of action.

Non-depolarizing – competitively bind to the nicotinic receptors blocking ACh. They also act on presynaptic receptors to prevent the entry of calcium thereby reducing ACh release. They can be further divided according to their chemical structure: benzyl-isoquinoliniums (e.g. atracurium and mivacurium) and steroidal compounds (i.e. rocuronium, vecuronium and pancuronium). All are highly ionized at body pH and are therefore poorly lipid soluble, with a small volume of distribution. They do not cross the blood–brain barrier so have no effect on the CNS. Offset occurs with time as ACh builds in the NMJ and displaces the agent from the nicotinic receptors. This can be potentiated with acetylcholinesterase inhibitors, e.g. neostigmine (a). The non-depolarizing agent is then metabolized either in the NMJ, blood or liver (b). Encapsulation of rocuronium and vecuronium with sugammadex will produce a very rapid offset (c).

Depolarizing – cause depolarization by mimicking the effect of ACh at the nicotinic receptor by non-competitively binding. However, they are not rapidly hydrolysed by acetylcholinesterases and therefore propagation of the action potential is prevented. The only clinically useful compound is suxamethonium. Fasciculations are seen due to an initial brief depolarization (phase I) followed by desensitization blockade (phase II), which continues for several minutes. Offset occurs with the metabolism of the agent by plasma cholinesterases.

4.16

Neuromuscular blocking agents – depolarizing

Suxamethonium is the only clinically relevant depolarizing NMBD. It mimics ACh at nicotinic cholinergic receptors causing membrane depolarization, but is not rapidly hydrolysed by acetylcholinesterases and therefore action potential propagation is prevented.

Chemical structure – dicholine ester of succinic acid; two ACh molecules joined through acetyl groups.

Presentation – clear colourless solution, $50\,mg.ml^{-1}$. Stored at 4°C.

Route of administration – intravenous (IV) or intramuscular (IM).

Dose – IV $1-2\,mg.kg^{-1}$, IM $3-4\,mg.kg^{-1}$.

Uses – rapid and short periods of muscle relaxation (rapid sequence induction), modification of seizures during electroconvulsive therapy.

Kinetics
- Onset of action approximately 30–60 seconds (IV).
- Rapid initial redistribution.
- Hydrolysed by butyryl (plasma) cholinesterase to succinylmonocholine (weakly active) and choline; further metabolized to succinic acid and choline. Only 20% (IV) reaches NMJ.
- Hydrolysis rate approximately $3-7\,mg.l^{-1}.min^{-1}$.
- 2–10% excreted unchanged in urine.
- Half-life 2.7–4.6 minutes.

Effects
- Muscarinic receptor stimulation at sino-atrial node causes sinus/nodal bradycardias and ventricular arrhythmias. More common in children and with repeated doses.
- Increased intracranial and intraocular pressure; potentially significant with already raised pressures or globe perforation.
- Raised intragastric pressure. Increased lower oesophageal sphincter tone.
- Elevation of serum potassium (approximately $0.2-0.4\,mmol.l^{-1}$) from cellular efflux following depolarization. Those with proliferation of extra-junctional ACh receptors are more susceptible (e.g. severe burns, neuromuscular disorders and paraplegia).
- Myalgia – particularly females and those ambulant early post-operatively.
- Malignant hyperthermia.
- Prolonged block ('sux apnoea') – genetic or acquired conditions causing reduced butyrylcholinesterase activity. Four genetic alleles (chromosome 3); usual $E1_u$ (normal), atypical $E1_a$ (dibucaine resistant), silent $E1_s$ (absent) and $E1_f$ (fluoride resistant). Acquired conditions include pregnancy, liver disease, renal failure, thyrotoxicosis and certain drugs.

Neuromuscular blocking agents – non-depolarizing

Agent	Dose (mg.kg⁻¹)	Speed of onset	Duration of action	Histamine release	Adverse effects
Atracurium	0.5	Medium	Medium	+	Histamine release
Mivacurium	0.2	Medium	Short	+	Prolonged degradation in some
Cisatracurium	0.2	Medium	Medium	–	Better side-effect profile than atracurium
Vecuronium	0.1	Medium	Medium	–	Prolonged action in renal failure
Rocuronium	0.6 (1.0 for RSI)	Dose-dependent	Medium	–	Prolonged action in renal failure
Pancuronium	0.1	Medium	Long	–	Prolonged action in renal failure

Non-depolarizing NMBDs are used to facilitate intubation, provide muscle relaxation during surgery and to increase compliance during mechanical ventilation.

Benzyl-isoquinoliniums
- Atracurium – a mixture of 10 stereoisomers due to 4 chiral centres. Minimally protein bound (15%) and broken down by ester hydrolysis (60%), by non-specific esterases, and Hofmann degradation (40%); a process of spontaneous degradation to laudanosine (an inactive metabolite which may cause seizures). These processes are independent of hepatic or renal function and therefore it is useful in patients with failure of these organs.
- Mivacurium – a mixture of 3 stereoisomers. Has a short duration of action due to rapid metabolism by plasma cholinesterases; it therefore may have prolonged action in individuals with low levels of this enzyme.
- Cisatracurium – one of the 10 stereoisomers of atracurium. 3–4 times more potent than atracurium and therefore has a slower onset time; this may be shortened by using higher doses. Similar properties to atracurium but with a low potential for histamine release and is broken down predominantly by Hofmann degradation.

Aminosteroids
- Vecuronium – monoquaternary analogue of pancuronium. Unstable in solution and therefore stored as a (yellow) powder for reconstitution. Has no effects on the cardiovascular system and does not cause histamine release. Metabolized in the liver by de-acetylation.
- Rocuronium – structurally similar to vecuronium. Excreted unchanged in the bile, undergoing some hepatic metabolism. Has low potency and therefore is given at higher doses to achieve similar clinical effects; this creates a higher concentration gradient at the NMJ producing favourable intubating conditions more rapidly.
- Pancuronium – bisquarternary aminosteroid. Causes tachycardia due to inhibition of cardiac muscarinic receptors and by preventing neuronal reuptake of noradrenaline. Metabolized in the liver producing some active metabolites.

4.18

Opioids – mode of action

Receptor subtype	Location	Effects	Side-effects with activation
μ, mu, MOP	• Throughout CNS – high density in spinal cord and brainstem • Peripheral sensory neurons • Gastrointestinal tract	Supraspinal analgesia, euphoria	Respiratory depression, inhibit gastrointestinal peristalsis, vomiting, pruritus, physical dependence
κ, kappa, KOP	• CNS – cerebral cortex and spinal cord • Peripheral sensory neurons	Analgesia, anticonvulsant	Sedation, dysphoria, diuresis No respiratory depression
δ, delta, DOP	• High densities in cerebral cortex • Spinal cord and peripheral sensory neurons	Spinal analgesia	Respiratory depression, inhibit gastrointestinal peristalsis
NOP	• CNS	Spinal analgesia	Supraspinal anti-analgesia, anxiety, depression

Strictly speaking, opiates are substances derived from opium. Opioids are any compound, natural or synthetic, that binds to opioid receptors to produce the characteristic effects of naturally occurring opiates. Opioids are reversed by naloxone.

Chemical structure – varies amongst opioids. These drugs may be classified into four chemical classes according to base structure.
- Phenanthrenes – the prototypical opioid composed of three fused benzene rings (e.g. morphine, codeine, buprenorphine).
- Piperidines – consist of a 6-membered ring (5 methyl bridges and 1 amine bridge) (e.g. fentanyl, alfentanil and remifentanil).
- Diphenylheptanes – e.g. methadone.
- Benzomorphans – e.g. pentazocine.

Tramadol, an atypical opioid, does not fit into this standard classification. It is a phenylpiperidine derivative of codeine.

Mode of action – opioid receptors are G-protein coupled, activating inhibitory G-proteins resulting in suppression of nociceptive neurotransmitter release (e.g. substance P and glutamate). Four receptor subtypes have been pharmacologically identified. Nomenclature has been controversial and changed numerous times. The current nomenclature approved by the International Union of Pharmacology is in keeping with the classical classification; μ, κ and δ. Opioid receptors are present in many regions of the nervous system. Supraspinal receptor localization is concentrated in the periaqueductal gray (primary control centre for descending pain modulation), amygdala and substantia nigra. Activation of spinal opioid receptors, within the substantia gelatinosa of the dorsal horn (region of spinal cord where sensory afferents synapse), inhibit both pre- and post-synaptic neurons to limit neurotransmitter release and neuronal excitability. Peripheral opioid receptors located outside the nervous system are responsible for some of the opioid associated side-effects: hypotension, constipation and pruritus.

While all classes of opioid have some analgesic activity, the most efficacious and widely used are those that act on the μ receptor.

Opioids – properties

Opioid	Effect at opioid receptor	pKa	Protein binding (%)	Terminal half-life (h)	Clearance (ml.min⁻¹.kg⁻¹)	Volume of distribution (L.kg⁻¹)	Relative lipid solubility
Morphine	μ – potent agonist κ – weak agonist	8.0	35	3	15–30	3–5	1
Codeine	μ – weak agonist κ – weak agonist	8.2	7–25	3	0.85	3.6	
Buprenorphine	μ – partial agonist κ – potent antagonist	8.3	96	20–75	20	2.8	
Alfentanil	μ – potent agonist	6.5	90	1.6	4–9	0.4–1.0	90
Fentanyl	μ – potent agonist	8.4	80	3.5	13	3–5	580
Remifentanil	μ – potent agonist	7.1	70	0.06	30–40	0.2–0.3	50

Kinetics

- Opioids are weak bases. At physiological pH, opioids with a pKa >7.4 predominantly exist in the ionized form. As alfentanil and remifentanil have a pKa <7.4, these drugs are largely unionized, attributing to a rapid onset of action.
- Distribution is determined by lipid solubility and plasma protein binding. Fentanyl is 500 times more lipid soluble than morphine. Its short duration of action at low doses (1–2 mcg.kg⁻¹) is explained by its rapid distribution, producing a dramatic decline in plasma concentration to subtherapeutic levels. After higher doses (or prolonged administration), distribution pathways become saturated, prolonging clinical effects. Duration of action is now dependent on elimination, not distribution.
- Opioid metabolism is largely hepatic, with generation of both active and inactive metabolites that are excreted in urine and bile. Extrahepatic metabolism is important for some opioids. Remifentanil is rapidly metabolized by non-specific plasma and tissue esterases resulting in a short elimination half-life. Due to the huge metabolic capacity, it is context insensitive.
- Opioid duration of action is determined by complex pharmacokinetic interactions that are not always evident from differences in clearance and half-life. Despite a similar terminal half-life as fentanyl, morphine demonstrates a significantly longer duration of action. Due to its low lipid solubility, onset of action is delayed as penetration of morphine across the blood–brain barrier is slow. Its effects persist due to the same principle, with release from the CNS being delayed.

Effects

Opioid pharmacodynamics are dependent on intrinsic activity of the drug. Opioids may be agonists, partial agonists or antagonists (see *Section 3.4 – Dose–response curves*).

Pure μ agonists are preferable for management of moderate or severe pain because no clinically relevant ceiling effect for analgesia exists, i.e. there is a dose-dependent relationship. As such, analgesic effects increase until analgesia is achieved or dose-limiting side-effects occur.

4.20

Paracetamol and NSAIDs

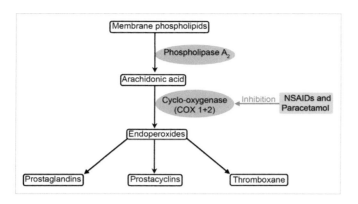

Paracetamol and non-steroidal anti-inflammatory drugs (NSAIDs) form the 'first step' of the WHO's analgesic ladder. Both exert their effects by inhibition of the cyclo-oxygenase (COX) enzymes, preventing the production of prostaglandins, prostacyclins and thromboxane.

Paracetamol

Paracetamol is an acetanilide derivative. It is thought to exert effects on both COX-1 and COX-2 enzymes, as well as on the serotonergic and cannabinoid pathways. In addition to analgesia, it also has an antipyretic effect.

Paracetamol can be administered orally, rectally or intravenously and is available in preparations containing other drugs, such as 'Cold and 'Flu' remedies.

Any person of >50 kg can be given 1 g every 4–6 hours, to a maximum daily dose of 4 g. Paediatric patients should receive 60–90 $mg.kg^{-1}.day^{-1}$, depending on age.

Paracetamol has good oral bioavailability and is minimally protein-bound in plasma. Approximately 90% is hepatically metabolized to a glucuronide form, before being actively excreted by the renal tubules. Elimination half-life is 2–4 hours.

In overdose, glutathione depletion can lead to hepatic damage by a toxic metabolite (N-acetyl-p-benzoquinone imine – NAPQI). This effect may be ameliorated by the administration of N-acetylcysteine (NAC).

NSAIDs

NSAIDs are a chemically diverse group of drugs with either non-specific inhibitory effects on COX (e.g. ibuprofen) or specific inhibition of COX-2 (e.g. parecoxib). They exert analgesic and anti-inflammatory effects.

NSAIDs can be orally, rectally and intravenously administered. They are highly protein-bound in plasma and have low volumes of distribution. NSAIDs are hepatically metabolized before being excreted in urine and bile.

As well as analgesic and anti-inflammatory effects, NSAIDs may cause gastric irritation and erosion, especially with prolonged use. This is due to reduced prostaglandin synthesis and thus reduced intestinal mucosal protective mechanisms. NSAIDs may also trigger acute severe asthma in up to 20% of asthmatics, impair renal function and impair platelet function.

4.21

Reversal agents

Neuromuscular blocking drug (NMBD) offset must have sufficiently occurred prior to meaningful spontaneous breathing and waking.

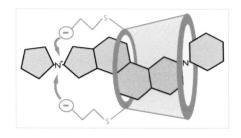

With depolarizing NMBDs (e.g. suxamethonium), this occurs with time due to hydrolysis by butyryl (plasma) cholinesterases. Non-depolarizing NMBDs are competitive antagonists at the nicotinic acetylcholine receptors. Offset occurs as acetylcholine builds in the neuromuscular junction (NMJ) and displaces the agent from the receptor. This can be potentiated with acetylcholinesterase inhibitors (e.g. neostigmine) and, in the case of aminosteroid compounds (e.g. rocuronium), rapid offset can be produced using encapsulation with sugammadex (see *Section 4.15 – Neuromuscular blockers – mode of action*).

	Neostigmine/glycopyrrolate	Sugammadex
Chemical structure	Neostigmine – quaternary amine anticholinesterase	Modified gamma cyclodextrin with lipophilic core and hydrophilic outer
	Glycopyrrolate – quaternary ammonium anticholinergic	1:1 encapsulation rendering NMBD inactive and generates concentration gradient between plasma and NMJ, increasing NMBD dissociation
Presentation	Clear colourless solution	Clear colourless to slightly yellow solution
	1 ml contains 2.5 mg neostigmine/ 0.5 mg glycopyrrolate	100 mg.ml^{-1} in 2 and 5 ml ampoules
Route of admin	Intravenous	Intravenous
Dose	Typically 2.5 mg/0.5 mg	16 mg.kg^{-1} – immediate reversal following administration of rocuronium
	Paeds – 50 mcg.kg^{-1}/10 mcg.kg^{-1}	2–4 mg.kg^{-1} – routine reversal (TOF ≥2)
Uses	Reversal of residual non-depolarizing neuromuscular blockade (≥2 twitches on TOF – see *Section 6.6 – Monitoring of neuromuscular blockade*)	Reversal of neuromuscular blockade by aminosteroid NMBDs
Kinetics	Neostigmine – hydrolysed by cholinesterases and metabolized in liver; excreted in bile and urine	Excreted unchanged in urine Elimination half-life 2 hours
	Glycopyrrolate – highly ionized at physiological pH with poor BBB and placental penetration; excreted in urine	
Effects	Glycopyrrolate reduces muscarinic side-effects of neostigmine (bradycardia, increased secretions, bronchospasm)	Bradycardia – vagal type response
		Interaction with progesterone – counsel those on oral contraceptive pill ('missed dose rules')
	Avoid use with suxamethonium (potentiates neuromuscular blockade)	Reported cases of anaphylaxis

4.22

Tranexamic acid

Tranexamic acid (TXA) is a synthetic derivative of the amino acid lysine. It binds to five lysine binding sites on plasminogen, competitively inhibiting plasmin formation and displaces plasminogen from the fibrin surface.

TXA's antifibrinolytic properties are useful in both the prevention and treatment of bleeding. The utility of TXA in decreasing mortality in trauma patients was demonstrated in the CRASH-2 study.

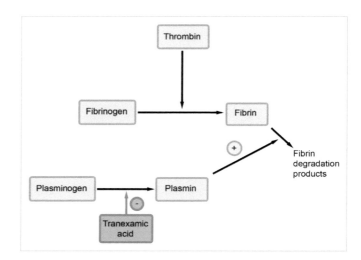

Chemical structure – stereoisomer of 4-(aminomethyl)cyclohexane-carboxylic acid.

Presentation – 500 mg tablets and 100 mg.ml⁻¹ colourless solution for intravenous (IV) injection (5 and 10 ml ampoules).

Route of administration – oral, intramuscular (IM) or IV.

Dose
- Oral dose: 15–25 mg.kg⁻¹ 2–3 times per day.
- IV: 0.5–1 g 3 times per day or initial 1 g slow bolus followed by 25–50 mg.kg⁻¹ by infusion over 24 hours.

Uses
- Prevention and treatment of excessive bleeding in both elective and emergency situations (including trauma, orthopaedic surgery, cardiac surgery, obstetrics, gynaecology and oral surgery).
- Prophylaxis of hereditary angioedema in elective procedures.

Kinetics
- Minimally (~3%) bound to plasma proteins.
- Less than 5% metabolized. Approximately 95% excreted unchanged via urine.
- Elimination half-life approximately 2 hours.

Effects
- Inhibition of plasminogen with reduction in bleeding.
- Side-effects include gastrointestinal disturbance (nausea, vomiting, diarrhoea) and seizures (at higher doses).

Use in trauma

Both the CRASH-2 study in 2011 and the CRASH-3 study in 2019 confirmed the safety and utility of TXA in trauma, including isolated traumatic brain injury (CRASH-3).

Volatile anaesthetic agents – mode of action

Anaesthetic agent	GABA$_A$ receptor	Potassium channel	Glycine receptor	NMDA receptor
Halogenated hydrocarbons	+	+	+	–
Nitrous oxide	0	+	+	–
Xenon	0	+	+	–
Propofol	+	0	+	–
Ketamine	0	0	0	–
Benzodiazepines	+	0	–	0
Barbiturates	+	0	+	–

GABA: gamma-aminobutyric acid; NMDA: N-methyl-D-aspartate.
+: potentiates; –: inhibits; 0: no effect.

How volatile anaesthetic agents work is uncertain. An attempt to produce a 'unitary theory' has been made but the picture is complex and it is likely there are multiple targets and mechanisms by which they produce anaesthesia. Various theories have been proposed.

The Meyer–Overton theory (see *Section 3.8 – Meyer–Overton theory*) – proposed that the potency of an anaesthetic agent is directly related to its lipid solubility. Suggested that with increased lipid solubility more anaesthetic agent molecules were dissolved in the lipid bilayer, and once sufficient numbers had dissolved, the resulting membrane disruption would result in anaesthesia. However, whilst an interesting observation, there are exceptions to this rule and the theory has become largely outdated. The correlation between potency and lipid solubility probably implies a hydrophobic site of action.

Critical volume hypothesis – proposed by Mullins, expands the Meyer–Overton theory by stating that absorption of anaesthetic molecules could expand the volume of the hydrophobic region within the cell membrane and distort the sodium channels, affecting sodium flux and therefore action potentials. Again, this theory is now largely redundant.

Protein targets (ion channels, receptors and intracellular enzyme systems) – CNS protein targets can be affected in a number of ways. These include disrupting normal synaptic transmission by changing the release of neurotransmitters pre-synaptically (either enhancing inhibitory or depressing excitatory transmission), by altering reuptake of neurotransmitters, changing their binding at the post-synaptic terminal or by changing ionic conductance. Possible targets include:
- Inhibitory ion channels
  - GABA$_A$ receptor-chloride channel – a ligand gated inhibitory complex that contains sites for propofol, benzodiazepines, barbiturates and volatile anaesthetics. Causes hyperpolarization of the neuronal membrane to reduce activity.
  - Glycine receptors.
  - Potassium channels.
- Excitatory ion channels
  - Glutaminergic ion channels.
  - NMDA receptor – nitrous oxide, xenon and ketamine preferentially act here.
  - Muscarinic complex.
  - Neuronal nicotinic ACh receptors.

4.24

Volatile anaesthetic agents – physiological effects

System	Variable	Desflurane	Isoflurane	Sevoflurane
CVS	HR	↑ (esp. >1 MAC)	↑	–
	BP	↓	↓	↓
	SVR	↓	↓	↓
	Contractility	–	↓	↓
	Catecholamine sensitivity	–	–	–
RS	Vt	↓	↓	↓
	RR	↑	↑	↑
	Bronchodilatation	Irritant	–	Yes
CNS	$CMRO_2$	↓	↓	↓
	CBF	↑	↑ (>1 MAC)	Autoregulation
	EEG	Burst suppression		
Muscles	Uterus	Some relaxation		
	Muscles	Significant relaxation		
Others	Special points	Needs heated vaporizer	?Coronary steal	Renal toxicity (fluorides and compound A)

BP – blood pressure, CBF – cerebral blood flow, $CMRO_2$ – cerebral metabolic rate for oxygen, CNS – central nervous system, CVS – cardiovascular system, EEG – electroencephalograph, HR – heart rate, RR – respiratory rate, RS – respiratory system, SVR – systemic vascular resistance, Vt – tidal volume.

The physiological effects of the commonly used volatile anaesthetic agents, desflurane, isoflurane and sevoflurane are summarized in the table and below.

Respiratory – all volatile anaesthetic agents cause dose-dependent respiratory depression, with a reduction in minute ventilation and a rise in P_aCO_2. They all cause bronchodilatation. Isoflurane and particularly desflurane have pungent odours and can cause upper airway irritability and breath-holding, making them less useful for inhalational induction of anaesthesia. Conversely, sevoflurane has a less pungent odour and is commonly used for inhalational induction.

Cardiovascular – the systemic vascular resistance falls with all the commonly used agents. A compensatory increase in heart rate is seen with isoflurane but not sevoflurane. This suggests that the carotid sinus reflex to a fall in blood pressure is preserved with isoflurane but not sevoflurane. Desflurane may produce cardiovascular stimulation over 1 MAC resulting in tachycardia and hypertension. None cause sensitivity to catecholamines. It has been proposed that isoflurane may have myocardial protective properties via its effects on ATP-dependent potassium channels.

CNS – all the agents cause a reduction in the cerebral metabolic rate ($CMRO_2$). They also reduce cerebral vascular resistance and may increase cerebral blood flow, potentially increasing intracranial pressure.

All agents cause a dose-dependent relaxation of the uterus and other muscle groups. They are all potential triggers for malignant hyperthermia.

4.25

Volatile anaesthetic agents – properties

Agent	Structure	MW (kDa)	BP (°C)	SVP at 20°C (kPa)	Blood:gas partition coefficient	Oil:gas partition coefficient	MAC (%)	Metabolites (% metabolized)
Nitrous oxide	N_2O	44	−88	5200	0.47	1.4	105	Nitrogen (<0.01)
Xenon	Xe	131	−108		14	1.9	71	
Des.	$CH(CF_3)_2OCH_2F$	168	23.5	89.2	0.45	29	6.6	Trifluoroacetic acid (0.02)
Iso.	$CF_3CHClOCF_2H$	184.5	48.5	33.2	1.4	98	1.17	Trifluoroacetic acid (0.2)
Enfl.	$CHFClCF_2OCF_2H$	184.5	56.5	23.3	1.8	98	1.68	Organic and inorganic fluorides, compound F (2)
Halo.	$CF_3CBrClH$	197	50.2	32.3	2.4	224	0.75	Trifluoroacetic acid (20)
Sevo.	$CF_3CFHOCF_2H$	200.1	58.5	22.7	0.7	80	1.8–2.2	Organic and inorganic fluorides, compounds A–E (3.5)

BP – boiling point, Des – desflurane, Enfl – enflurane, Halo – halothane, Iso – isoflurane, MAC – minimum alveolar concentration, MW – molecular weight, Sevo – sevoflurane, SVP – saturated vapour pressure.

Sevoflurane – a liquid at room temperature and stable in light. It undergoes hepatic metabolism to a greater extent than many of the other volatile agents by cytochrome P450 (isoform 2E1).

Isoflurane – a liquid at room temperature and stable in light. It is minimally metabolized with no known toxic metabolites.

Desflurane – a liquid at room temperature but unstable in light. It is extremely volatile (boiling point is 23.5°C and has an SVP at room temperature of 89.2 kPa). It therefore requires a special vaporizer for safe administration. It has a low blood:gas partition coefficient and therefore fast onset and offset. It is minimally metabolized.

With a move away from soda lime CO_2 absorbers, the issues with potential production of carbon monoxide and compound A are no longer a problem. Newer CO_2 absorbers, such as lithium-containing absorbers, eliminate these concerns.

All volatile anaesthetic agents are halogenated hydrocarbons and have the potential to act as potent greenhouse gases with significant global warming potential. Given the minimal metabolism of these agents during clinical use, they are exhaled and vented into the outside environment virtually unchanged. A global consensus statement from the World Federation of Societies of Anesthesiologists has recommended use of environmentally preferable medications (i.e. the agent with the lowest global warming potential – sevoflurane before isoflurane before desflurane). The EU has formulated a proposal to ban desflurane, or at least severely restrict its use, by January 2026 and the UK intends to do this by early 2024.

5.1

Avogadro's law

$$V = kn$$

$$k = \frac{RT}{P}$$

V = volume of gas (l)

k = constant

n = amount of substance of the gas (mol)

R = universal gas constant

T = temperature (K)

P = pressure (kPa)

Avogadro's law is a component of the ideal gas law. Avogadro's law states that 'equal volumes of gases at the same temperature and pressure contain the same number of molecules regardless of their chemical nature and physical properties'. Rearranging the ideal gas equation, for a constant temperature and pressure, the volume of a gas maintained at constant temperature and pressure is directly proportional to the number of moles of the gas. At 273K and 1 atmosphere (standard temperature and pressure, STP), 22.4 l of any gas contains 6.02×10^{23} gas molecules. Avogadro's number of 6.02×10^{23} equates to one mole.

Applications

Estimation of the volume of nitrous oxide in a cylinder – nitrous oxide stored at room temperature is below its critical temperature (36.5°C) and can therefore be liquified by compression. As such, cylinders contain saturated vapour in equilibrium with liquid. At a constant temperature, the saturated vapour pressure does not decrease until all of the liquid has evaporated. The gauge on the cylinder is therefore not necessarily representative of the cylinder contents. To estimate the volume of nitrous oxide, the cylinder must be weighed.

$$\frac{V_1}{m_1} = \frac{V_2}{m_2}$$

m = mass (kg)

$$\frac{22.4 l}{0.044 \, kg} = \frac{V_2}{mass \ of \ fluid \ in \ cylinder}$$

$$V_2 = mass \ of \ fluid \ in \ cylinder \times \frac{22.4 l}{0.044 \, kg}$$

Using Avogadro's law, one mole of nitrous oxide, with a molecular weight of 0.044 kg, occupies 22.4 l. With the mass of fluid within the cylinder known (actual weight – tare weight), the volume of nitrous oxide remaining in the cylinder can be calculated.

5.2

Beer–Lambert law

$$l = l_0 . e^{-(LC\beta)}$$

l = emergent light

l_0 = incident light

e = Euler's number

L = path length

C = concentration

β = molar extinction coefficient

The Beer–Lambert law is a combination of two laws that describe the absorption of monochromatic light by a transparent substance.

- Beer's law states that the absorbance of light passing through a medium is proportional to the concentration of the medium; as the concentration of the medium increases, the amount of light absorbed will also increase. If described in terms of emergent light, the intensity will decrease exponentially as the concentration of the medium increases.
- Lambert's law states that the absorbance of light passing through a medium is proportional to the length of the path it takes; as the path length increases, the amount of light absorbed will increase. Again, in terms of emergent light, the intensity will decrease exponentially as the path length increases.

The equation combines the two laws. The molar extinction coefficient is a measure of how avidly the medium absorbs light. A practical application of the Beer–Lambert law is in the understanding of how a pulse oximeter calculates peripheral arterial oxygen saturation (see *Section 6.9 – Pulse oximeter*). With the concentration and molar extinction coefficient remaining constant, the only variable becomes the path length which alters as arterial blood expands the vessels in a pulsatile way.

Critical temperatures and pressure

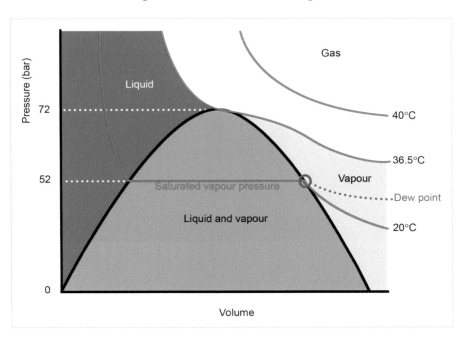

Isotherms are lines of constant temperature that depict the relationship between the pressure and volume of a substance at that temperature. A common example used (as illustrated above) is nitrous oxide; at 40°C (above its critical temperature of 36.5°C and therefore in gaseous form) the line is a rectangular hyperbola demonstrating that as the pressure doubles, the volume halves (see *Section 5.10 – Gas laws – Boyle's law*). At 36.5°C, as pressure increases, the line climbs as a rectangular hyperbola until it reaches a midpoint with a small flattened portion where a small amount of gas is liquefied. After this, the line rapidly climbs as all the vapour becomes liquid and incompressible. At 20°C, the line curves up initially, becoming horizontal as it crosses the liquid–vapour curve and thereafter rises rapidly as all the vapour becomes liquid.

Critical temperature is the temperature above which a substance cannot be liquefied, regardless of the pressure applied. Vapour is matter in the gaseous form below its critical temperature, i.e. particles may enter the liquid phase. Critical pressure is the vapour pressure of a substance at its critical temperature (an alternative definition is the lowest pressure needed to liquefy a gas at critical temperature).

When substances are mixed their critical properties may change. The pseudocritical temperature applies to a mixture of gases, and is the temperature at which it separates into its constituent parts.

Entonox (50% nitrous oxide (N_2O) and 50% oxygen) is produced by bubbling oxygen gas through liquid N_2O causing it to vaporize and creating a gaseous N_2O/oxygen mix (the Poynting effect). The critical temperature of N_2O changes from 36.5°C to a pseudocritical temperature of −5.5°C (at 117 bar). There is therefore a risk of separation, with liquid phase formation (lamination), if the temperature falls below this. Consequently, a hypoxic mixture may be delivered when the oxygen becomes depleted.

5.4

Diathermy

Diathermy is used during surgery to cut or coagulate tissues. It works on the principle of current density (current per unit area). When a current is applied over a small area the density is high and a heating effect occurs; conversely when that same current is applied over a large area the density is low and no heating occurs.

There are two main types.
- **Monopolar** – consists of a small pointed electrode with a high current density allowing accurate cutting or coagulation and a fixed second indifferent electrode with a large surface area (low current density).
- **Bipolar** – has both electrodes mounted on the same device, both with a small surface area and high current density. Has the advantage of preventing the flow of current through other tissues of the body and focuses just on the tissue in the surgical field.

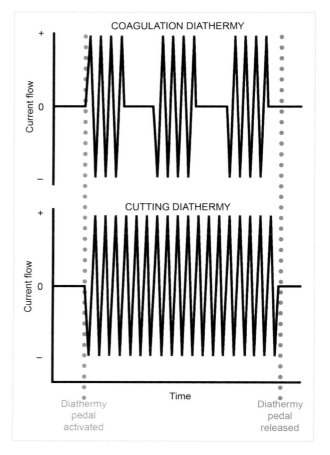

When a voltage is applied across the body current will flow through it. The frequency of that current will determine the effect that it has. At low frequencies it will have effects proportional to the current size; initially tingling and pain, increasing to muscle stimulation and eventually to ventricular fibrillation. Surgical diathermy uses a very high frequency current (0.5–1 MHz) that produces only heating effects with no stimulation.

Diathermy equipment may be set to cutting or coagulation depending on the surgical need. Cutting diathermy is high energy and delivers a sustained high frequency AC waveform that is able to cut tissues. Coagulation diathermy has a different waveform, delivering bursts or pulses of high frequency AC current interrupted by periods of no current flow. This cauterizes the tissue and causes less destruction than the cutting waveform.

Disadvantages of diathermy include:
- Monitoring interference.
- Burns.
- Disruption of pacemaker function.
- Pollution from vaporized tissue.

Doppler effect

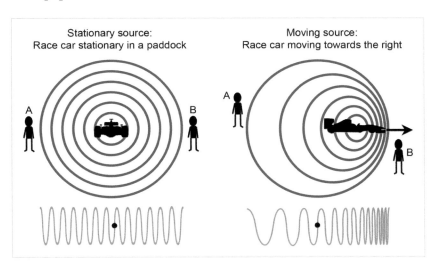

The Doppler effect is the perceived change in frequency of waves emitted by a source moving relative to the observer. Sound waves are longitudinal waves that travel outwards in all directions from the source producing a series of concentric circles. As a wave moves through a medium, each medium particle vibrates at the same frequency. This creates alternating high- and low-pressure disturbances of medium particles at a given frequency. Pitch is a measure of the frequency of a sound wave; high pitch signifies high frequency while low pitch signifies low frequency.

Stationary source

The source is stationary with respect to observers A and B. As wave velocity is fixed for a given medium (e.g. air), both observers will perceive the sound at the same pitch.

Moving source

The source is moving towards observer B at a fixed velocity.
- **Moving towards observer B** – as the source moves, each consecutive disturbance originates from a point nearer to observer B. The wavelength in the direction of source motion is thus shortened, while the wave velocity remains fixed. Therefore, a shorter wavelength results in a higher frequency. As such, observer B perceives the sound wave as higher in pitch.
- **Moving away from observer A** – conversely, as the source moves away from observer A, the wavelength increases. The observed frequency is reduced with observer A perceiving a lower pitch sound.

The Doppler principle is utilized in oesophageal cardiac output monitoring. Ultrasound waves emitted at fixed frequency reflect off moving red blood cells (RBCs) in the descending aorta. If the RBCs are moving towards the probe, the wavelength of reflected waves is reduced and frequency is increased. The opposite occurs if RBCs are moving away from the probe. Analysis of the reflected frequencies determines descending thoracic aortic blood flow, allowing cardiac output to be derived.

5.6
Electrical safety

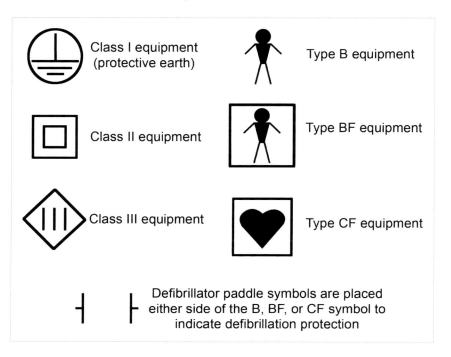

Electrical equipment is classified according to International Electrotechnical Commission standards (IEC 61140), with further regulation for medical appliances (IEC 60601-1-1).

- Class I – consists of earthed equipment and fuses. Any conducting part that could come into contact with a user is connected to an earth to protect against electrocution. Fuses exist to add extra safety if a short-circuit occurs. Not considered safe for direct connection to the heart.
- Class II – double insulated so it is impossible for a user to come into contact with the live wire. Not earthed.
- Class III – called safety extra-low voltage (SELV) as it does not need an electrical supply exceeding 24 volts AC. Risk of micro-shock still exists. Internally powered, e.g. with batteries.

Class I, II and III equipment may also contain floating circuits that are not earthed but are isolated from the rest of the circuit by transformers. Leakage currents can still occur through inductive or capacitive effects and can lead to micro-shock if the equipment is in close contact with the heart.

Electrical equipment can also be classified according to the risk of leakage currents:

- Type B – may be class I, II or III equipment and has a low leakage current even in the presence of a fault. Can be safely connected to the patient either internally or externally but is not considered safe for direct connection to the heart.
- Type BF – similar to type B but is safer because the patient is isolated via a floating circuit. Maximum permitted leakage current is 100 µA but still not considered safe enough to be connected directly to the heart.
- Type CF – considered safe for direct connection to the heart because the leakage current is very small (less than 10 µA). Used for thermodilution catheters, ECG leads and pressure transducers.

5.7

Electricity

Variable	Description	Derived units
Electric charge	Quantity of electricity	Coulomb (C) = A.s
Current	Flow of charge	Ampere (A) = C.s⁻¹ (the ampere is a base SI unit)
Electric field	Force per unit charge	Newtons per coulomb (N.C⁻¹)
Voltage	Electric potential	Volt (V) = J.C⁻¹
Electric potential difference	Work done per unit charge	Volt (V) = J.C⁻¹
Electrical power	Rate of work	Watt (W) = J.s⁻¹
Electrical resistance	Resistance to flow of charge	Ohm (Ω) = V.A⁻¹

Electricity is a form of energy resulting from the existence of charged particles (e.g. protons and electrons). If an atom has equal numbers of protons and electrons, it is electrically neutral. If it has an unequal number of protons and electrons, it becomes electrically charged. The quantity of electricity is the amount of electric charge. Current is defined as the flow of electric charge.

Electrically charged particles are surrounded by an electric field that exerts a force on other electrically charged particles. The force exerted by the electric field is the voltage. Voltage, also called electric potential, is the force required to make electric current flow. Electric potential energy is the potential energy of a charged particle that results from the presence of voltage. A force is required to displace a charged particle from one position to another; this is work (see *Section 5.29 – Work*). Energy is required to do work. This energy is transferred to the charged particle as electric potential energy. Electric potential difference is the difference in electric potential (voltage) between two positions. It represents the work done to move a charged particle between two points.

Power is the rate of work done. Therefore, electrical power is a product of the electric potential difference and the amount of charge passing a given point per unit time (i.e. the current).

Electrical resistance is the resistance to flow of charge in an electric circuit. Resistance is directly proportional to the length of wire and inversely proportional to the cross-sectional area of the wire. Materials that are inherently better conductors of charge will exhibit a lower resistance.

Current, resistance and electric potential are related by Ohm's law (see *Section 1.2.6 – Ohm's law*). Current will increase when a greater force (voltage) is applied to the charged particles. As resistance to flow of charge increases, current will decrease.

5.8

Exponential function

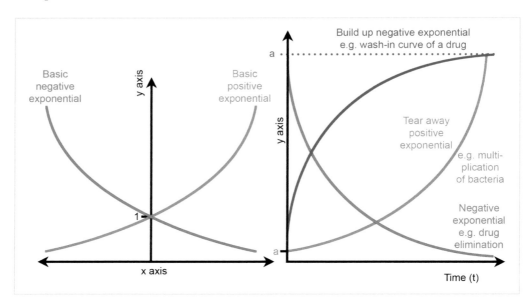

An exponential function is a condition where the rate of change of the function is proportional to the value of the variable at that point in time. An everyday example would be that the rate of decrease in temperature of a cup of coffee is proportional to the temperature of the coffee at that time point. There are many exponential functions in anaesthesia, an example being that the rate of decline in drug plasma concentration is proportional to the concentration of the drug itself.

Euler's number, or 'e', is seen in the exponential function equations. It is called a transcendental number and represents the value 2.71828... It is the limit of $(1 + 1/n)^n$ as n approaches infinity and can also be defined as the base of the natural logarithm.

The graphs show a series of exponential relationships.
- The basic positive exponential ($y = e^x$) is asymptotic with the x-axis and crosses the y-axis at 1 (as any number to the power 0 is equal to 1).
- The corresponding negative exponential ($y = a^{-x}$) has similar features but is a mirror image of the positive version.
- A tear away exponential, an example of which could be multiplication of bacteria, has the equation $y = a.e^{kx}$ and crosses the y-axis at a.
- A build-up negative exponential ($y = a - b.e^{-kx}$) is seen as a wash-in curve during drug administration. It is a negative exponential because the rate of increase in y is reducing exponentially as time, t (x), increases.
- Lastly, a negative exponential ($y = a.e^{-kx}$), seen clinically during drug elimination, declines exponentially as time increases.

Fick's law of diffusion

$$\text{Rate} \propto \frac{A\left[C_1 - C_2\right]}{D}$$

Rate = rate of diffusion

A = area of membrane

$C_1 - C_2$ = concentration gradient

D = membrane thickness

Fick's (first) law of diffusion can be used to describe certain characteristics of a membrane that will facilitate diffusion of a substance across it. The rate of diffusion across a membrane is directly proportional to its area, the concentration gradient across it and inversely proportional to its thickness.

Adolf Fick described two laws related to diffusion in 1855. His work was inspired by the earlier work done by Thomas Graham that related molecular weight to the rate of diffusion (see *Section 5.14– Graham's law*). The first law relates diffusion of a substance to the concentration gradient under the assumption of steady state. It describes movement of molecules in high concentration to regions where they are in a lower concentration; the magnitude of which is proportional to the concentration gradient. Fick's second law describes how diffusion causes the concentration to change with time.

When applied to the lung, the surface area for gas transfer across the alveoli is large and the membrane across which transfer of gases occurs is incredibly thin; this provides a very efficient gas exchange interface. Certain pathological conditions interfere with this process, e.g. the presence of pulmonary oedema will increase the membrane thickness, thus slowing the rate of diffusion. Similarly, in disease states such as emphysema a reduction of the surface area for gas transfer will also reduce the rate of diffusion. Fick's law can also be applied to induction of anaesthesia using a volatile agent ('gas induction'); a high alveolar concentration of the volatile agent will create a large concentration gradient, encouraging uptake into the blood and speeding the onset of anaesthesia.

5.10

Gas laws – Boyle's law

$$V \propto \frac{1}{P} \text{ at constant temperature}$$

$$PV = nRT$$

$$PV = \text{constant}$$

P = pressure (Pa)

V = volume (m³ or l)

N = number of moles (mol)

R = universal gas constant = 8.314 m³.Pa.K⁻¹.mol⁻¹

T = temperature (K)

Boyle's law states that 'for a fixed mass of gas at constant temperature, the volume is inversely proportional to the pressure'. This principle may be expressed mathematically using the ideal gas equation, substituting 'nRT' for a constant. The pressure of a gas within a container is the result of gas molecules colliding with the container walls. As the volume becomes smaller, gas molecules collide with the container more frequently. As such, the pressure increases. If the volume of a container is halved, the pressure exerted by the gas doubles. Boyle's experiment demonstrated this relationship in the opposite order. Using a J-shaped tube of glass, oxygen was trapped at the sealed short limb. Maintaining the gas at a constant temperature, Boyle added increasing amounts of mercury to the tube, resulting in an increasing amount of pressure being applied to the oxygen. By increasing the pressure of this fixed amount of gas, the volume reduced at a constant rate.

Applications

- Syringe – pulling back on the plunger of a syringe increases the volume of the container. The resultant drop in pressure draws liquid into the syringe.
- Estimation of volume of pressurized gas when exposed to atmospheric pressure – an E sized oxygen cylinder, as stored on the back of an anaesthetic machine, stores oxygen at a pressure of 137 bar and has a water capacity of 4.7 l. Boyle's law can be used to determine the volume of oxygen gas available when it is exposed to atmospheric pressure.

$$V_1 \times P_1 = V_2 \times P_2$$

$$V_2 = \frac{4.7 \ l \times 137 \ bar}{1 \ bar} = 644 \ l$$

Gas laws – Charles' law

$$V \propto T \text{ at constant pressure}$$
$$PV = nRT$$
$$V = constant \times T$$

P = pressure (Pa)

V = volume (m^3 or l)

N = number of moles (mol)

R = universal gas constant = 8.314 m^3.Pa.K^{-1}.mol^{-1}

T = temperature (K)

Charles' law states that 'for a fixed mass of gas at constant pressure, the volume is directly proportional to absolute temperature'. In this circumstance, nR/P is replaced by a constant. If the temperature of a fixed mass of gas is increased, the velocity of the gas molecules will increase leading to an increase in frequency of molecular collision with the container walls. A transient increase in pressure results in an increase in container volume to maintain a constant pressure. The converse is true with regards to the volume–temperature relationship of a gas. As the volume of a fixed amount of gas increases, the frequency with which gas molecules collide with the container walls reduces, leading to a transient reduction in pressure. An increase in temperature increases the molecular kinetic energy of the gas, subsequently increasing the frequency of collision and restoring pressure.

Applications

- Hot air balloon – gas within the hot air balloon is heated. As the temperature increases, the pressure increases transiently. To restore a constant pressure, the volume of the gas (and balloon) increases. Density of a gas is equal to the mass of the gas divided by its volume. As the mass of gas is fixed, an increase in volume will reduce gas density. The gas within the hot air balloon is now less dense than the surrounding air, thus allowing the balloon to rise.
- Heat loss by convection – this is a similar principle to the hot air balloon. The body heats the air immediately next to it. This increases the kinetic energy leading to an increase in volume. This less dense air rises being replaced with cooler, denser air. This movement of gas contributes to the development of convection currents.

5.12

Gas laws – Gay-Lussac's (Third Perfect) law

P ∝ T at constant volume

$PV = nRT$

P = constant × T

P = pressure (Pa)

V = volume (m³ or l)

N = number of moles (mol)

R = universal gas constant = 8.314 m³.Pa.K⁻¹.mol⁻¹

T = temperature (K)

Gay-Lussac's law, or the Third Perfect gas law, states that 'for a fixed mass of gas at constant volume, pressure is directly proportional to absolute temperature'. This law is founded on the kinetic molecular behaviour of gases. As the temperature of a fixed mass of gas increases, kinetic energy also increases leading to a rise in pressure when volume is constant.

When applying proportionality relationships described by the gas laws, absolute temperature (K) must be used. Doubling of room temperature (21°C or 294 K) is not 42°C (315 K) but actually 315°C (588 K). Failure to convert to absolute temperature would clearly introduce significant error into any calculations. Similarly, for Charles' and Gay-Lussac's gas laws, which employ temperature as a variable factor, using negative Celsius temperatures would generate nonsensical negative volume or pressure calculations.

Applications

- Tyre pressure – the most accurate measure of tyre pressure is performed when the tyres are cold. With driving, the tyres heat due to friction. As the temperature rises, the kinetic energy of the air inside the tyre rises, resulting in an increase in pressure.
- Storage of compressed gas cylinders – storage requirements state that temperature should not exceed that recommended by the gas supplier. If temperature rises above a defined value, gas pressure within the cylinder increases, potentially leading to explosion.

5.13

Gas laws – ideal gas law and Dalton's law

$$PV = nRT$$

P = pressure (Pa)

V = volume (m³ or l)

N = number of moles (mol)

R = universal gas constant = 8.314 m³.Pa.K⁻¹.mol⁻¹

T = temperature (K)

The ideal gas law relates pressure, temperature and volume of an ideal gas. This law is a combination of all the simple gas laws: Boyle's law, Charles' law, Gay-Lussac's law and Avogadro's law. Mathematically, the ideal gas law may be expressed as the ideal gas equation. An ideal gas is a theoretical gas that upholds a number of assumptions:

- A gas comprises a large number of tiny particles so small that their size is negligible.
- All collisions between molecules or atoms are perfectly elastic.
- No intermolecular forces exist.
- At any given time, there is a wide range of molecular kinetic energies. However, the average kinetic energy is proportional to the absolute temperature.

Most gases do not fulfil these assumptions, however, the ideal gas law and its component laws provide a reasonable approximation of gas behaviour.

The identity of a gas is not required to apply the gas laws. This means that a gas mixture behaves in exactly the same fashion as a pure gas.

The universal gas constant (R) is a proportionality constant relating energy to temperature. It is common for all gases. The value of R depends on the units used for pressure, volume and temperature.

Dalton's law

$$P_{total} = P_1 + P_2 + P_3... P_n$$

P = partial pressure of gas (kPa)

Dalton's law states that the total pressure of a gas mixture in a container is the sum of the partial pressures of its individual components. This law assumes that the gases within the mixture behave independently. Using the ideal gas law, at a constant temperature and volume, the pressure exerted by a gas is proportional to the number of moles. This concept holds true regardless of the identity of the gas/gases present. As gases are added together to create a mixture, the pressure increases directly proportionally to the increase in the total number of moles of gas.

5.14

Graham's law

For one gas:

$$Rate \propto \frac{1}{\sqrt{MW}}$$

Rate = rate of diffusion (volume or number of moles per unit time)

MW = molecular weight

For two gases:

$$\frac{Rate_1}{Rate_2} \propto \sqrt{\frac{MW_2}{MW_1}}$$

Graham's law states that the rate of diffusion of a gas is inversely proportional to the square root of its molecular weight; the higher the molecular weight, the slower the rate of diffusion. If the molecular weight of one gas is four times that of another, it will diffuse at half the rate of the other.

Thomas Graham, a Scottish physical chemist, proposed his law in 1848. It is also known as Graham's law of effusion; effusion relating to both the direction and the rate of change of diffusion. It can be applied to two gases and helps to explain the second gas effect, seen when nitrous oxide is used with a volatile anaesthetic agent. In the case of two gases, the rate of effusion of the first gas, divided by that of the second is equal to the square root of the second gas' molecular weight, divided by that of the first. If the molecular weight of the first gas is much smaller than that of the second it will effuse out of the alveoli more quickly. Proportionally more of the second gas will be left in the alveoli and therefore its concentration will increase. This effect is seen with nitrous oxide because it has a smaller molecular weight than the volatile agents. The increased concentration of volatile agent in the alveoli speeds its onset of action.

Graham's Law can also be used to find the approximate molecular weight of a gas in a mixture of two gases. If the weight of the second gas and the specific ratios of diffusion of the two gases are known, the equation can be rearranged to solve the unknown molecular weight.

5.15

Heat

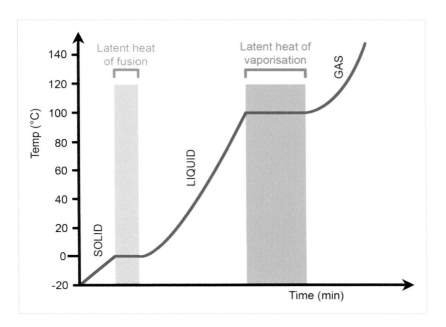

Heat is a form of energy associated with movement of molecules; it can be transferred from one site to another owing to a temperature difference between the two sites (temperature gradient). It is measured in joules or calories; 1 calorie is the amount of heat required to raise the temperature of 1 g of water by 1°C; 1 calorie equals 4.16 joules.

Temperature is a measure of the thermal state of an object and describes how hot or cold it is. Heat energy passes down a gradient from high to low temperature; the temperature of the object receiving the heat energy therefore increases. Addition or removal of heat energy can cause a change in physical state, with the amount needed varying according to pressure. At 1 atmosphere the freezing point of water is 0°C, however, this decreases with increasing pressure.

Latent heat is the energy required to change the state of a substance without a change in its temperature; it is measured in joules per kilogram ($J.kg^{-1}$). Latent heat of vaporization is the change from a liquid to a gas, or vice versa; latent heat of fusion is the change of a solid to a liquid, or vice versa. Specific latent heat is the heat required to convert 1 kg of a substance from one phase to another at a given temperature. It is greater at lower temperatures and falls as temperature increases until it reaches zero at the critical temperature, i.e. the lower the temperature the more latent heat is needed to vaporize a substance.

Volatile anaesthetic agents require latent heat for vaporization. Vaporizers must compensate for this (usually with a heat sink): if the temperature of the liquid is allowed to fall it becomes less volatile, lowering its saturated vapour pressure and reducing the amount of anaesthetic vaporized.

5.16

Henry's law

$$P_{gas} = k_H \times C$$

P_{gas} = partial pressure of gas above solution (atm)

k_H = Henry's law constant (l.atm.mol^{-1})

C = concentration of dissolved gas (mol.l^{-1})

Henry's law describes gas solubility, stating that 'at constant temperature, the amount of a given gas that dissolves in a given type and volume of liquid is directly proportional to the partial pressure of that gas in equilibrium with that liquid'. For example, if the partial pressure of an anaesthetic agent in the alveoli is doubled, once equilibrated the partial pressure and quantity dissolved in the blood would also double.

Gases dissolve in liquids, forming solutions. An equilibrium constant relates the solubility of a gas in a liquid to the partial pressure of that gas above the liquid, when the system is in equilibrium. The equilibrium constant is known as Henry's law constant (k_H); it is dependent on temperature and the nature of the gas and liquid.

Gas solubility is dependent on:
- Temperature – as temperature increases, solubility decreases. An increase in temperature increases the kinetic energy of molecules. This increase in molecular motion facilitates intermolecular bonds to break and gas molecules to escape from solution.
- Pressure – as gas partial pressure increases, solubility increases. An increase in gas partial pressure increases the frequency with which gas molecules collide with the solution's surface. More gas molecules are forced into the solution, relieving the applied pressure and restoring equilibrium.

Applications
- Carbonated drinks – dissolved carbon dioxide stays in solution in a closed container where the partial pressure of carbon dioxide is high. When the container is opened, the partial pressure drops dramatically and dissolved carbon dioxide escapes from solution.
- Decompression sickness ('the bends') – deep sea divers inhale highly compressed air at depth. This increase in alveolar partial pressure increases the solubility of air into the capillaries, tissue and joints. If the diver returns to the surface rapidly, partial pressure reduces, and nitrogen solubility rapidly decreases, forming gas bubbles in tissues or blood.

5.17

Humidity

Humidity describes the amount of water vapour present in the atmosphere. Absolute humidity is the mass of water vapour present in a given volume of air expressed in $mg.l^{-1}$ or $g.m^{-3}$. Relative humidity is the ratio of the mass of water vapour in a given volume of air to the mass required to saturate that given volume of air at the same temperature; it is usually expressed as a percentage.

A hygrometer is an instrument used to measure humidity; most measure relative humidity. Examples include:

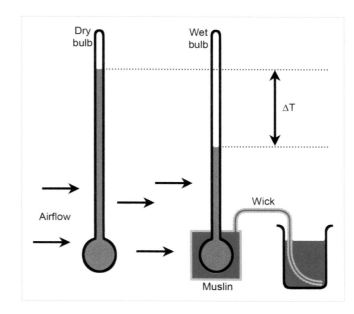

- Hair hygrometer – gives a direct reading of relative humidity. Consists of a pointer attached to a human hair; as humidity increases the hair lengthens.
- Wet and dry hygrometer (shown above) – measures relative humidity. Consists of two bulb thermometers, one dry and the other wrapped in a wet wick. The dry bulb reads true ambient temperature. The wet bulb reads at a lower temperature due to the cooling effect from the evaporation of water from the wick surrounding the bulb and the consequent loss of latent heat of vaporization. The temperature difference between the two bulbs is related to the rate of evaporation, which in turn depends on the ambient humidity. Relative humidity can be determined from a set of tables.
- Regnault's hygrometer – consists of a silver tube containing ether, which is cooled by blowing air through it with a rubber bulb. When condensation appears on the outside, the air is saturated with water at that temperature, i.e. the dew point. From a graph of saturated air water content against temperature, water content at the dew point temperature can be determined. This gives a measurement of absolute humidity; relative humidity can then be calculated.
- Absolute humidity can also be measured by transducers, mass spectrometry and ultraviolet light absorption hygrometers.

5.18

Laser

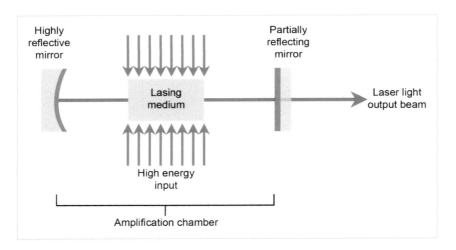

Laser stands for **l**ight **a**mplification by **s**timulated **e**mission of **r**adiation. They consist of an energy source, lasing medium (which may be solid, liquid or gas) and an amplification chamber. The laser is usually named according to its lasing medium.

The light emitted, through a process of amplification based on the stimulated emission of electromagnetic radiation, is:

- Monochromatic, consisting of a single wavelength.
- Coherent, in phase.
- Collimated with little divergence from the point of origin.

When energy is applied to an atom, it can be absorbed and electrons may jump from their ground state to an excited state. Some of the excited electrons will spontaneously return to their ground state, releasing the absorbed energy in the form of a photon. This is known as a 'spontaneous emission' and the photon's wavelength will be dependent on the energy difference between the ground and excited state. The emitted photon may then collide with one of the mirrors in the amplification chamber and reflect back to the lasing medium causing further collision with other excited atoms. They may then return to their ground state releasing 2 photons, identical in direction, phase and wavelength. This cascade effect is known as 'amplification'. Energy input from the energy source maintains 'population inversion' – where most of the atoms are in their excited state.

Some of the photons escape from the lasing medium through a partially reflecting mirror (output coupler) and produce the laser light in the visible, infrared or ultraviolet spectrum. Fibre-optic guides can be used to target the delivery of the laser light.

Examples of medical lasers include:

- CO_2 laser – far-infrared (10 600 nm), cutting and coagulation of soft tissue.
- NdYAG – near-infrared (1060 nm), cutting and coagulation, tattoo removal.
- Argon – blue–green (400–600 nm), used in retinal surgery and vascular malformations.

Metric prefixes

Prefix name	Prefix symbol	Value	
Yotta	Y	10^{24}	Septillion
Zetta	Z	10^{21}	Sextillion
Exa	E	10^{18}	Quintillion
Peta	P	10^{15}	Quadrillion
Tera	T	10^{12}	Trillion
Giga	G	10^{9}	Billion
Mega	M	10^{6}	Million
Kilo	k	10^{3}	Thousand
Hecto	h	10^{2}	Hundred
Deca	da	10^{1}	Ten
		10^{0}	One
Deci	d	10^{-1}	Tenth
Centi	c	10^{-2}	Hundredth
Milli	m	10^{-3}	Thousandth
Micro	μ	10^{-6}	Millionth
Nano	n	10^{-9}	Billionth
Pico	p	10^{-12}	Trillionth
Femto	f	10^{-15}	Quadrillionth
Atto	a	10^{-18}	Quintillionth
Zepto	z	10^{-21}	Sextillionth
Yocto	y	10^{-24}	Septillionth

In the metric system of measurement, multiples or fractions of a basic unit of measure are expressed by combining the unit of measure with a prefix. The International System of Units (SI) specifies 20 prefixes. Each prefix is represented by a unique symbol corresponding to a specific power of ten and should not be used in combination. This applies to all units of measurement, including mass where the SI base unit is the kilogram. Multiples of the kilogram are named utilizing 'gram' as the base unit.

For a given unit of measurement, the commonly used prefixes are dependent on the most plausible or frequently encountered values, international guidance and specific scientific field practice. Terms outside of this prefix system are also commonly used, e.g. the micron is frequently used instead of the micrometre. Similarly, international bodies advise against the use of prefixes with time-related units representing time greater than 1 second. Here, minutes, hours, days, etc. are generally used.

5.20

Power

$$\text{Work (J)} = \text{Force} \times \text{Distance} = \text{N.m} = \text{kg.m}^2.\text{s}^{-2}$$

$$\text{Power (W)} = \frac{\text{Work}}{\text{Time}} = \text{J.s}^{-1} = \text{kg.m}^2.\text{s}^{-3}$$

J = joules

N = newtons

m = metres

kg = kilograms

s = seconds

W = watts

Knowledge of simple mechanics is important for anaesthetists because many of the concepts can help explain physiological mechanisms that are relevant to practice, including many found in the cardiovascular and respiratory systems.

Work is defined as the product of the force exerted on an object and the distance moved in the direction of that force; it is measured in joules (J). One joule is the work expended by a one newton force (N) through a distance of one metre (m). Power, in mechanical terms, is the rate at which work is done; it is measured in watts (W). One watt can be defined as the power expended when one joule of energy is consumed in one second.

Applied to physiology, it is possible to calculate the power needed to maintain a physiological system. In the body, work is done when the displacement of fluid or gas occurs, which requires shortening or lengthening of a muscle. Work performed is force multiplied by distance (N.m) which has the same units as pressure multiplied by volume (N.m^{-2} × m^3 = N.m). It is therefore possible to calculate the work of breathing or work done by the heart during contraction. Having calculated the work per cycle, the power required can also be calculated by measuring the rate at which work is done, e.g. by measuring respiratory rate or heart rate (see *Section 1.3.25 – Work of breathing*).

Pressure

$$F\ (N) = ma = kg.m.s^{-2}$$

$$P\ (Pa) = \frac{F}{A} = N.m^{-2} = kg.m^{-1}.s^{-2}$$

F = force	N = newtons
m = mass	kg = kilograms
a = acceleration	s = seconds
P = pressure	Pa = pascals
A = area	m = metres

Force is that which changes, or tends to change, the state of motion or rest of an object; it is measured in newtons (N). Pressure is defined as the force applied over an area; it is measured in pascals (Pa).

One newton is the force that will give a mass of one kilogram an acceleration of one metre per second per second. One pascal is defined as the force of one newton acting over one square metre. In practical terms, one pascal is very small, so kilopascals (kPa) are more commonly used.

There are many different units used to represent pressure, the following are all equivalent values:
- 100 kPa.
- 1 bar.
- ~1 atmosphere (atm) (0.987 bar).
- 750 mmHg and torr.
- 1020 cm H_2O.
- 14.5 lb.inch^{-2} (psi).
- 100 000 N.m^{-2} and kg.m^{-1}.s^{-2}.

The measurement of pressure may be referred to as:
- **Atmospheric** – which is approximately 1 bar (and atm) at sea level.
- **Gauge pressure** – the pressure relative to atmospheric pressure (i.e. above or below it). Zero-referenced against atmospheric pressure. Also defined as absolute pressure minus atmospheric pressure.
- **Absolute pressure** – atmospheric plus gauge pressure. Zero-referenced against a perfect vacuum.

Gauge pressure is used for the measurement of airway pressure during ventilation, arterial and venous pressure measurements and in gas cylinder pressure measurements. Atmospheric pressure is variable with altitude and weather. If the absolute pressure remains constant, the gauge pressure of a fluid will vary as the atmospheric pressure changes, e.g. the gauge pressure will read slightly higher at high altitude (lower atmospheric pressure).

Various techniques are used to measure pressure; examples include:
- Hydrostatic – mercury column, piston, liquid column.
- Aneroid – Bourdon gauge (see *Section 6.1 – Bourdon gauge*), diaphragm, bellows.
- Electrical – strain gauge, capacitive, magnetic, optical.
- Ionization gauge – hot and cold cathode.

5.22

Raman effect

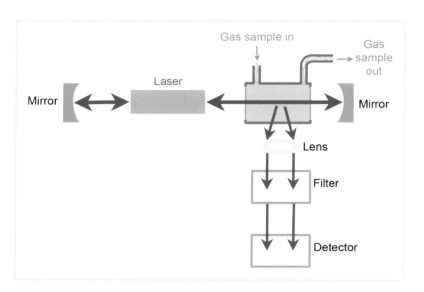

When light encounters molecules in a gas medium, the light beam deviates from its straight trajectory; this is called scattering. The predominant pattern of light scatter is elastic, where photon energy remains constant but travels in a different direction (Rayleigh scattering). One in every 30 million photons scatter inelastically (Raman scattering). When these photons collide with gas molecules, they induce a vibrational/rotational state in the gas molecule. As a result of a partial transfer of energy, frequency and wavelength of the scattered photon are altered. Most commonly energy is transferred from the photon to the gas molecule. This in turn causes a decrease in the photon's electromagnetic frequency and an increase in wavelength. Different gas molecules produce characteristic changes to photon frequency and wavelength.

Raman spectroscopy utilizes inelastic light scattering to provide breath-to-breath analysis of the constituents of a gas mixture. As the Raman effect is a relatively rare phenomenon, an intense light source, such as a laser beam, must be used to generate a measurable signal. The laser beam is focused on a sample chamber positioned between two high reflectance mirrors that concentrate the beam. Optical filters allow photons of a specific wavelength to pass through to a photodetector. Each gas molecule of interest is measured independently using a specific filter for that gas.

A Raman spectrum is produced as a plot of the intensity of Raman scatter against the wavenumber shift. A wavenumber is the inverse of the wavelength and the wavenumber shift represents the difference between the wavelength of scatter light and the incident beam. The Raman spectroscopy units are more expensive than infrared spectroscopy systems. However, they exhibit several advantages, including faster response time and the ability for multi-gas analysis. Unlike infrared spectroscopy, Raman spectroscopy is not limited to gas molecules having dissimilar atoms. As such, oxygen and nitrogen, which do not show infrared absorption, can be measured.

5.23

Reflection and refraction

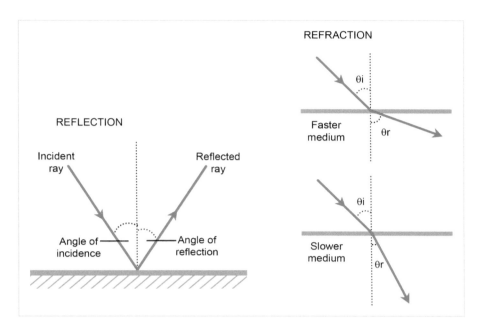

Reflection

Defined as the change in wave direction at an interface of two different media, returning the wave into the medium from which it originated. This principle applies to different wave types, such as light, sound and water.

The law of reflection states that the angle of incidence equals the angle of reflection.
- Angle of incidence lies between the incident/incoming wave and the normal.
- The normal is a line drawn at right angles to the reflector at the point where the incident wave contacts the reflector surface.
- The angle of reflection lies between the reflected wave and the normal.

A requirement of this law is that the normal, incident and reflected waves all lie within the same plane. If the reflecting surface is perfectly smooth, wave reflection is mirror-like. For light, this produces a mirror image and for sound, an echo. If the reflecting surface is irregular, waves are scattered in differing directions. However, each single point of the reflecting surface follows the law.

Refraction

Defined as bending of a wave due to a change in medium. As the physical characteristics of the medium are responsible for wave velocity, this change in direction results from a change in wave velocity. As a wave passes across the boundary from a medium in which it has high velocity into a medium in which its velocity is slower, the wave bends towards the normal, reducing the angle of refraction (θr) to less than the angle of incidence (θi). Refraction of light is a fundamental concept for image formation by a lens. A lens is a transparent, curved device used to refract light. A double convex lens, as found in the eye, is a converging lens that refracts light to intersect at the focal point, allowing projection of an image.

5.24

SI units

Unit	Measure	Symbol	Definition
Kelvin	Temperature	K	Numerical value of the Boltzmann constant k to be 1.38×10^{-23} when expressed in the unit $J.K^{-1}$ (equal to $kg.m^2.s^{-2}.K^{-1}$). [Pre-2019: 1/273.16 of the thermodynamic temperature of the triple point of water]
Second	Time	s	Unperturbed ground-state hyperfine transition frequency of the caesium-133 atom when expressed in Hz (equal to s^{-1})
Mole	Amount	mol	1 mole contains 6.02×10^{23} elementary entities. This is the numerical value of the Avogadro constant, N_A, when expressed in mol^{-1} (the Avogadro number). [Pre-2019: amount of substance that contains as many elementary entities as there are atoms in 0.012 kg of carbon-12]
Ampere	Current	A	Numerical value of the elementary charge e to be 1.60×10^{-19} when expressed in C (equal to $A.s$). [Pre-2019: current that would produce a force of 2×10^{-7} $N.m^{-1}$ between two parallel conductors of infinite length placed 1 metre apart in a vacuum]
Metre	Distance	m	Numerical value of the speed of light in vacuum c to be 3.00×10^8 when expressed in $m.s^{-1}$
Candela	Luminous intensity	cd	Numerical value of the luminous efficacy of monochromatic radiation of frequency 540×10^{12} Hz, K_{cd}, to be 683 when expressed $lm.W^{-1}$ (equal to $cd.sr.W^{-1}$ or $cd.sr.kg^{-1}.m^{-2}.s^3$)
Kilogram	Mass	kg	Numerical value of the Planck constant h to be 6.63×10^{-34} when expressed in $J.s$ (equal to $kg.m^2.s^{-1}$). [Pre-2019: based on an international prototype kilogram]

The International System of Units, or Le Système International d'Unités (SI), comprises a system of measurement used worldwide. It is built around seven base units, from which other units are derived. Since 2019 all SI units are defined in terms of constants that describe the natural world. Prefixes (see *Section 5.19 – Metric prefixes*) are often used because many of the base units are in the wrong order of magnitude for common use.

There are many derived units based on the SI base units including area (m^2), volume (m^3), velocity ($m.s^{-1}$) and acceleration ($m.s^{-2}$). Some derived units have their own symbols (expressed in terms of other SI units and with SI base units in brackets):
- Frequency – hertz, Hz (s^{-1}).
- Force – newton, N ($kg.m.s^{-2}$).
- Pressure – pascal, Pa ($N.m^{-2} = kg.m^{-1}.s^{-2}$).
- Work and energy – joule, J ($N.m = kg.m^2.s^{-2}$).
- Power – watt, W ($J.s^{-1} = kg.m^2.s^{-3}$).
- Electrical charge – coulomb, C ($A.s$).
- Potential difference – volt, V ($W.A^{-1} = kg.m^2.s^{-3}.A^{-1}$).
- Capacitance – farad, F ($C.V^{-1} = kg^{-1}.m^{-2}.s^4.A^2$).
- Resistance – ohm, Ω ($V.A^{-1} = kg.m^2.s^{-3}.A^{-2}$).
- Absorbed dose – gray, Gy ($J.kg^{-1} = m^2.s^{-2}$).

The SI was established in 1960 at the 11th General Conference on Weights and Measures (CGPM – Conférence Générale des Poids et Mesures). The CGPM is an international organization tasked with disseminating and modifying the SI as necessary. It was created in Paris in 1875 by a diplomatic treaty called the Meter Convention. The 9th edition of the SI brochure is the most recent, being published in 2019 and updated in 2022.

Triple point of water and phase diagram

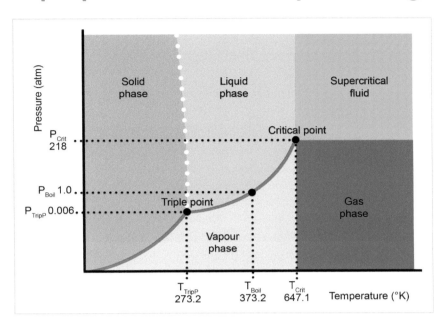

A phase diagram is a graphical representation of the physical phases of a substance under varying conditions of temperature and pressure. Phase boundaries are lines marking the conditions where two phases exist in equilibrium.

Water has a complex phase diagram. The phase boundary between solid and vapour phases represents sublimation. The boundary between liquid and solid marks the process of melting/freezing. For most substances, this phase boundary is sigmoid in shape, representing the increased temperature required to melt a substance at a higher pressure. However, water demonstrates anomalous behaviour where ice is easily liquefied with the application of increased pressure. This is represented graphically by a vertical melting/freezing phase boundary. The phase boundary between liquid and vapour phases represents vaporization.

The triple point of a substance is the temperature and pressure at which the three phases coexist in equilibrium. This point is depicted as the intersection of all three phase boundaries. The triple point of water occurs at exactly 273.16 K (0.01°C) and a partial pressure of 0.618 kPa (0.00610 atmospheres – atm). Under these conditions, water exists as a vapour, liquid and solid in equilibrium. The triple point of water is used to define the SI unit of temperature, the Kelvin (see *Section 5.24 – SI units*).

The critical point of a substance is the temperature and pressure above which distinct liquid and gas phases do not exist; the intersection of the critical temperature and pressure. For water, this occurs at 647 K and 22 089 kPa (218 atm). Under temperatures or pressures exceeding the critical point, a single phase exists as a homogenous supercritical fluid. A supercritical fluid demonstrates properties between those of a gas and a liquid. Through manipulation of pressure and temperature, supercritical fluid properties can be altered to make them more gas- or liquid-like.

5.26

Types of flow

$$Re = \frac{\rho v d}{\eta}$$

Re = Reynolds number

ρ = fluid density

v = fluid velocity

d = vessel diameter

η = fluid viscosity

Flow is defined as the volume of fluid passing a point per unit time. Flow may be described as laminar, turbulent or mixed. Reynolds number (Re) is a dimensionless number calculated to characterize flow type. A Reynolds number of less than 2000 indicates laminar flow, while turbulent flow is observed when Re is greater than 4000. When Re lies between 2000 and 4000, flow is transitional, demonstrating both laminar and turbulent characteristics.

Laminar flow is characterized by parallel layers of fluid motion with little disruption between them. Conversely, turbulent flow describes fluid motion that has local velocities and pressures that fluctuate randomly, resulting in disorganized flow and eddy currents. It occurs when fluid moves through an orifice (an opening where the diameter is many times greater than the length the fluid passes through) or past sharp edges and may also occur in a tube if flow exceeds the critical velocity. Because turbulent flow is variable, no equation exists to calculate flow. However, it is proportional to the square of the radius and square root of the pressure gradient, while being inversely proportional to tube length and fluid density.

Flow measurement, for clinical use, is made through indirect means by calculating a variable that changes in parallel with flow.

Pressure related
- Constant orifice, variable pressure (e.g. pneumotachograph). A pressure transducer converts the pressure difference across a fixed resistance to an electrical signal that is proportional to flow.
- Variable orifice, constant pressure (e.g. rotameter). As flow increases, the orifice area also increases to decrease the resistance. This maintains a constant pressure across the bobbin.

Mechanical movement – rotation of a vane (e.g. spirometer). Calculates flow in relation to kinetic energy of the fluid.

Heat transfer – (e.g. hot-wire anemometer). A heated wire element is cooled as gas flows past it. The subsequent change in resistance of the wire is proportional to flow.

5.27
Wave characteristics

A wave is defined as a disturbance propagating through space, transferring energy from one point to another without transferring matter. Mechanical waves, e.g. sound, require a medium for transfer.

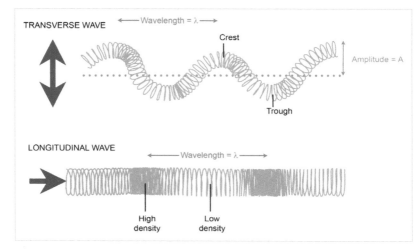

Electromagnetic waves, e.g. light and radiation, are capable of transmission through a vacuum (e.g. outer space). Waves may be classified according to the direction of the disturbance in relation to wave movement.

- **Longitudinal/compression wave** – medium displacement is along the same axis as the direction of wave movement (e.g. sound). Waves consist of regions of high and low density.
- **Transverse wave** – medium displacement is perpendicular to the direction of the wave movement (e.g. wave on a string).

Periodic waves are generated by a series of disturbances. Periodic waves have a number of characteristics that define their behaviour.

- Amplitude (A) – maximal displacement of a wave medium from its resting position. For transverse waves this is represented by the distance from baseline to crest or trough. For longitudinal waves, the amplitude relates to rise and fall of pressure within the medium. Amplitude corresponds to wave energy.
- Wavelength (λ) – distance between the same points on successive waves.
- Period – time it takes a wave to complete one cycle or oscillation, expressed in units of time.
- Frequency (f) – number of cycles or oscillations per second. The SI unit is the hertz, defined as one cycle per second. Frequency is the inverse of the period.
- Velocity (v) – speed with which a wave is moving in a specified direction.

Wavelength, frequency and velocity of a wave are related mathematically.

$$v = \lambda \times f$$

v = velocity
λ = wavelength
f = frequency

The velocity of a wave is determined by the physical characteristics of the medium. As such, velocity is fixed for a given medium. Frequency and wavelength are, therefore, inversely proportional, i.e. higher frequencies correspond to shorter wavelengths.

5.28

Wheatstone bridge

The Wheatstone bridge, or resistance bridge, is an electrical circuit that is used to measure an unknown resistance by balancing a system of known resistances. It is a common component of transducers used in invasive pressure monitoring devices.

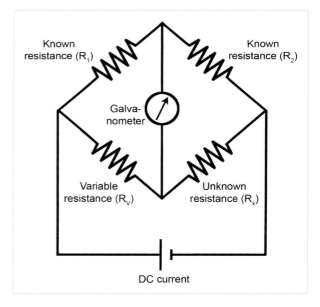

The circuit of the Wheatstone bridge consists of a common electrical source, a galvanometer and four resistors; two have fixed known resistances (R_1 and R_2), one has a variable known resistance (R_v) and the other has an unknown resistance (R_x). They are arranged in two parallel branches each with two resistors, one fixed and the other either variable or unknown. If the branches are unbalanced, current will flow across the galvanometer causing the dial to move. The variable resistor is adjusted to achieve null deflection (balancing or zeroing the system); at this point the resistances of three resistors are known and from the equation below the unknown resistance can be deduced.

$$\frac{R_v}{R_1} = \frac{R_x}{R_2}$$

$$R_x = \frac{R_v}{R_1} \times R_2$$

R = resistance

v = variable

x = unknown

The invasive measurement of arterial blood pressure is based around the movement of a diaphragm within a transducer, which is in contact with the arterial blood via a column of fluid. A strain gauge (commonly a pattern of metallic foil wire on an insulated backing) is attached to the diaphragm; its resistance changes as the diaphragm is stretched with the pulsatile movement of the arterial blood. The strain gauge forms the unknown resistance in the Wheatstone bridge. With the bridge 'zeroed', any change in the strain gauge resistance will cause a deflection of the galvanometer; this is amplified and converted to a blood pressure reading.

Work

$$W = FD$$

$$P = \frac{F}{A}$$

$$W = PAD = PV$$

W = work (J or N.m)

F = force (N)

D = distance (m)

P = pressure (Pa)

A = area (m²)

V = volume (l or m³)

Work is done when a force acts upon an object to cause displacement of the object. The SI unit of work is the joule. One joule (J) is equivalent to one newton of force (N) causing a displacement of one metre (m); work is therefore sometimes described in terms of newton metres (N.m). Substituting force for a rearranged pressure equation gives rise to an alternative work equation, where work is the product of pressure and volume.

Mechanical energy is the capacity for doing work. The SI unit of energy is also the joule because energy must be expended to do work; to accomplish 50 J of work, 50 J of energy must be expended.

Myocardial work

Stroke work is a measure of mechanical work performed by the ventricle with each contraction. It is used as an index for myocardial contractility, defined as work done by the heart for a given pre- and afterload. The two main components of stroke work are:

- Pressure–volume work – work done to push the stroke volume (SV) into the arterial system. This is the primary component of stroke work and is best estimated by generation of a ventricular pressure–volume (PV) loop (see *Sections 1.1.23* and *1.1.24 – Ventricular pressure–volume loops*). Pressure–volume work is represented by the area contained within the PV loop and may be calculated as the product of intraventricular pressure and SV.
- Kinetic energy work – work done by ventricular contraction to move the ejected blood at a certain velocity.

As kinetic energy work is negligible under normal cardiac output conditions, stroke work is calculated using mean pulmonary artery pressure or mean aortic pressure as an estimate of right and left intraventricular pressure, respectively. Conditions that increase SV or mean pressures generated by the ventricles increase myocardial work.

6.1

Bourdon gauge

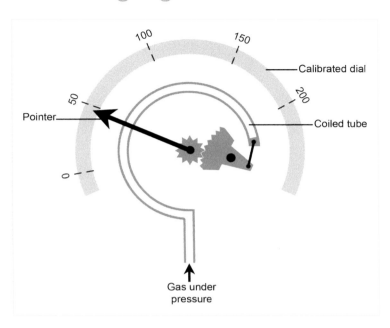

The Bourdon gauge can be used to measure pressure or, indirectly, temperature. It was patented by a French watchmaker in 1849 and is an example of an aneroid gauge (Greek – without fluid). It is robust and can be used to measure high pressures where a manometer would be inappropriate (for example, a mercury manometer would need to be 103 m high to measure an oxygen cylinder pressure of 13 700 kPa). It consists of a robust and flexible coiled metal tube linked to a cog and pointer. The coiled tube is flattened and oval in cross-section. When high pressure gas enters one end of the tube, it uncoils, moving the pointer across a calibrated scale indicating the pressure. The amount of movement of the tube is dependent on the compliance of the tube; more rigid tubes are therefore used for higher pressures.

In anaesthesia, Bourdon gauges are often used to measure cylinder or pipeline gas pressures. The gauges are calibrated and colour-coded to the particular gas they are measuring. In an oxygen cylinder at room temperature, the pressure indicates the available contents in the cylinder as it is entirely in its gaseous form (having a critical temperature of −118.6°C) and so obeys Boyle's law. However, nitrous oxide is a mixture of vapour and liquid at room temperature (as it has a critical temperature of 36.4°C); the pressure therefore, will not indicate the available contents until all the liquid has been vaporized.

It may also be used to measure temperature; the hollow tube can be attached at one end to a temperature-sensing bulb containing a volatile liquid or vapour. This will expand as the temperature increases, causing the tube to uncoil and move the pointer. In this instance the scale will be calibrated for temperature rather than pressure.

6.2
Clark electrode

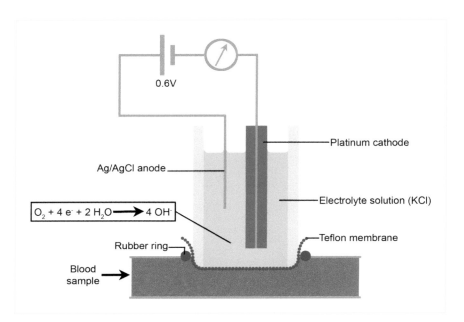

0.6V

Platinum cathode

Ag/AgCl anode

Electrolyte solution (KCl)

$O_2 + 4\,e^- + 2\,H_2O \longrightarrow 4\,OH^-$

Teflon membrane

Rubber ring

Blood sample

The partial pressure of oxygen (PO_2) may be measured via the Clark electrode (polarographic oxygen electrode), fuel cell or paramagnetic analyser. All three techniques may be used for oxygen analysis in a gas mixture. The Clark electrode is commonly used to measure PO_2 in blood gas analysers.

The Clark electrode comprises several components.
- **Anode** – silver (Ag) anode is immersed in electrolyte solution, commonly potassium chloride (KCl), to produce the following reaction:

$$4KCl + 4Ag \rightarrow 4AgCl + 4K^+ + 4e^-$$

- **Cathode** – platinum cathode utilizes electrons produced at the anode to combine with oxygen from sample blood to produce hydroxyl ions (OH^-). Electron consumption at the cathode produces a current proportional to sample PO_2. The more oxygen in the sample, the greater the flow of electrons and the greater the current.
- **Electrolyte solution** – bathes the electrodes and serves as a source of chloride ions.
- **Thin oxygen-permeable membrane** – allows diffusion of gases, separates the cathode from the blood sample to prevent build-up of protein that would impair function.
- **External power source** – applies a voltage between 0.4 and 0.8 V to the electrodes. Within this range of voltages, current is solely dependent on the rate of oxygen diffusion to the cathode.

The Clark electrode is temperature sensitive because solubility of oxygen in solution is significantly affected by temperature. For a given partial pressure of a gas, solubility will be inversely proportional to temperature; at lower temperatures, oxygen solubility is increased. Blood gas analysers measure partial pressures at 37°C. Clinical implications arise as blood taken from a hypothermic patient is warmed to 37°C by the analyser. A rise in temperature reduces oxygen solubility, leading to a higher measured PO_2 than is present *in vivo*. Blood gas analysers use algorithms to correct measured values to the actual body temperature.

Damping

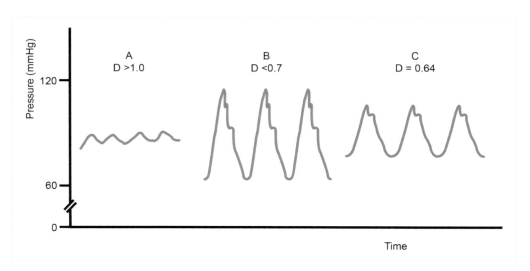

Damping describes a decrease in the amplitude of an oscillating system as a result of energy lost from resistive forces. A degree of damping is desirable in a system, however, the output is adversely affected by either excessive or insufficient damping. Most damping in a system such as an arterial line originates from frictional forces, however, overdamping is also caused by:

- air bubbles and clots
- narrow, long or compliant tubing
- compliant diaphragm
- kinks in the cannula or tubing
- three-way taps.

The damping coefficient (D) of a system is an index of the tendency for it to resist oscillations. It is proportional to the friction coefficient and inversely proportional to the mass of the oscillating object. Overdamping (D >1.0 – trace A) causes the systolic pressure to under-read and the diastolic pressure to over-read – the mean pressure will be unaffected. The system shows a slow blunted response to change and therefore causes some inaccuracy. An underdamped system (D <0.7 – trace B) will lead to over-reading of the systolic and under-reading of the diastolic – again the mean will be generally unaffected. After flushing, an underdamped system will overshoot and will be unable to prevent oscillations.

A critically damped system (D = 1.0) allows the most rapid attainment of a new input value with no overshoot, but is slow to respond. A compromise is therefore found at which the system is said to be optimally damped. The system will have a rapid response to a change in input but with minimal overshoot. The damping coefficient for an optimally damped system is 0.64 (trace C). It corresponds to 2–3 oscillations in the arterial baseline trace following the system being flushed.

6.4

Depth of anaesthesia monitoring

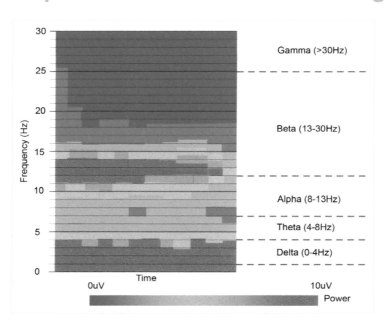

Electroencephalogram (EEG) waveforms (See *Section 1.4.5 – Electroencephalogram waveforms*) progressively and predictably change during different depths of anaesthesia, as follows.

- Light – decreased beta activity, increased alpha and delta activity.
- Intermediate – further decrease in beta activity, further increase in alpha and delta activity.
- Deep – periods of flat waveform alternating with burst of alpha and beta activity (i.e. burst suppression).
- Profound – completely flat waveform.

EEG electrical signal, measured via forehead surface electrodes, is amplified, filtered, and processed into a clinically usable measure of depth of anaesthesia. Many commercial devices exist (e.g. E-Entropy, Bispectral Index (BIS), Narcotrend), each with their own proprietary and confidential algorithms. All devices simplify EEG signal to a single dimensionless number on a scale of 0 (cortical electrical silence) to 100 (fully awake). Target ranges during general anaesthesia differ according to device.

In addition to displaying the numerical value of depth of anaesthesia (scale 0–100), most monitors will display at least one EEG waveform for visual analysis.

A spectrogram, displayed as a heat map, is a visual representation of the spectrum of signal frequencies over time. EEG spectrograms display the relative proportion of waveforms (i.e. power) within each EEG frequency band occurring in an EEG signal. Information is derived from EEG pattern and feature analysis. The power of the EEG signal is colour-coded and integrated into a 2-dimensional plot of EEG frequency (y-axis) over time (x-axis). Warmer colours are used to depict higher power which means a greater proportion of waveforms within that frequency band are present in the EEG signal.

Electromyography (EMG) is a common confounding factor that can interfere with EEG signals. Depth of anaesthesia monitors measure EMG activity and, using signal processing, can minimize EMG interference to provide a more reliable measure of anaesthetic depth.

Fuel cell

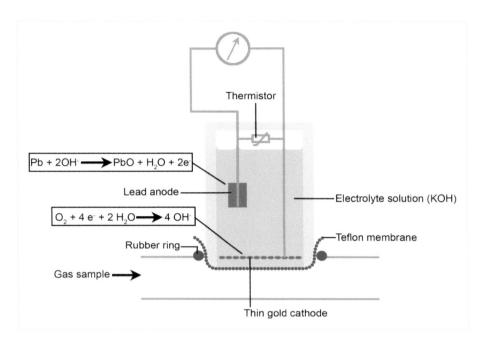

$$Pb + 2OH^- \longrightarrow PbO + H_2O + 2e^-$$

Lead anode

$$O_2 + 4e^- + 2H_2O \longrightarrow 4OH^-$$

Rubber ring

Gas sample

Thermistor

Electrolyte solution (KOH)

Teflon membrane

Thin gold cathode

The fuel cell measures the partial pressure of oxygen in a gas mixture using principles similar to the Clark electrode (see *Section 6.2 – Clark electrode*). Component parts include the following.

- **Anode** – at the lead anode, electrons are produced by a reaction of the anode with potassium hydroxide electrolyte solution.
- **Cathode** – electrons travel through a circuit from the anode to the thin gold cathode. At the cathode, gold acts as a catalyst for electrons to combine with oxygen molecules diffused into the cell from the gas sample. This process generates a flow of electrons proportional to the partial pressure of oxygen in the sample.
- **Electrolyte solution** – bathes the electrodes and is specifically designed to allow ions to travel between the electrodes. In the fuel cell, hydroxyl ions (OH^-) produced at the cathode travel back to the anode allowing further electron production. The electrolyte solution is continuously replenished by the reaction at the cathode.
- **Thermistor** – usually incorporated to allow temperature compensation. As all diffusion processes are temperature sensitive, the current produced by the fuel cell would vary with temperature if no compensation measures were employed.

Unlike the Clark electrode, the fuel cell does not require an external power source. The described chemical reactions create a predictable voltage within the cell, usually about 0.7 V. At this voltage, current is proportional to the rate of oxygen diffusion to the cathode.

Fuel cells exhibit a finite lifespan due to exhaustion of the cell components, namely the lead anode. Its lifespan depends on the rate at which the lead anode material is consumed. This, in turn, is related to the concentration of oxygen to which it is exposed and the duration of exposure.

Response time for the fuel cell is slow, taking approximately 30 s. Therefore, this system cannot be used for breath-to-breath oxygen analysis.

6.6

Monitoring of neuromuscular blockade

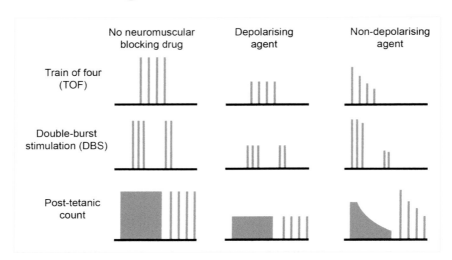

Peripheral nerve stimulators evaluate the degree of neuromuscular blockade (NMB) through monitoring transmission across the neuromuscular junction.

Patterns of stimulation

Train of four (TOF) – four stimuli applied at a frequency of 2 Hz. The TOF count describes the number of muscle twitches following stimulation. The TOF ratio is the ratio of the fourth twitch amplitude compared to the first. Subjective evaluation of TOF ratio is inaccurate. Objective measurement is achieved through acceleromyography. Muscle acceleration is proportional to force of contraction and measurement at the adductor pollicis muscle correlates well with upper airway tone. To minimize risk of residual NMB, and ensure sufficient return of pharyngeal muscle function, current research suggests an objective TOF ratio >0.9 is necessary prior to tracheal extubation.

Administration of a non-depolarizing muscle relaxant produces a predictable TOF pattern. Initial amplitude reduction of muscular twitches is observed with the fourth twitch most affected. Incremental reduction in amplitude is known as fade. With increasing intensity of NMB, the fourth twitch is lost (75–89% NMB), followed by loss of the third (85% NMB), second (90% NMB) and then first twitch (98–100% NMB). The reverse pattern is observed during blockade recovery. Depolarizing muscle relaxants do not demonstrate fade.

Double-burst stimulation (DBS) – two 50 Hz bursts of stimuli are applied with a 750 ms interval between them. Each burst consists of 2 or 3 impulses, usually in a 3:3 or 3:2 pattern. These stimuli manifest as two separate muscle contractions. The ratio of twitch amplitude is related to the TOF ratio. DBS improves visual detection of fade.

Post-tetanic count – a 50 Hz tetanic stimulation is applied for 5 s followed by 1 Hz supramaximal stimuli after a 3 s pause. The number of post-tetanic twitches correlates inversely with time to recovery of the first TOF twitch, allowing assessment of deep NMB.

Oximetry – paramagnetic analyser

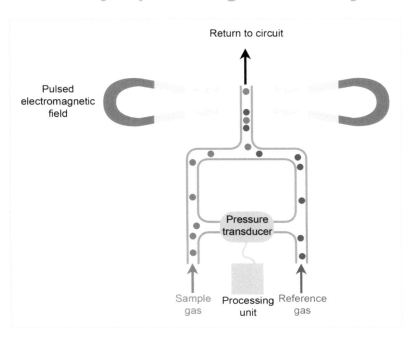

The paramagnetic analyser can perform oxygen analysis of inhaled and exhaled gases. It works on the principle that oxygen is a paramagnetic gas and is therefore attracted into a magnetic field due to unpaired electrons in its outer ring. Nitric oxide is also paramagnetic. Most other gases in anaesthesia are diamagnetic, i.e. they are repelled by a magnetic field.

The traditional paramagnetic analyser consists of a gas-tight chamber containing two glass spheres in a dumbbell arrangement and containing nitrogen, suspended by a filament in a non-uniform magnetic field. Oxygen is then introduced into the chamber and is attracted towards the magnetic field, displacing the glass spheres; the degree of displacement is proportional to the oxygen concentration. The degree of displacement can be measured by adding a mirror and using the reflection of a beam of light as a marker of oxygen concentration on a scale. Alternatively, photocells can be used to detect the beam of light and then modulate an opposing magnetic field in order to keep the dumbbell in steady state. The amount of current needed to do this is proportional to the oxygen concentration in the sample.

Modern systems use a switched electromagnetic field that creates a pressure differential between a reference sample and the patient's sample. A transducer detects the pressure fluctuations and converts them into a DC voltage, which is directly proportional to the oxygen concentration.

The paramagnetic analyser has a fast response time allowing breath-to-breath analysis of oxygen so that inspired and expired concentrations can be measured. Its accuracy can be affected by the presence of nitrous oxide or water vapour in the sample. Water vapour may be removed by passing the sample through a drying agent such as silica gel before analysis.

6.8

pH measuring system

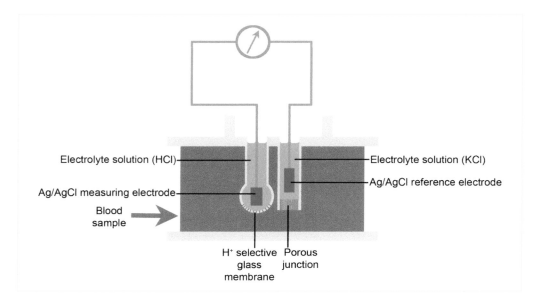

Electrolyte solution (HCl)

Ag/AgCl measuring electrode

Blood sample

Electrolyte solution (KCl)

Ag/AgCl reference electrode

H⁺ selective glass membrane

Porous junction

The pH measuring system calculates hydrogen ion concentration ([H^+]), and thus pH, through measurement of an electrical potential difference between two electrodes.

- A pH electrode is the measuring electrode used to determine the pH of an aqueous solution. It consists of a glass bulb with a hydrogen-selective glass tip, a silver/silver chloride (Ag/AgCl) internal electrode and a buffer solution (hydrogen chloride). The buffer solution maintains a constant [H^+] within the electrode. If the [H^+] of the sample passing the measuring electrode is different from that within the electrode, an electrical potential difference develops between the inner and outer surfaces of the glass membrane. The magnitude of this potential difference is proportional to the difference in pH between the inner buffer and sample.
- A reference electrode, with a similar internal Ag/AgCl electrode immersed in an electrolyte solution (potassium chloride), provides electrical contact with the sample. This interface is achieved via a porous junction present at the bottom of the electrode, allowing measurement of the electrical potential of the sample.

The electrical circuit between the electrodes is completed through connection of both electrodes to a galvanometer. The potential difference between the measuring and reference electrodes is a function of the pH of the sample solution.

Modern pH measuring systems are manufactured as a combination electrode, housing both the measuring and reference electrodes within one unit.

Pulse oximeter

The pulse oximeter is a non-invasive device used to measure the percentage of haemoglobin saturated with oxygen in peripheral arterial blood (SpO_2) and the pulse rate. The amount of light absorbed by oxygenated and deoxygenated forms of haemoglobin

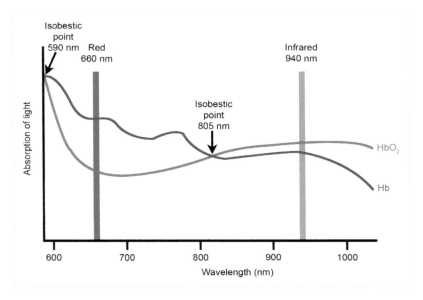

differs. The probe has two light-emitting diodes, producing beams in the red (660 nm) and infrared (940 nm) range, and opposite them a photodetector. The diodes flash approximately 30 times per second in sequence, with a pause when both are off to compensate for ambient light. The amount of light that is absorbed (and therefore reaching the photodetector) at the two wavelengths varies as vessels expand and contract with the arterial pulse. A microprocessor analyses the changes, ignoring the non-pulsatile component from tissues and venous blood.

The Beer–Lambert law (see *Section 5.2 – Beer–Lambert law*) enables estimation of the SpO_2 based on the amount of light absorbed. Compared to deoxygenated haemoglobin, oxygenated haemoglobin absorbs more infrared than red light (and vice versa). The ratio of the amount of light reaching the photodetector for each wavelength allows the microprocessor to calculate the SpO_2. The isobestic point is the point at which oxygenated and deoxygenated haemoglobin absorb a certain wavelength of light to the same extent; this occurs at 590 and 805 nm. These can be used as reference points because light absorption is independent of the degree of saturation. Dark skin, anaemia and jaundice do not affect accuracy, however, inaccuracy may be caused by:

- poor peripheral perfusion
- carboxyhaemoglobin – overestimates the reading
- methaemoglobin – readings tend towards 85% regardless of the true saturation
- methylene blue – reads lower than true saturation
- venous congestion
- pulsatile venous flow, e.g. tricuspid regurgitation
- bright ambient light
- diathermy
- shivering/patient movement
- nail varnish.

6.10

Severinghaus carbon dioxide electrode

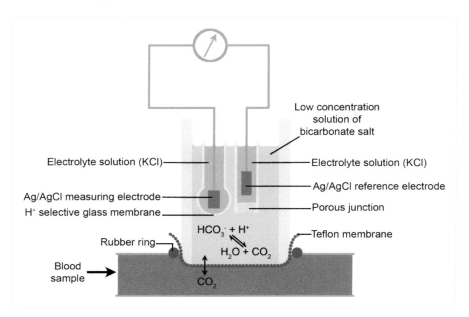

The Severinghaus electrode is used to directly measure the partial pressure of dissolved carbon dioxide (CO_2) in a solution. This device is a modified pH measuring system with CO_2 measurement being based on the electrode's hydrogen ion concentration ($[H^+]$).

When CO_2 is dissolved in an aqueous solution, it exists in chemical equilibrium.

$$CO_2 + H_2O \leftrightarrow H_2CO_3 \leftrightarrow H^+ + HCO_3^-$$

CO_2, but not hydrogen ions, from the sample diffuses across a Teflon semi-permeable membrane into the sodium bicarbonate solution of the Severinghaus electrode. The amount of CO_2 diffusing into the electrode is in accordance with Henry's law (see *Section 5.16 – Henry's law*). Within the bicarbonate solution, CO_2 combines with water to form carbonic acid with a proportion of this dissociating into hydrogen and bicarbonate ions. Hydrogen ion production is proportional to the amount of dissolved CO_2 present. The change in $[H^+]$ causes a resultant change in pH of the bicarbonate solution. The $[H^+]$ is measured by the measuring electrode that is separated from the bicarbonate solution by a hydrogen ion selective glass membrane. The bicarbonate solution is in direct contact with the reference electrode. The potential difference between the measuring and reference electrode is measured by the galvanometer and converted to partial pressure of CO_2.

Blood gas analysers

Blood gas measurement is a collective term applied to measurement of blood sample pH, partial pressure of oxygen (PO_2) and partial pressure of CO_2 (PCO_2). Automated analysers utilize the glass pH electrode, Clark electrode and Severinghaus electrode for measuring pH, PO_2 and PCO_2, respectively. The pH electrode is the most reliably accurate of the three electrodes, with an accuracy of pH measurement within +/- 0.01 units. Variation in PO_2 and PCO_2 measurements should be less than 3 mmHg and 1 mmHg, respectively.

6.11

Temperature measurement

Temperature has many definitions including:
- A measure of the average kinetic energy of the particles in a sample of matter.
- A measure of the ability of a substance or, more generally, any physical system to transfer heat to another physical system.

Heat is the form of energy that may be transferred between two samples of matter due to their temperature difference.

The SI unit for temperature is the Kelvin (K) (see *Section 5.24 – SI units*). The celsius scale is also internationally approved.

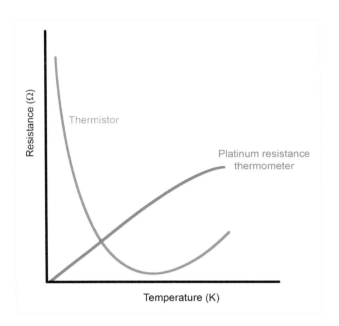

Non-electrical temperature measurement

These techniques exploit the predictable change in physical properties various substances undergo with a change in temperature. Examples include mercury and bimetallic strip thermometers.

Electrical temperature measurement

Resistance thermometer (resistance temperature detector – RTD) – electrical resistance of a pure metal increases linearly with a rise in temperature. Platinum resistance thermometers (PRTs) are the most accurate. RTDs are most commonly used in industrial settings because the temperature range over which they measure is vast (i.e. 10–1335 K).

Thermistor – electrical resistance in semiconductors (rather than pure metal) falls with a rise in temperature. The semiconductor material is a mixture of metal oxides pressed into a bead. Temperature curves deviate widely from linearity, except over narrow ranges. Thermistor sensitivity is very high compared to RTDs, demonstrating high resolution and accuracy. Thermistors lend themselves well to medical use for the following reasons:
- compact size for use in small probes
- fast response due to low thermal mass
- temperature measurement is over a narrow range and therefore thermistors may be chosen to provide a linear signal in this range
- highly sensitive.

Thermistors are commonly employed in a number of medical devices including thermodilution cardiac output monitors and blood gas analysers.

Thermocouple – based on the Seebeck effect (see *Section 6.12 – Thermocouple and Seebeck effect*).

6.12

Thermocouple and Seebeck effect

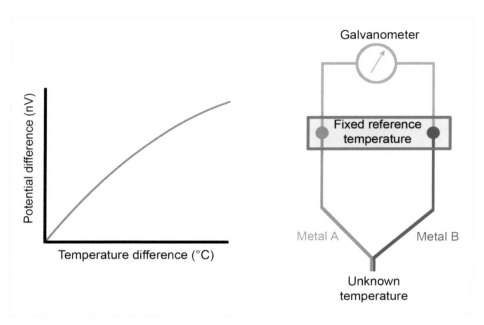

The thermocouple is a device used to measure temperature. It utilizes the Seebeck effect (Seebeck – Estonian–German physicist); the generation of an electromotive force that occurs when two different metals are joined to form two separate but identical junctions, which are then exposed to different temperatures. The electromotive force produces a potential difference between the two junctions, the magnitude of which is proportional to the temperature difference between them. The order of magnitude for the potential difference generated is dependent on the metals used and the temperature difference the thermocouple is exposed to; for medical devices, potential difference is usually measured in nV.

It produces an essentially linear curve of potential difference against temperature difference. The curve passes through zero as no potential difference will be generated if there is no temperature gradient between the junctions.

Copper, iron or chromel (nickel–chromium alloy) is commonly combined with constantan, a copper–nickel alloy containing 40% nickel. The metal wires are joined to form a circuit consisting of a reference and sensing junction with a galvanometer between them. The reference junction is maintained at a known temperature, while the temperature at the sensing junction can be determined using the galvanometer to measure the potential difference generated.

The advantages of the thermocouple are:
• Small – each metal can be made into fine wires.
• Accurate.
• Rapid response time – although slower than the thermistor.
• Cheap.

Disadvantages include:
• The system requires signal amplification and processing.

Bag valve mask resuscitator

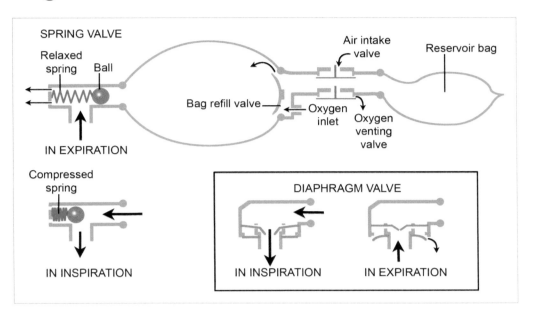

Bag valve mask (BVM) system components

Inflatable bag – oxygen inlet allows adjustable flow rates of supplemental oxygen. An oxygen reservoir increases the potential fraction of inspired oxygen. A unidirectional air intake valve allows entrainment of room air if fresh gas flow is less than the patient's minute volume.

- Self-inflating bag – automatically re-expands after manual compression due to sub-atmospheric pressure within the bag. This negative pressure opens the unidirectional bag refill valve allowing entrainment of room air (via air intake valve), reservoir oxygen or a combination of both. These bags are commonly utilized in the pre-hospital and in-hospital emergency settings because controlled ventilation is possible in the absence of a pressurized supplemental gas source.

Non-return valve – directs fresh gas flow to the patient and prevents rebreathing. BVMs may be classified by the type of valve they employ.

- Spring-loaded valve – consists of a disk/ball supported by a spring. With bag compression, a positive pressure is applied to the valve, occluding the exhalation port. As positive pressure ceases, the spring returns the disk/ball to the resting position, allowing exhaled gas to be vented externally.
- Diaphragm valve – application of positive pressure opens the orifice between the valve leaflets while simultaneously forcing them against the exhalation port. When flow ceases, negative pressure within the bag causes the diaphragm to move away from the exhalation port. Valve leaflets return to the closed position, preventing exhaled gases from entering the bag.

The standardized 15 mm internal diameter patient port allows connection of the system to facemasks, supraglottic airways or endotracheal tubes. Paediatric systems employ a smaller volume of bag and must incorporate a pressure-limiting valve (e.g. pop-off valve) to minimize the risk of barotrauma.

7.2

Breathing circuits – circle system

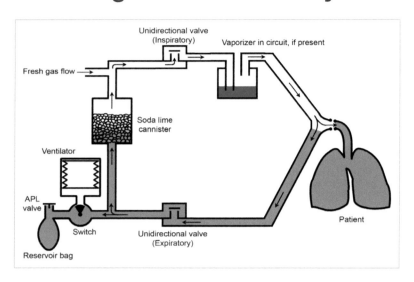

The circle system describes a closed breathing system in which gases are recycled during ventilation, with carbon dioxide (CO_2) being removed by CO_2 absorbers. The important features of the system include:
- unidirectional valves – inspiratory and expiratory
- reservoir bag
- Y connector
- fresh gas supply
- adjustable pressure limiting (APL) valve
- CO_2 absorber, e.g. soda lime or baralyme
- vaporizer – in or out of circuit.

During inspiration, the expiratory valve closes and gas flows from the bag to the patient via the inspiratory tubing. On expiration, the inspiratory valve closes and gas flows into the bag. The expired CO_2 is absorbed and excess gas is vented via the APL valve.

The position of the bag and APL valve may vary in relation to the absorber, but there are important features that must be present to prevent rebreathing:
- Unidirectional valves must exist between the patient and the bag on both inspiratory and expiratory limbs.
- The APL valve must not be positioned between the inspiratory valve and the patient.
- The fresh gas flow must not enter between the expiratory valve and the patient.

Advantages of the circle system include warming and humidification of inspired gas and reduction in atmospheric pollution from efficient scavenging. They are also economical; anaesthesia can be maintained using low fresh gas flows ($0.5–1$l.min^{-1}), minimizing the amount of anaesthetic vapour needed. However, the volume of oxygen entering the system must at least equal the patient's oxygen consumption, otherwise a hypoxic mixture could be delivered (especially if nitrous oxide is also used).

During low flow anaesthesia, changes in inspired anaesthetic concentration will be slow to change. Additionally, the unidirectional valves may become stuck in the open position due to water vapour condensation, causing reduced efficiency of the system and rebreathing of CO_2.

Breathing circuits – Mapleson's classification

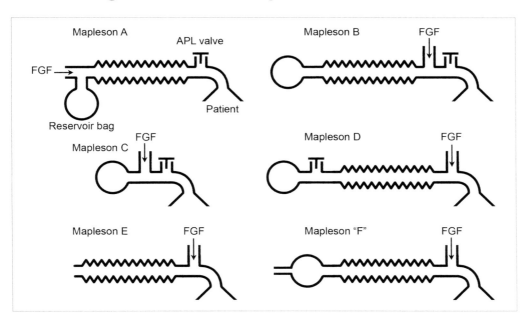

This classification groups breathing systems depending on the circuit position of the fresh gas flow (FGF), reservoir bag, tubing, expiratory valve and facemask. It also defines the FGF needed to prevent rebreathing with spontaneous and controlled mechanical ventilation (SV and CMV, respectively). Each provides good inspired anaesthetic concentration control because fresh gas is delivered with each breath. However, they are less economical than circle systems because FGF normally needs to be at least that of minute ventilation (M_v) to prevent rebreathing.

- **A** – Magill and Lack (co-axial). On expiration, gas moves back towards the reservoir (anatomical dead space gas first) that is being filled with fresh gas. As pressure builds, the expiratory valve opens, allowing exhaled gas to escape (alveolar first). The expiratory pause allows fresh gas to fill the circuit. On inspiration, fresh and dead space gas is inspired. Efficient for SV but inefficient for CMV. To prevent rebreathing; for SV the FGF must equal the M_v (approximately 70 ml.kg^{-1}.min^{-1}) and for CMV the FGF must be 2–3 times the M_v.
- **B** – FGF enters at patient end, before the expiratory valve. To prevent rebreathing; for both SV and CMV the FGF must be twice the M_v.
- **C** – Water's circuit, similar to B but with shorter tubing.
- **D** – Bain (co-axial). FGF via inner tube and exhaled gas vents through outer tube. During the expiratory pause, FGF from the inner tube flushes exhaled gas from outer tube. Fresh gas is then inspired from the outer tube. Inefficient for SV but more efficient for CMV. To prevent rebreathing; for SV the FGF must be twice the M_v and for CMV the FGF must equal the M_v.
- **E** – Ayre's T-piece, useful in paediatrics because minimal dead space and resistance (no valves)
- **"F"** – not originally classified by Mapleson, Jackson–Rees' modification of Ayre's T-piece with addition of a two-ended bag to expiratory limb.

7.4

Bronchoscope

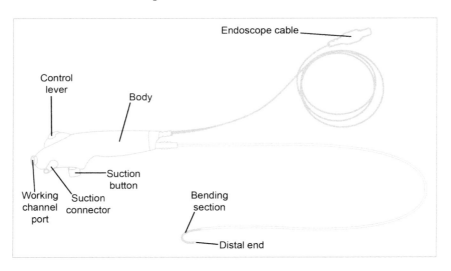

Bronchoscopes may be classified as rigid or flexible.

A rigid bronchoscope is a straight, hollow metal tube used to visualize the trachea and proximal bronchi. Rigid bronchoscopy is performed to diagnose and manage central airway pathology. The large lumen facilitates airway intervention such as foreign body removal, stent insertion and endoluminal therapy (e.g. laser treatment).

A flexible bronchoscope is a long, thin device capable of accessing the upper and lower airways. Indications for use are as follows.

Diagnostic
- Diagnose diseases of the tracheobronchial tree.
- Obtain lung samples (e.g. bronchoalveolar lavage specimens).

Therapeutic
- Difficult intubation.
- Guide placement of percutaneous tracheostomy.
- Suctioning of lower airways.
- Treatment of specific disorders (e.g. control bleeding of focal lesions).

Traditionally, flexible bronchoscopes employed fibreoptic technology. More modern devices, including single-use bronchoscopes, use video or hybrid systems.

Key components of a video flexible bronchoscope are outlined below:
- Distal tip – contains camera, LED light source, and working channel exit.
- Bending section – manoeuvrable portion of the bronchoscope.
- Control lever – moves the distal tip up and down in a single plane through movement of the bending section.
- Working channel port – allows for instillation of fluids (e.g. local anaesthetic).
- Suction connector – allows for connection of suction tubing.
- Suction button – activates suction when button depressed.
- Endoscope cable – transmits live video image from the distal tip to the display unit.

7.5

Cleaning and decontamination

Method	Technique	Specific points
Cleaning	Manual	Washing (<45°C)
	Automated	Ultrasonic baths
Disinfection	Chemical	High level – glutaraldehyde, hydrogen peroxide, peracetic acid, chlorine and chlorine-releasing compounds
		Low level – alcohol, sodium hypochlorite and iodophore solutions
	Pasteurization	Temperature of 77°C for 30 min
Sterilization	Steam	121°C for 15 min or 134°C for 3 min
	Chemical	Ethylene oxide (at 29–65°C for 0.5–2 hours), 2% glutaraldehyde (>2 hours)
	Gas plasma	Ionized gas for 75 min
	Radiation	Gamma irradiation

Precautions to protect against the transmission of disease between patients via anaesthetic equipment should be part of everyday practice. A cycle exists for the management of contaminated medical items – the item is cleaned, disinfected, inspected, packaged, sterilized and stored ready for its next use. Some items are single use and therefore will not undergo the cleaning process and should be discarded.

- Cleaning involves the physical process of removing any foreign material from an item including infectious agents and organic matter. It does not necessarily destroy these agents but lowers the burden of biological material for subsequent disinfection or sterilization. It usually involves washing with cool water and detergent.
- Decontamination removes contaminants so that they are unable to reach a susceptible site in sufficient quantities to cause an infection. It involves cleaning followed by disinfection and/or sterilization.
- Disinfection renders equipment free from all pathological organisms except bacterial spores. It usually involves liquid chemicals or pasteurization.
- Sterilization renders equipment completely free of all viable infectious material including bacterial spores. Methods include steam sterilization, chemical, gas plasma and radiation.

Prions are misfolded protein molecules that if transmitted into a healthy organism can induce normal proteins to become misfolded. They cause the transmissible spongiform encephalopathies. As the protein is the infective agent, sterilization requires denaturation of the protein to prevent transmission. However, prions are relatively resistant to proteases, heat, radiation and aldehydes. The World Health Organization suggests a number of processes that can be used to denature the infective protein. One of these involves immersing the instrument in a pan of sodium hydroxide and heating in an autoclave to 121°C for 30 minutes before rinsing and performing routine sterilization. Alternatively, single use instruments can be used.

7.6

Continuous renal replacement therapy – extracorporeal circuit

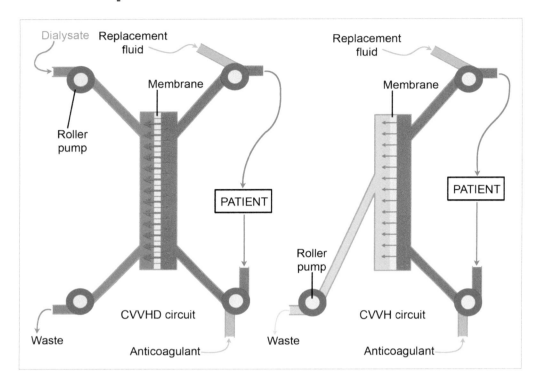

Circuit components

- Blood access – achieved acutely via a large-bore double lumen catheter inserted into a central vein.
- Blood tubing – conveys blood to and from the semipermeable membrane.
- Blood pump – provides controlled flow of blood to the membrane.
- Semipermeable membrane/filter – hollow fibre structure allowing blood to flow through a series of small tubes increasing the membrane surface area. Membrane properties such as charge, wall thickness and pore size affect function.
- Dialysis and/or replacement fluids – prepared bags of balanced salt solutions containing a buffer, usually bicarbonate.
- Effluent collection system.
- Anticoagulation – passage of blood through extracorporeal circuits activates coagulation pathways, affecting filter performance and risking loss of blood contained in a clotted circuit. Unfractionated heparin is the mainstay of anticoagulation for continuous renal replacement therapy. However, regional anticoagulation of the circuit is becoming more popular (e.g. with citrate) and is the preferred method in those patients with coagulopathy or bleeding disorders.
- Safety features – air bubble traps, safety alarms.

Continuous renal replacement therapy – modes

CRRT mode	Therapeutic goal	Primary indication	Principle used
SCUF	Fluid volume management	Fluid overload without electrolyte imbalance	Ultrafiltration
CVVH	Solute removal and fluid volume management	Uraemia, severe acid–base or electrolyte disturbance Removal of medium-sized solute	Convection
CVVHD	Solute removal and fluid volume management	Uraemia, severe acid–base or electrolyte imbalance	Diffusion
CVVHDF	Solute removal and fluid volume management	Uraemia, severe acid–base or electrolyte disturbance Removal of medium-sized solutes	Diffusion and convection

Continuous renal replacement therapy (CRRT) allows slow, balanced fluid and/or solute removal with less haemodynamic instability compared to intermittent techniques. CRRT may be classified in terms of solute removal.

Convection – one-way movement of solutes resulting from bulk movement of fluid, also called solvent drag. Movement of fluid occurs secondary to a pressure gradient across a membrane, known as the transmembrane pressure (TMP). This principle of ultrafiltration is similar to the function of the glomerulus in the kidney. The primary determinant of convection is the ultrafiltration rate. This is influenced by membrane water permeability, membrane surface area, TMP and colloid osmotic pressure gradient (impedes filtration).

Dialysis – defined as diffusion of solutes across a semi-permeable membrane down their concentration gradients. Fluid moves along an osmotic gradient created by solute movement. During dialysis, electrolyte fluid (dialysate) flows in a countercurrent direction to blood, which is separated by a semipermeable membrane, allowing equilibration of plasma and dialysate solute concentrations. The rate of diffusion is primarily determined by solute concentration gradients. Other factors include solute characteristics, membrane permeability and the rate of solute delivery (blood and dialysate flow rates).

Modes of CRRT
- Continuous veno-venous haemodialysis (CVVHD) – most effective mode for removal of solutes of small molecular weight (e.g. urea, creatinine, potassium).
- Slow continuous ultrafiltration (SCUF) – effective for safe management of fluid removal but does not allow significant convective solute clearance due to small filter pore size.
- Continuous veno-venous haemofiltration (CVVH) – similar clearance of small molecular weight solutes compared to CVVHD. Enhanced clearance of medium molecular weight solutes (e.g. cytokines, complement). Net fluid removal possible depending on the amount of replacement fluid infused.
- Continuous veno-venous haemodiafiltration (CVVHDF) – combination of diffusion and convection enhances solute clearance of both small and medium molecular weight substances.

7.8

Gas cylinders

Gas	Symbol	Cylinder body colour	Cylinder shoulder colour	Pressure (kPa) (std valve)	Physical state in cylinder	Pin index position
Oxygen	O_2	Black (green in USA)	White	13700	Gas	2 and 5
Nitrous oxide	N_2O	French blue	French blue	4400	Liquid/vapour	3 and 5
Carbon dioxide	CO_2	Grey	Grey	5000	Liquid/vapour	1 and 6
Air	–	Grey	Black/white	13700	Gas	1 and 5
Entonox	N_2O/O_2	Blue	Black/white	13700	Gas	7
Helium	He	Brown	Brown	13700	Gas	None
Heliox	He/O_2	Black	White/brown	13700	Gas	2 and 4

Medical gas cylinders are made from a molybdenum steel alloy, which is stronger and lighter than its carbon steel predecessor. The neck of the cylinder ends in a tapered screw-threaded block into which a valve may be fitted. The seal between the block and cylinder is made of a material (Wood's metal) that will melt if the cylinder is exposed to high temperatures, reducing the risk of an explosion.

Manufacturers regularly test cylinders; the plastic disc around the neck details the year it was last examined. Engraved on the cylinder are details of the tests undertaken.
- Internal endoscopic examination.
- Pressure testing.
- Tensile testing (1 in 100 cylinders).
- Flattening, bend and impact testing (1 in 100 cylinders).

Different sized cylinders are manufactured: A to J. Size E cylinders are usually attached to the anaesthetic machine; they can release 680 l of oxygen or 1800 l of nitrous oxide. Size J cylinders are used for cylinder manifolds. Lightweight cylinders made from aluminium alloy with a fibreglass covering can be used for transportation.

The filling ratio describes the weight of the fluid in the cylinder divided by the weight of water required to fill the cylinder; in the UK it is 0.75, however, in hotter countries it is 0.67 to reduce the risk of explosion.

Marks and labels on the cylinder include:
- details of testing (see above)
- name, chemical symbol, pharmaceutical form, specification, licensing
- tare weight (empty weight)
- hazard and safety notices
- cylinder size code
- filling date, expiry date
- directions for use, storage and handling
- nominal cylinder contents and maximal pressure.

Safety features include colour coding and the pin index system, a non-interchangeable safety system used to prevent the accidental connection of a cylinder to the wrong anaesthetic machine yoke.

7.9

Glucometer

Self-monitoring of blood glucose (SMBG) most commonly involves pricking a finger with a lancet-type device. Capillary blood is then applied to a reagent strip inserted into a glucometer. An automated, single time-point reading is obtained.

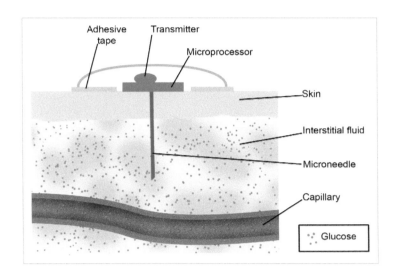

Continuous glucose monitoring (CGM) uses a small, wearable device that measures the glucose concentration in the interstitial fluid. Glucose is transferred from capillary blood to the interstitial fluid by simple diffusion in the setting of a concentration gradient. Interstitial glucose concentrations may be affected by the metabolic rate of cells adjacent to the sensor as well as localized blood flow. An average lag time of 8–10 minutes accounts for the time required for glucose diffusion. Worn on the arm or abdomen, a CGM device comprises a:

- subcutaneous microneedle sensor
- receiver – a monitor that displays glucose measurements; separate from sensing device
- transmitter – transmits the sensor data to the receiver.

Readings are automatically transmitted to the receiver (e.g. every 5 minutes). A display shows the latest reading and measurement trend. Alarms may be set to alert the user if glucose concentrations are measured outside a selected range. Some devices require daily calibration with capillary blood (via SMBG).

Flash glucose monitoring (FGM) is similar to CGM with an integral sensor that measures glucose concentration in the interstitial fluid. Glucose levels are measured regularly and stored in the sensor. Intermittent scanning of the sensor with a reader device allows 'on-demand' transmission of measurements. FGM devices undergo factory calibration, negating the need for calibration with capillary blood.

Perioperative management of CGM and FGM:
- Device safety with diathermy use – manufacturer guidance recommends sensor and transmitter removal.
- Accuracy of measurements – caution recommended in situations with rapidly changing glucose levels and fluid/electrolyte shift, and in patients treated with vasoactive agents or poor tissue perfusion. Device accuracy unclear in the setting of electromagnetic interference.

7.10

Humidifier

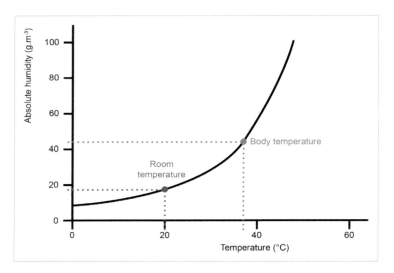

As temperature increases, humidity increases. The absolute humidity at various important temperatures is:

- Room temperature (20°C) – 17 g.m⁻³.
- Upper trachea (34°C) – 34 g.m⁻³.
- Body temperature (37°C) – 44 g.m⁻³.

There are various ways to humidify inspired gases.

Passive

- **Cold water bath** – dry gas is bubbled through water at room temperature. Inefficient, achieving only 30% humidity. Efficiency decreasing further as the loss of latent heat of vaporization cools the water.
- **HME** – heat and moisture exchanger. May reach 70% efficiency. Contains a hygroscopic element (such as calcium chloride). Exhaled gases cool as they pass through the element so water vapour condenses. The element is warmed by both the specific heat of the exhaled gas and the latent heat of water. On inspiration, the water evaporates and warms the gases achieving a humidity of up to 25 g.m⁻³.

Active

- **Hot water bath** – dry gas is bubbled through water at approximately 60°C. Over 90% efficient but risks include microbial contamination and thermal injury to the airway.
- **Cascade humidifier** – variation on the hot water bath. Gas bubbles through a perforated plate, improving efficiency by increasing the surface area that is exposed to water.
- **Nebulizers** – gas-driven devices; high pressure gas stream entrains water by the Venturi effect creating a fine spray that is directed at an anvil producing smaller droplets. Ultrasonic devices; a plate vibrating at ultrasonic frequencies produces droplets of less than 1–2 μm in size. Extremely efficient. Can deliver gas with a relative humidity greater than 100%, potentially leading to fluid overload.

The effects of breathing dry gases include:

- drying of secretions causing mucus plugging and difficulty expectorating
- damage to cilia
- keratinization of epithelium
- heat loss via latent heat of vaporization as dry gases are humidified in the respiratory tract.

7.11

Intra-aortic balloon pump

The intra-aortic balloon pump is an endovascular device that aims to improve coronary perfusion whilst reducing left ventricular work. The primary goal in optimizing myocardial oxygen–demand balance is to improve ventricular performance and cardiac output.

The balloon catheter is sausage-shaped, with a selection of appropriate balloon sizes correlating to patient height. The catheter is inserted into the femoral artery via standard percutaneous Seldinger technique, and advanced until the tip is just distal to the aortic arch. Helium is

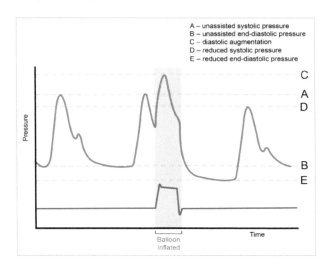

A – unassisted systolic pressure
B – unassisted end-diastolic pressure
C – diastolic augmentation
D – reduced systolic pressure
E – reduced end-diastolic pressure

used for balloon inflation because the lower gas density allows rapid inflation and deflation due to improved flow characteristics (see *Section 1.2.3 – Hagen–Poiseuille equation*).

Intra-aortic balloon pump use is based on the principle of counter-pulsation, where balloon inflation/deflation is timed to occur during different phases of the cardiac cycle. Modern devices utilize fibreoptic technology, allowing cardiac cycle monitoring, to achieve appropriate triggering of the device.

- Balloon inflation – onset of diastole after aortic valve closure, corresponding to dicrotic notch on arterial pressure waveform. Results in partial occlusion of the descending aorta. Aortic diastolic pressure is augmented (label C), increasing driving pressure into the coronary arteries. Blood is displaced proximally and distally in the aorta; the intended benefits are an increase in coronary blood flow and improved systemic perfusion, respectively.
- Balloon deflation – immediately before opening of the aortic valve, corresponding to the point just before upstroke on arterial pressure waveform. Aortic pressure is markedly reduced during systole (label D). Ejection of blood into a lower pressure system reduces left ventricular work and end-diastolic pressure (label E), leading to an improvement in stroke volume.

Insertion of an intra-aortic balloon pump is a temporary strategy of myocardial support to facilitate definitive treatment or recovery. Indications for use include:

- Cardiogenic shock.
- Refractory unstable angina.
- Acute myocardial infarction.
- Cardiomyopathy.
- Sepsis.
- Post-cardiac surgery for weaning from cardiopulmonary bypass.

7.12

Laryngoscopes

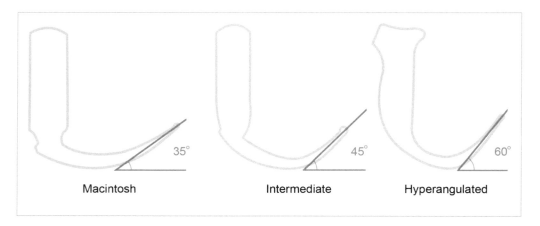

Macintosh   35°

Intermediate   45°

Hyperangulated   60°

Direct laryngoscope (DL) – non-video enabled laryngoscope, typically using a Macintosh or Miller blade. Facilitates direct laryngoscopy where visualization of the glottis occurs under direct vision.

Video laryngoscope (VL) – describes a large number of devices that facilitate indirect laryngoscopy. Most devices use a camera, positioned near the distal end of the blade, to provide an indirect view of the glottis that is displayed on an external screen. Video laryngoscope blades may be classified according to blade shape as follows:

- Macintosh geometry (Mac-VL) – uses similar technique and optimizing manoeuvres as DL. May be used to facilitate direct and/or indirect laryngoscopy.
- Hyper-angulated or hyper-curved (HA-VL) – facilitates indirect visualization ('around the corner' view) of the glottic opening. Direct laryngoscopy is not feasible. Often achieves a superior view to DL or Mac-VL. Endotracheal tube passage may be challenging, despite good glottic visualization, and requires use of a stylet. May be further classified as:
  - non-channelled – independent steering of tracheal tube towards and through the glottic opening
  - channelled – includes an integrated channel in the blade to guide tracheal tube delivery into the glottis.
- Intermediate geometry – blade curvature/angulation is in between DL and HA-VL. Use of a stylet or tracheal tube introducer (e.g. bougie) is recommended.

Use of video laryngoscopy vs. direct laryngoscopy

Much research is published on this topic. Studies include known difficult airways as well as airway management occurring outside of the operating room. Multiple blade types have been evaluated.

Systematic review of evidence demonstrates reduced rates of failed intubation and higher first-pass success compared to direct laryngoscopy for all adults undergoing tracheal intubation.

Routine use of a video laryngoscope has been recommended, whenever feasible, by the Project for Universal Management of Airways.

7.13

Oxygen delivery systems – Bernoulli principle and Venturi effect

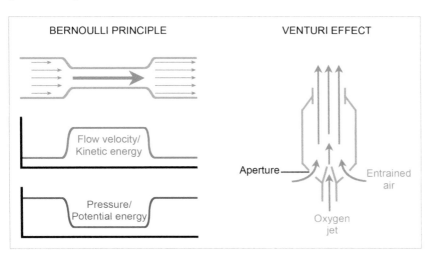

Fixed performance devices deliver a constant and predictable fractional inspired oxygen concentration (FiO_2).

Venturi masks are an application of two principles:
- The Bernoulli principle – describes conservation of energy in flowing fluids, stating that an increase in fluid velocity (kinetic energy) is associated with a simultaneous decrease in pressure (potential energy).
- The continuity equation – describes continuity of mass flow as fluids flow through pipes of varying diameters; as the cross-section of flow decreases, velocity of flow increases.

Combining these principles gives rise to the Venturi effect. A Venturi device has a constriction through which supplemental oxygen flows. Entrainment of ambient air occurs due to a drop in pressure distal to the constriction. The degree of air entrainment and, therefore, FiO_2 is dependent on aperture size. To ensure accuracy, oxygen must be supplied at the calibrated flow rate for each specific device. Even at low oxygen flow rates, Venturi devices provide high total fresh gas flow rates due to combined flows of oxygen and entrained air. These high flows exceed peak inspiratory flow rates making performance consistent despite variability in patient factors and ensure that expired gases are vented rapidly.

Variable performance devices deliver a fluctuating FiO_2 depending on:
- Device factors – supplemental oxygen flow rate, how tightly the device is fitted.
- Patient factors – peak inspiratory flow rate, minute ventilation, ventilatory pattern.

Hudson face masks are basic reservoir systems. Oxygen is delivered at flow rates less than the peak inspiratory flow rate. During inspiration, ambient air is entrained through holes in the mask, diluting the supplied oxygen. Continuous oxygen flow assists venting exhaled gases. During the expiratory pause, the mask body acts as an oxygen reservoir.

Nasal cannulae utilize nasopharynx dead space as an oxygen reservoir. During inspiration, entrained ambient air mixes with reservoir air, increasing the FiO_2.

7.14

Piped gases

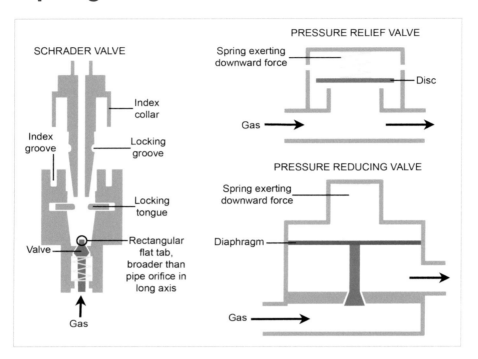

SCHRADER VALVE
- Index collar
- Index groove
- Locking groove
- Locking tongue
- Valve
- Rectangular flat tab, broader than pipe orifice in long axis
- Gas

PRESSURE RELIEF VALVE
- Spring exerting downward force
- Disc
- Gas

PRESSURE REDUCING VALVE
- Spring exerting downward force
- Diaphragm
- Gas

Piped gas can be supplied from several sources:
- Cylinder manifold.
- Vacuum-insulated evaporator (VIE).
- Oxygen concentrator.
- Compressed air supply.

Gases are supplied from their central store via colour-coded pipelines that terminate in Schrader sockets. Pressure reducing and pressure relief valves ensure the pipeline pressure is 4 bar. The gas can then be supplied to the anaesthetic machine via flexible hoses with the following features:
- Schrader probe – prevents misconnection of gases. Each gas supply has a unique indexing collar with a unique diameter to fit into the corresponding socket for that gas.
- Flexible hose – colour-coded and reinforced to prevent damage.
- Non-interchangeable screw thread connection – each gas supply has a probe that is specific for each gas (however, the nut and thread are actually the same for all the gases). A one-way valve ensures unidirectional flow.

Medical air is obtained from the atmosphere near to the site of compression taking care to avoid contamination from pollutants. It is compressed to 13 700 kPa and passed through columns of alumina (aluminium oxide) to remove water. It is supplied at a pressure of 4 bar to the anaesthetic machine (for use as both a ventilator driving gas and for delivery to patients) and at 7 bar to drive surgical tools. The terminal outlets (Schrader sockets) of the two supplies are different to prevent misconnection.

The VIE (see *Section 7.17 – Vacuum-insulated evaporator*) stores liquid oxygen for supply to large hospitals. The inner shell is made from stainless steel and is separated from the outer carbon steel shell by an insulating gas with a vacuum of 0.15–0.3 kPa. The contents are at high pressure (1050 kPa) and low temperature (−160 to −180°C), which is below the critical temperature of oxygen (−118.6°C).

7.15

Scavenging

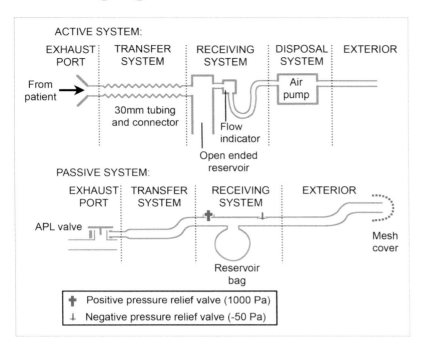

ACTIVE SYSTEM:

EXHAUST PORT | TRANSFER SYSTEM | RECEIVING SYSTEM | DISPOSAL SYSTEM | EXTERIOR

From patient

30mm tubing and connector

Air pump

Flow indicator

Open ended reservoir

PASSIVE SYSTEM:

EXHAUST PORT | TRANSFER SYSTEM | RECEIVING SYSTEM | EXTERIOR

APL valve

Mesh cover

Reservoir bag

✝ Positive pressure relief valve (1000 Pa)
↓ Negative pressure relief valve (-50 Pa)

Scavenging system components
- **Collection system** – a shroud connected to the adjustable pressure limiting valve or ventilator expiratory valve. Use of a 30 mm connector prevents misconnection with breathing system connectors.
- **Transfer system** – conveys waste gases from the breathing system to receiving reservoir. Tube diameter should differ from the breathing system to avoid misconnection. Tube length should be less than 1 m, minimizing the risk of kinking.
- **Receiving system** – a reservoir system that protects against excess pressures through the use of pressure relief valves. Excessive pressures may occur with blockage of system components. The positive pressure relief valve guards against pressures exceeding 1000 Pa. The negative pressure relief valve is set at −50 Pa. Receiving systems may be open or closed.
  - o Closed – a reservoir bag is flanked with positive and negative pressure relief valves. This system is uncommon in developed world anaesthesia.
  - o Open – the reservoir consists of a tube open to the atmosphere.
- **Disposal system** – vents waste gases to the atmosphere.

The ideal scavenging system should not affect ventilation or oxygenation of the patient. Nor should it affect breathing system dynamics.

Scavenging systems may be classified as passive or active.
- **Passive** – rely on the patient's expiratory effort or the ventilator for the flow of waste gases. The transfer system should be short and wide bore to minimize resistance. The disposal system outlet should be protected from the elements to minimize pressure fluctuations within the system.
- **Active** – a constant vacuum, generated by a fan or pump, is applied to the system. Active systems should only employ open receiving systems.

7.16

Ultrasound

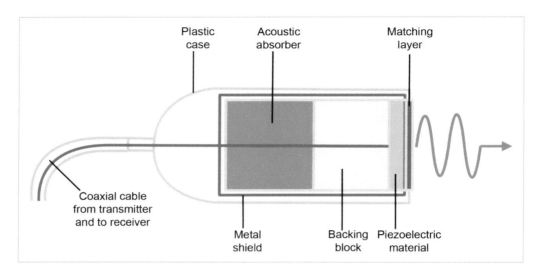

Sound travels as a mechanical longitudinal wave. Humans can hear sound with frequencies between 20 and 20 000 Hz. Ultrasound is high frequency sound with frequencies greater than 20 kHz.

Ultrasound waves may be generated by piezoelectric materials, such as lead zirconate titanate (PZT) or quartz. These materials exhibit a piezoelectric effect where applied mechanical stress (e.g. compression or stretching) creates an electrical potential difference (i.e. voltage).

A transducer is a device that converts one form of energy to another. Ultrasound transducers contain a plate of piezoelectric material. These transducers transmit ultrasound waves via the reverse piezoelectric effect, converting electrical energy into mechanical energy (e.g. sound). The same transducer receives reflected ultrasound waves, converting these mechanical waves into an electric signal, which is processed and displayed as an image on the screen.

A basic transducer has the appearance of a cylindrical tube. Component parts include:
- Case – protects the internal components from damage. Also insulates the patient from electrical shock.
- Electrical shield – a thin metallic barrier lining the inside of the case. Prevents electrical noise, present in the air, from contaminating electrical signals within the transducer.
- Acoustic absorber – a thin barrier of cork or rubber that insulates internal components. Prevents vibrations in the case from inducing electrical voltage in the piezoelectric material.
- Piezoelectric material (e.g. PZT) – shaped like a coin. Characteristics of the sound beam are determined by the dimensions of the piezoelectric material.
- Coaxial cable – provides electrical energy to the piezoelectric material, causing crystal vibration and generation of ultrasound waves.
- Matching layer – positioned in front of the piezoelectric material. Increases efficiency of sound energy transfer between the piezoelectric material and the body.
- Backing block – bonded to the back of the piezoelectric material. Controls the deformation of the piezoelectric material when electrical energy is applied. The sound wave produced is dampened, which shortens duration and length.

7.17

Vacuum-insulated evaporator

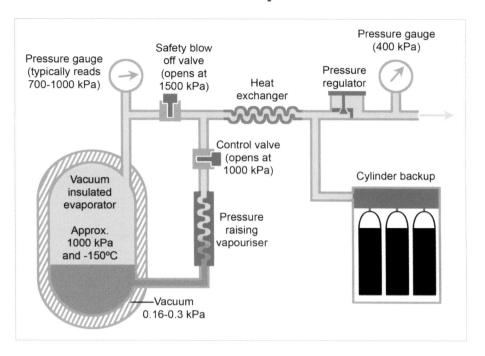

A vacuum-insulated evaporator (VIE) is the main storage vessel for bulk medical oxygen supply. As one litre of liquid oxygen is equivalent to 840 l of gaseous oxygen, bulk storage of oxygen in liquid form is the most economical and convenient option. A specific container for liquid oxygen storage is required to maintain a temperature below its critical temperature of −118°C.

The VIE chamber comprises two shells of steel separated by an insulating gap with a vacuum of 0.16–0.3 kPa. Up to 1500 l of liquid oxygen is stored at a temperature between −150°C and −170°C at a pressure of 500–1000 kPa. Under these conditions, oxygen exists as a vapour in equilibrium with its liquid state. The vacuum shell helps to maintain chamber temperature. With oxygen use, oxygen vapour is drawn from the gaseous layer via a withdrawal point above the liquid. This reduces the vapour pressure allowing further oxygen evaporation. Evaporation of liquid oxygen requires heat. This latent heat of vaporization is sourced from the internal chamber system, thereby assisting temperature control. All outgoing gases are warmed to ambient temperature by a heat exchanger and pressure is reduced to 400 kPa before entering the hospital piped gas system.

A differential pressure gauge measures the pressure difference from the top and bottom of the chamber from which contents can be calculated.

Low oxygen demand or high ambient temperature raises the temperature and pressure of the liquid oxygen. A pressure relief valve opens at 1500 kPa allowing venting into the environment. High oxygen use or cold ambient temperature reduces liquid oxygen temperature and pressure. This fall in pressure opens a valve allowing liquid oxygen to pass through a pressure-raising vaporizer. Gaseous oxygen returns to the chamber, restoring pressure within the system.

7.18

Vaporizer

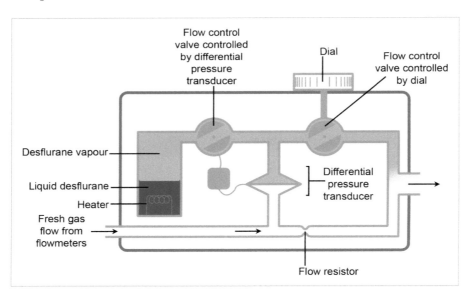

Vaporizers deliver a controlled and predictable amount of anaesthetic agent to the fresh gas flow (FGF) of an anaesthetic circuit.

Plenum vaporizers split FGF into two streams: one passes through the vaporization chamber containing liquid anaesthetic and becomes completely saturated, while the other bypasses it. Chamber gas agent concentration can be calculated from its saturated vapour pressure (SVP). It is mixed with the anaesthetic-free bypass gas in proportions dependent on the position of the control dial.

The vaporization chamber contains wicks and baffles to increase the surface area and assist mixing, respectively. Cooling of the anaesthetic agent occurs during vaporization, from loss of latent heat, making it less volatile. To compensate the vaporizer is made of material with high density, specific heat capacity and thermal conductivity, e.g. copper, to act as a heat sink. It also contains a bimetallic strip that acts as a temperature-sensitive valve and adjusts the splitting ratio according to the temperature; if it falls, more flow is directed into the vaporization chamber.

Safety features include a key filling system, colour-coding and interlocking mechanisms that prevent more than one agent being used if there are multiple vaporizers on the back bar of the anaesthetic machine.

Desflurane has a boiling point of 23.5°C and needs a specific vaporizer to prevent small changes in temperature causing large changes in SVP. The Tec 6 vaporizer has two circuits acting in parallel: FGF and vapour. Desflurane is heated within a chamber to 39°C (producing an SVP of 1500 mmHg) and injected into the FGF. The FGF is restricted by a flow resistor so that pressure becomes proportional to flow. A differential pressure transducer detects this pressure and adjusts a valve so that vaporizing chamber outflow pressure equals FGF pressure. The control dial then adjusts a second valve, which regulates the output of the desflurane gas.

Ventilation – pressure-controlled

Mechanical ventilation allows manipulation of pressure, volume and flow variables to support gas exchange and respiratory function.

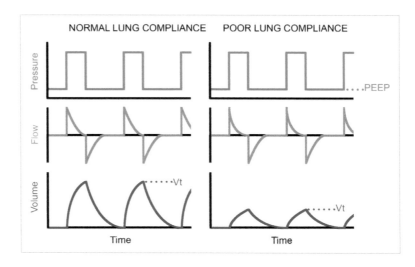

NORMAL LUNG COMPLIANCE   POOR LUNG COMPLIANCE

Pressure

Flow

Volume

....PEEP

······Vt

······Vt

Time   Time

- Control/ independent variable – used as the feedback signal to control inspiration; either pressure or volume.

This preset variable remains constant even in the setting of changing lung compliance or resistance. Only one variable may be controlled at a given time. The control variable may be determined by examining the flow–time curve.

- Dependent variables – vary with changes in lung mechanics.

Pressure-controlled ventilation

During pressure-controlled ventilation (PCV), pressure is the control variable with two pressure levels being kept constant: peak inspiratory pressure (P_{insp}) and positive-end expiratory pressure (PEEP). A pressure-limited breath is delivered at a set respiratory rate. During breath delivery, flow rises rapidly at the start of inspiration, with gas flowing into the chest down a pressure gradient. An increase in alveoli volume rapidly increases airway pressure, reducing the pressure gradient. Gas flow reduces exponentially until delivered pressure equals airway pressure. At this point, flow ceases. The flow–time curve illustrates this exponentially decreasing flow pattern.

Tidal volume and flow rate are dependent variables, changing in response to variations in lung resistance and compliance. Increased airway resistance or reductions in compliance lower the delivered tidal volume.

Benefits of PCV.
- Lower peak airway pressures are required to deliver the same volume.
- As pressure is the constant variable, peak inspiratory pressure is tightly controlled.
- Improved volume distribution within the lungs, especially with regionally reduced pulmonary compliance. The exponentially decreasing flow pattern allows ventilation of less compliant lung units and may reduce overventilation of more compliant lung parenchyma.

These benefits minimize barotrauma risk, conferring favour for use in patients requiring protective ventilatory strategies.

Disadvantages of PCV.
- Tidal volume delivery will fluctuate with changes in airway compliance. As such, minute ventilation may also vary.

7.20

Ventilation – volume-controlled

During volume-controlled ventilation (VCV), tidal volume is the constant variable. The ventilator generates a pressure necessary to achieve a predetermined tidal volume for each mandatory breath. During breath delivery, the inspiratory flow rate instantly rises to a preset value

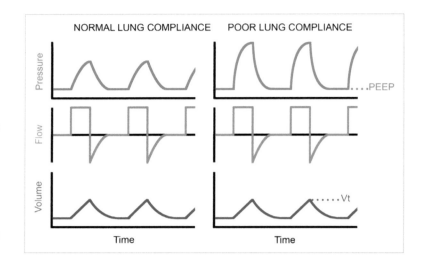

and remains constant for the duration of the inspiratory time, creating a square waveform on the flow–time curve.

As tidal volume is delivered, airway pressure rises. At the start of inspiration, pressure rises dramatically due to resistance of the system. Pressure continues to rise in a linear fashion to peak inspiratory pressure, the pressure at which the set tidal volume is achieved. At this point, flow ceases. Airway pressure quickly falls to plateau pressure, defined as the pressure applied to small airways and alveoli. Plateau pressure is representative of compliance of the respiratory system and is measured during an inspiratory pause on the ventilator. Inspiratory pressure is the dependent variable of VCV, changing in association with dynamic lung mechanics. Increased airway resistance or reductions in lung compliance will lead to an increase in airway pressure.

Benefits of VCV.
- Direct control of tidal volume and minute ventilation, allowing tight control of arterial partial pressure of carbon dioxide (P_aCO_2).

Disadvantages of VCV.
- Constant flow may cause high peak pressures increasing the risk of barotrauma. Peak pressure alarms should be set within acceptable limits.

Pressure-controlled ventilation with volume guarantee (PCV–VG)

By combining PCV and VCV the benefits of both ventilatory methods may be exploited. The PCV–VG pattern may be described as pressure-limited ventilation with tidal volume targeting. A preset tidal volume is delivered with an exponentially decreasing flow at the lowest peak inspiratory pressure. This ventilatory pattern allows breath-to-breath dynamic changes of the inspiratory pressure, within the maximum pressure limit, in response to compliance. The goal is to minimize variation in the tidal volume delivered.

7.21

Viscoelastic tests of clotting

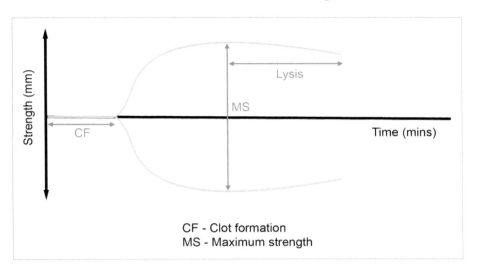

CF - Clot formation
MS - Maximum strength

Traditional coagulation tests are based on the classic cascade model of coagulation (see *Section 1.11.2 – Coagulation – cascade (classic) model*) and may not reflect haemostatic events occurring *in vivo* (see *Section 1.11.3 – Coagulation – cell-based model*).

Viscoelastic tests (VETs) of coagulation provide a more comprehensive, 'whole blood', integrated assessment of haemostasis. Designed as point-of-care tests, VETs allow convenient, rapid assessment. The two most common assays in current practice are thromboelastography (TEG) and rotational thromboelastometry (ROTEM).

VETs assess clot characteristics during the transition of whole blood from a liquid to gel state. As a clot forms, blood becomes increasingly elastic and resists deformation under shearing forces. Exposure of blood to different reagents evaluates relative contribution of plasma (e.g. clotting factors) and cellular (e.g. platelets) components on coagulation.

- Original VETs – measure clot strength via immersion of a pin in a whole blood sample contained in a cup. Depending on the measurement system used, either the cup or pin oscillates. As clot forms and strengthens, rotational force is applied to the pin. Characteristics of clot strength are represented by the degree of pin rotation plotted against time. Testing requires pipetting of blood sample and reagents.
- Modern VETs – employ cartridge-based systems which contain all necessary reagents. Some devices continue to utilize pin/cup technology. Other systems employ sonographic techniques whereby blood is exposed to vibration over a spectrum of frequencies. Motion of the blood meniscus is assessed because the resonant frequency of a sample changes with clot formation.

Measurements are device-specific but broadly measure clot strength over time. Functional parameters are displayed as numerical results as well as a graphical trace.

- Time to initial clot formation reflects, predominantly, coagulation factor activity and the presence of inhibitory substances (e.g. heparin).
- Maximum clot strength is represented by the maximum amplitude of the graphical trace. This parameter reflects platelet activity and fibrin strength.
- Clot lysis is the degree of fibrinolysis observed 30–60 minutes following maximum clot strength.

Mean, median and mode

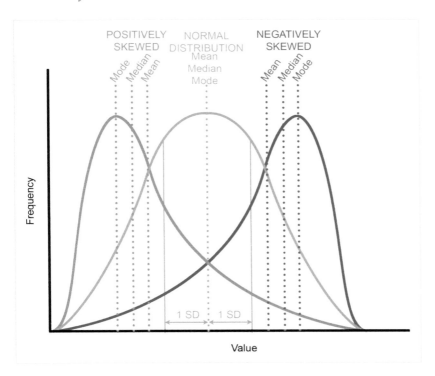

Various terms are used to describe the central tendency of data and the spread of data around it. The mean, median and mode are ways of measuring that central tendency.

The mean is the arithmetical average of the values – the sum of the data values divided by the total number of data points. It is frequently used when describing data that have a normal distribution. Although all data points are used for its calculation one of the main disadvantages is it is heavily influenced by outliers and skewed data.

The median gives the middle value in a series of data, where half the values lie above, and half below it. It is affected less by skewed data and outliers.

The mode is the most frequently occurring value in a set of data. However, there can be multiple modes in a set of data and it is a poor measure of central tendency.

In data that are normally distributed, the mean, median and mode will all be the same value. In data that are positively skewed, the values will separate so that the mean > median > mode and the mean is found closest to the tail of the curve. Conversely, in negatively skewed data, the mean < median < mode, again the mean is closest to the tail.

The spread of data around the mean can be described in terms of the variance (the average of the squared differences from the mean) or standard deviation. The standard deviation (SD) is the square root of the variance and is described more often due to its convenience; 68% of a normally distributed population will fall within 1 SD either side of the mean, 96% within 2 SD and 99% within 3 SD.

8.2

Normal distribution

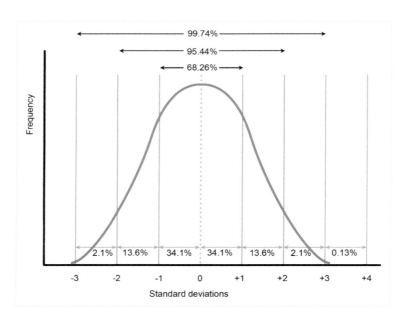

Determination of data set distribution is essential for determining the correct statistical technique for data analysis. Many statistical tests assume that data to which they are applied follow a 'normal' distribution. A normal distribution is a unimodal (one value for the mode) symmetric distribution for a continuous variable. There are two parameters that describe a normal distribution; the mean (see *Section 8.1 – Mean, median and mode*) and standard deviation. The mean provides information on the location of the central peak, whilst the standard deviation describes the spread of the sample distribution.

Assessing normality

Graphical

- A histogram plots the frequency of data observations in successive numerical intervals (range of values of equal width). A normal distribution has a central peak with the curve descending symmetrically on either side. However, histograms rarely depict the classic bell-shaped curve and are a relatively subjective assessment of normality.
- A quantile–quantile (Q–Q) plot compares two distributions by plotting their quantiles (subgroups of the total amount) against each other. If the plot is linear, the data are normally distributed.

Statistical tests – statistical programs can perform a goodness of fit test for a normal distribution. The Kolmogorov–Smirnov test compares sample data with the distribution expected if the data were normally distributed.

Parametric statistical tests make assumptions about the defining parameters of the population. Commonly used parametric tests are the *t*-test and analysis of variance (ANOVA). These tests assume that the sample being analysed is from a population with a normal distribution. If these tests are used for a sample from a population that is not normally distributed, the *P*-value (probability of rejecting the null hypothesis) may be inaccurate, especially for small sample sizes. Non-parametric tests are described as distribution-free tests because they make no assumptions on the distribution of the data being analysed.

8.3

Number needed to treat

$$NNT = \frac{1}{ARR}$$

NNT = number needed to treat

$$ARR = \left(\begin{array}{c} \text{event rate in} \\ \text{control group} \end{array}\right) - \left(\begin{array}{c} \text{event rate in} \\ \text{treatment group} \end{array}\right)$$

ARR = absolute risk reduction

The number needed to treat (NNT) can be used as a measure of effectiveness of an intervention. It gives the average number of patients that need to have an intervention to prevent one outcome event occurring. The NNT is easy to comprehend and allows comparison to be made between different interventions. The NNT calculated from systematic reviews provides the highest level of evidence due to the number of trials and patients involved in the analysis.

The NNT is the inverse of the absolute risk reduction (the numerical difference between the event rate in the treatment and control groups). The units for event rates (also described as the probability of an outcome) are number of events per patient; therefore the units for NNT are number of patients per event.

There is no absolute number for a NNT that defines whether a treatment is effective or not. The best NNT would be 1, where everyone receiving the treatment would have a favourable outcome; as the treatment becomes less effective the NNT becomes higher. If there were no difference between the treatment and control groups the NNT would increase to infinity.

The NNT can drop below zero suggesting that the intervention is actually doing harm, but rather than using a negative value the term number needed to harm (NNH) is used. In a similar way to NNT, the NNH can range from 1 to infinity; the lower the NNH, the worse the risk factor and at a value of 1, on average, every patient treated is harmed.

It is important to remember that NNT is treatment- and time-specific in achieving a particular outcome, i.e. if a study took x years to find the NNT for an intervention the yearly NNT would be x.NNT.

8.4

Odds ratio

	Group 1 (intervention)	Group 2 (control)
Outcome 1	a	c
Outcome 2	b	d

$$OR = \left(\frac{a}{b}\right) \Big/ \left(\frac{c}{d}\right)$$

$$RR = \left(\frac{a}{a+b}\right) \Big/ \left(\frac{c}{c+d}\right)$$

OR = odds ratio

RR = relative risk

The odds ratio (OR) and relative risk (RR) are statistical measures of the relative likelihood of an outcome occurring in two sample groups. The OR is the ratio of the odds of an outcome in the intervention group compared to the odds of an outcome in the control group. The RR is the rate (or risk) of an occurrence in the intervention group compared with that in the control group.

Both the OR and RR may be used when data relate to a prospective study, whereas only the OR can be calculated for retrospective case–control studies. This is because the total number of individuals at risk in each group needs to be known when calculating the RR. In a prospective study, the total number of patients at risk of an outcome is known whereas in a retrospective study, the outcome is the starting point and the total number of patients at risk is unknown.

An OR or RR greater than 1 indicates an increased likelihood of the stated outcome being achieved in the intervention group. However, if the OR or RR is less than 1 it is more likely to occur in the control group, and at 1 there is no outcome difference between both groups. These values should be reported with confidence intervals (CI) in order to give the precision of intervention effect. The 95% CI of a study estimate will be the range in which it is 95% certain that the true population intervention effect will lie; the wider the interval, the less the precision. If the CI crosses 1 (e.g. 0.89–1.05), then there is not a statistically significant difference between the two groups. If it does not cross 1, there is said to be a statistically significant difference.

8.5

Predictive values

	Disease	Disease-free
Positive test result	a	b
Negative test result	c	d

$$PPV = \frac{a}{(a+b)}$$

$$NPV = \frac{d}{(c+d)}$$

PPV = Positive predictive value

NPV = Negative predictive value

An ideal diagnostic test will always give a positive result with disease and a negative result without disease. In reality, this is not the case. The probability that a diagnostic test will give the correct diagnosis is known as the predictive value and assesses the usefulness of a test.

- Positive predictive value (PPV) – the proportion of patients with a positive test result who actually have the disease. The PPV may also be defined as the post-test probability of disease given a positive test. A PPV of 0.65 means a person with a positive test has a 65% chance of having the disease.
- Negative predictive value (NPV) – the proportion of patients with a negative test result who do not have the disease. The NPV represents the post-test probability of not having the disease given a negative test.

Predictive values may be calculated from a 2×2 table (as illustrated).

The usefulness of a test is influenced by the prevalence of the disease in the tested population. Prevalence is the proportion of a population who have a disease at a given time. Considering predictive values, prevalence may be considered as the pre-test probability of having the disease.

Exercise stress testing for diagnosis of coronary artery disease has a mean sensitivity and specificity of 68% and 77%, respectively. Used as a general screening test, where disease prevalence is 10%, a low PPV of 25% deems this test unreliable for disease detection. However, a high NPV of 96% allows its use as a screening test for ruling out those without disease. Applying this same test to a high-risk population, with a higher prevalence, will result in an increase in true positives and PPV. Performing multiple screening tests, as part of a diagnostic algorithm, allows the PPV of the tests to be combined, resulting in greater disease detection.

8.6

Sensitivity and specificity

	Disease	Disease-free
Positive test result	a	b
Negative test result	c	d

$$\text{Sensitivity} = \frac{a}{(a+c)}$$

$$\text{Specificity} = \frac{d}{(b+d)}$$

- The **sensitivity** of a test is the proportion of the true positives, i.e. those patients who test positive for a condition and actually have it.
- The **specificity** is the proportion of true negatives, i.e. those who don't have the condition and test negative for it.

The sensitivity can be calculated by dividing the number of patients who have the disease and test positive (**a** in the table) by the total number of patients with the disease. If a test has a high sensitivity, a negative test result is useful for ruling out the disease; at 100% it will identify all patients with the disease, i.e. there will be no false negatives (**c** in the table). However, it is not useful for ruling in disease, because it does not take into account the false positives (**b** in the table). A test with a high sensitivity is said to have a low type II error rate (see *Section 8.9 – Type I and Type II errors*).

The specificity can be calculated by dividing the number of patients without the disease and who test negative (**d** in the table) by the total number of disease-free patients. A positive result in a test with a high specificity is useful for ruling in disease; at 100% it will read negative for all patients without the disease, i.e. there will be no false positives. However, it is not useful for ruling out disease, because it does not take into account the false negatives. A test with high specificity is said to have a low type I error rate.

Sensitivity and specificity are prevalence-independent, because their values are intrinsic to the test and are not dependent on the disease prevalence in the population. They should not be confused with positive and negative predictive values (see *Section 8.5 – Predictive values*).

Significance tests

Data type					
Quantitative				**Qualitative (non-parametric)**	
Parametric (normally distributed)		**Non-parametric**			
2 groups	>2 groups	2 groups	>2 groups	1×2 2×2	>2×2
Paired – paired t-test	Paired – two-way ANOVA	Paired – Wilcoxon signed-rank	Paired – Friedman	Fisher's exact	Chi square
Unpaired – unpaired t-test	Unpaired – one-way ANOVA	Unpaired – Mann–Witney U (Wilcoxon rank-sum)	Unpaired – Kruskal–Wallis		

A significance test, or statistical hypothesis test, uses the sample data to assess the probability (P-value) of a specified null hypothesis (H_0) being correct. The H_0 states that there is no difference between groups. When deciding which test to apply to a set of data, ask:
- Are the data quantitative or qualitative?
- Are the data parametric or non-parametric?
- How many groups are there?
- Are the data paired or unpaired?

Quantitative data are numerical measurements based around a scale measure, e.g. temperature (°C) and height (m). They may be discrete or continuous. Qualitative (or categorical) data are measurements expressed in natural language descriptions rather than numbers, e.g. hair or eye colour. They may be ordinal (where the variables are ordered, and may have a numbering system attributed to them) or nominal (where there is no natural ordering, e.g. race or gender).

Continuous quantitative data can be analysed using parametric and non-parametric tests. Both these definitions are hard to understand unless you have an in depth knowledge of statistics. However, parametric tests are based on assumptions about the population from which the samples were taken; the most common being that the population is normally distributed. Non-parametric tests do not rely on these assumptions, but are often of a lower power than a parametric test for the same sample size, if the data are normally distributed.

Data may also be described as paired or unpaired depending on the way data were obtained. Paired data sets can either be from a single group that has data points taken on two separate occasions (frequently before and after an intervention, e.g. blood pressure before and after administration of an antihypertensive drug) or from two (or more) groups that are matched. Unpaired data are obtained from two or more groups that are unmatched.

8.8

Statistical variability

$$s^2 = \frac{\Sigma(x-\mu)^2}{n-1}$$

$$SD = \sqrt{s^2}$$

s^2 = sample variance (σ^2 for population variance)

x = data value

μ = sample mean

n = number of values in sample

SD = standard deviation

Statistics is divided into two major categories:
- Descriptive statistics – used to organize and summarize a data set. Can only be used to describe the study group.
- Inferential statistics – allows inferences to be made about a population from analysis of a sample taken from that same population.

Statistical variability is the spread of data in a distribution. A measure of variability usually accompanies a measure of central tendency (i.e. mean, median). Variability may be used as a descriptive statistic to describe the spread of data about the central tendency. In inferential statistics, it provides a measure of how accurately any individual data point represents the entire population. When statistical variability is small, data are clustered about the central tendency. As such, any individual value will provide a good representation of the entire population from which the sample is drawn.

Statistical variability may be measured with:
- Range – difference between the largest and smallest observed value.
- Interquartile range (IQR) – difference between the upper and lower quartiles (75th and 25th percentiles, respectively). As it measures the spread of the central 50% of data, the IQR is less sensitive to outliers. Uses the median as the central tendency.
- Variance – average of the squared differences from the mean. As such, considers all data set values to produce a measure of spread. Divided by n if working with a complete population or n–1 (Bessel's correction) to produce an unbiased estimation of population variance from a sample.
- Standard deviation (SD) – square root of the variance. The SD is only used to measure variability about the mean. SD is sensitive to outliers, potentially distorting the picture of spread. When analysing data with a normal distribution, approximately 68% of data lie within +/– 1 SD, 95% within +/– 2 SD and 99% within +/– 3 SD.

Type I and type II errors

	Null hypothesis is true	Null hypothesis is false
Rejects null hypothesis	False positive	True positive
	Type I (α) error	Correct outcome
Accepts null hypothesis	True negative	False negative
	Correct outcome	Type II (β) error

In statistical terms, the null hypothesis (H_0) states that there is no difference between two measured phenomena. The H_0 may be true (there is no difference) or false (there is a difference) and statistical tests are used to try to determine which is correct. However, they may lead to the rejection of the H_0 when in fact it is true (a false positive result); in other words, the test shows a difference when there isn't one. Conversely, statistical tests may accept the H_0 when in fact it is false (a false negative result), i.e. they show no difference when there is one.

A false positive result is called a type I error and a false negative result a type II error. As an example:
- a type I error occurs if a test result for a disease is positive when the patient is disease free
- a type II error occurs when a test fails to detect the presence of a disease in a patient who actually has it.

The α-risk and β-risk are the probabilities that a type I and type II error occur, respectively; these terms are used interchangeably.

Any statistical test will have a probability of making these errors; often efforts to reduce one result in an increased likelihood of the other occurring. The only way to reduce both error rates is to increase the sample size. Statistical power is the ability of a test to detect an effect, if the effect actually exists. Power analysis determines the smallest sample size needed to confidently detect an effect of a given size. Power is equal to $1 - \beta$ and a value of 0.8 is often used; it implies a 4:1 weighting for β- and α-risk ($\beta = 0.2$ and $\alpha = 0.05$ are commonly used values).

ASA classification

ASA PS classification	Description	Clinical example(s)
ASA 1	A normal healthy patient	
ASA 2	A patient with mild systemic disease	Current smoker, uncomplicated pregnancy, obesity BMI <40
ASA 3	A patient with severe systemic disease	End-stage renal failure, poorly controlled diabetes or hypertension
ASA 4	A patient with severe systemic disease that is a constant threat to life	Recent MI or CVA (<3 months ago), ongoing cardiac ischaemia or severe valve dysfunction, severe reduction of ejection fraction
ASA 5	A moribund patient who is not expected to survive without the operation	Ruptured abdominal aneurysm, major trauma, intracranial bleed with mass effect
ASA 6	A declared brain-dead patient whose organs are being removed for donor purposes	

The ASA classification (American Society of Anesthesiologists Physical Status Classification System) was first described in 1941. It had originally been hoped that it would aid statistical modelling of operative risk. However, even the original authors realized this was impossible without also including other factors, including specific physiological and operative variables (e.g. age, frailty, type of surgery).

The ASA classification does provide a simple way of both assessing and communicating a patient's pre-anaesthesia medical co-morbidities.

Since the original publication there have been several iterations of the ASA classification.

Currently there are 6 categories (ASA 1 to ASA 6). If the patient is undergoing an emergency operation (defined when a delay in treatment would lead to a significant increase in the threat to life or a body part) then an 'E' is added to the category.

Of note, if a pregnant patient is undergoing surgery, even if uncomplicated, then due to the significant alteration to the parturient's normal physiological state this is assigned ASA 2.

There is good evidence that there is significant inter-observer variability and therefore subjectivity in the application of ASA scoring. This variability may be even more pronounced when applied to the paediatric population. This raises concerns regarding its scientific applicability in medical research.

The ASA physical status classification has been incorporated into several systems that calculate post-operative mortality, including the National Emergency Laparotomy Audit (NELA) score and the American College of Surgeons National Surgical Quality Improvement Program (ACS NSQIP) surgical risk calculator. Combining ASA with other parameters (including frailty score) improves outcome prediction in the preoperative patient population.

9.2

Clinical frailty scale

Category/ score	Descriptor	Inpatient mortality (%)
1	**Very fit** – robust, energetic, active	2
2	**Fit** – no active disease but less fit than category 1	2
3	**Managing well** – well-controlled medical problems but not active beyond routine walking	2
4	**Living with very mild frailty** – not dependent on others but symptoms limit activity	3
5	**Living with mild frailty** – need help with high order activities (e.g. heavy housework, finances)	4
6	**Living with moderate frailty** – need help with all outside activities and with keeping house	6
7	**Living with severe frailty** – completely dependent for personal care	11
8	**Living with very severe frailty** – completely dependent for personal care and approaching end of life	24
9	**Terminally ill** – life expectancy of less than 6 months who are not otherwise living with severe frailty	31

Adapted from Rockwood *et al*. A global clinical measure of fitness and frailty in elderly people. *CMAJ* 2005;173:489.

Frailty, defined by an international expert group at the Frailty Consensus Conference in 2012, is a medical syndrome with multiple causes and contributors that is characterized by diminished strength, endurance, and reduced physiological function that increases an individual's vulnerability for developing increased dependency and/or death. Frailty is a dynamic condition that may improve or worsen with time.

Around 10% of people aged over 65 years have frailty, rising to between 25% and 50% for those over the age of 85. Whilst there is often overlap between frailty, multimorbidity and disability, it is important to distinguish between them.

There are several scoring systems to quantify the degree of frailty. The most ubiquitous is the Clinical Frailty Scale (CFS) developed at Dalhousie University in Canada. This uses a 9-item scale ranging from fit and managing well (1–3), those living with mild/moderate frailty (4–6), to those living with more advanced frailty (7–8), and terminally ill patients (9).

A CFS score can be calculated by any appropriately trained healthcare professional and should be based on the patient's capability 2 weeks prior to the time the assessment is performed. It is important to carefully differentiate between a CFS score of 6 and 7 because there is a significant increase in all-cause inpatient mortality between the two scores. A CFS has not been validated in a younger (i.e. those less than 65 years of age) population nor has it been validated in those with learning difficulties.

Frailty is an independent predictor of adverse surgical outcome. Unfortunately, there is currently little evidence to show that single or multiple interventions are proven to modify the syndrome of frailty or to impact on post-operative outcomes in frail individuals.

Cormack and Lehane classification

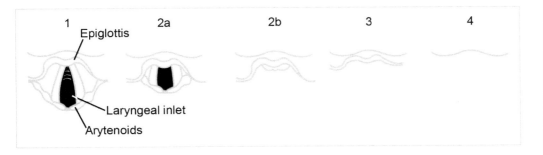

The Cormack and Lehane system classifies the view obtained by direct laryngoscopy based on the visualized structures. It was initially described by R.S. Cormack and J. Lehane in 1984 as a way of simulating potential scenarios that trainee anaesthetists may encounter. Initially a 4-grade classification, a modified version that subdivided grade 2 was described in 1998.

Grade	Description
1	Full view of the glottis
2a	Partial view of the glottis
2b	Posterior extremity of glottis seen or arytenoid cartilages
3	Epiglottis seen but no view of the glottis
4	Neither glottis nor epiglottis seen

The higher the grade, the more likely the possibility of a difficult intubation.

The grade described should be the 'best' grade viewed and can be after airway manoeuvres, such as external manipulation and BURP (backward, upward, rightward pressure), are performed.

The incidence of a true grade 4 view is extremely low (less than 1%). This incidence is further reduced, even in patients with anticipated difficult airway, using a video laryngoscopic technique.

Even though the Cormack and Lehane classification system is ubiquitous in current anaesthetic practice, knowledge of its detail is poor amongst anaesthetists, thus raising concerns regarding its reproducibility. In addition, the skill and experience of the anaesthetist has a significant effect on the grade described, so inter-clinician variability is important to acknowledge. However, the Cormack and Lehane classification provides a simple means of communicating and documenting the presence of a potentially difficult intubation.

9.4

Mallampati classification

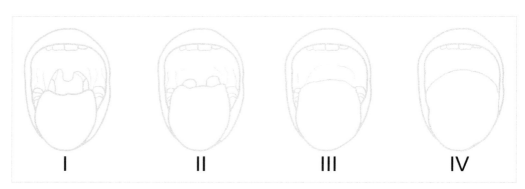

First published in 1985 by Dr Seshagiri Mallampati, the original 3-grade classification showed that the size of the base of the tongue was important in the determination of the difficulty of direct laryngoscopy.

The grading system described the ability to visualize the faucial pillars, soft palate, and the base of the uvula. The higher the grade, the greater the chance of difficult laryngoscopy.
- Class 1 – faucial pillars, soft palate, and uvula.
- Class 2 – faucial pillars and soft palate.
- Class 3 – soft palate.

In 1987 the original classification was modified by the addition of a 4th grade. A useful mnemonic 'PUSH' may aid recollection:
- Class 1 – faucial **P**illars, **U**vula, **S**oft palate, **H**ard palate: 'PUSH'
- Class 2 – **U**vula, **S**oft palate, **H**ard palate: 'USH'
- Class 3 – **S**oft palate, **H**ard palate: 'SH'
- Class 4 – **H**ard palate only: 'H'

Both Mallampati and modified Mallampati scores should be assessed with the patient in a seated position, the head held in a neutral position, the mouth wide open, and the tongue protruding to its maximum.

Mallampati testing should be used in conjunction with other predictors of difficult laryngoscopy, including previous difficult intubation, thyromental distance <6 cm, sternomental distance <12 cm, inadequate mandibular protrusion, neck circumference >40 cm, and reduced (<4 cm) inter-incisor or inter-gingival gap.

Scoring systems

Types of medical scoring systems	Example(s)
Anatomical	Injury Severity Score (ISS), Abbreviated Injury Score (AIS)
Organ-specific	Sequential Organ Failure Assessment (SOFA)
Physiological assessment	Acute Physiology and Chronic Health Evaluation (APACHE)
	Intensive Care National Audit & Research Centre (ICNARC)
Disease-specific	Model for End-Stage Liver Disease (MELD)
Therapeutic weighted scores	Therapeutic Intervention Scoring System (TISS)

Several scoring systems are in use in perioperative and critical illness populations. Originally created to grade illness severity, they now have a number of other uses, including:
• Comparison of predicted and observed outcomes.
• Stratification of patients for use in research.
• Resource management.
• Inter-hospital comparison.

An ideal scoring system should include the following characteristics:
• Free and available to all.
• Reliable and objective.
• Sequential (allowing collection of multiple data points).
• Reproducible across patient populations.
• Able to discriminate acute versus chronic organ dysfunction.
• Able to predict mortality/functional status/quality of life post-ICU.

Scoring systems in critical care

Most scoring systems incorporate physiological data obtained on the first day of ICU admission. Other frequently used parameters include:
• Pre-existing health conditions (e.g. metastatic disease, liver disease or immunodeficiency).
• Age and frailty.
• Source of, diagnosis on, and reason for admission.

Of the scoring systems employed in current UK practice, the two most common are the APACHE (Acute Physiology and Chronic Health Evaluation) score and the ICNARC (Intensive Care National Audit & Research Centre) model.

APACHE, introduced in 1981, has undergone multiple modifications to improve discrimination and model calibration. The current version (APACHE IV) uses acute physiological variables combined with chronic health information and ICU admission data to predict in-hospital mortality. Use of APACHE IV has been validated in multiple critically ill populations across multiple countries.

The ICNARC model (currently version ICNARC h-2018) was developed for use with the UK ICU Case Mix Programme. It uses physiological parameters obtained within the first 24 hours of admission combined with other data, including age, past medical history, dependency prior to hospital admission, cardiopulmonary resuscitation prior to admission, source of admission and primary reason for admission. Critical care units receive cumulative Quarterly Quality Reports which identify trends over time, assisting each unit in understanding the care they deliver.